July, 2006

To Patti,

Thanks for all of your help in getting the Neuro Spine Service up and running. I really appreciate all of your help and hard work. I know I am not the easiest person to have in the room. Thanks for your patience and your sarcastic humor!

Warm Regards,

[illegible]

Atlas of Cervical Spine Surgery

Atlas of Cervical Spine Surgery

Mark R. McLaughlin, MD
Princeton Brain and Spine Care
Princeton, New Jersey
Langhorne, Pennsylvania

Regis W. Haid, Jr., MD
Atlanta Brain and Spine Care
Atlanta, Georgia

Gerald E. Rodts, Jr., MD
Emory University
Atlanta, Georgia

Illustrator: **William Winn, MS, FAMI**
Atlanta, Georgia

ELSEVIER
SAUNDERS

ELSEVIER
SAUNDERS

1600 John F. Kennedy Blvd.
Ste 1800
Philadelphia, PA 19103-2899

ATLAS OF CERVICAL SPINE SURGERY ISBN 0-7216-9429-2

Library of Congress Cataloging-in-Publication Data
McLaughlin, Mark R.
Atlas of cervical spine surgery / Mark McLaughlin, Regis Haid, Gerald Rodts.—1st ed
p. cm
ISBN 0-7216-9429-2
1. Cervical vertebrae-Surgery-Atlases. I. Haid, Regis W. II. Rodts, Gerald E. III. Title.

RD533.M354 2005
617.4′71-dc22 2004066010

Acquisitions Editor: Rebecca S. Gaertner
Project Manager: David Saltzberg
Cover Art: William Winn

Printed in the United States of America

Last digit is the print number: 9 8 7 6 5 4 3 2 1

Dedication

This book is dedicated to my Grandfather, who taught me how to be a Physician.
And to my Parents, who taught me how to be a Person.
Mark R. McLaughlin, MD

To my family, to whom I owe everything.
Regis W. Haid, Jr, MD

This book is dedicated to my grandfather, Adolph H. Sellmann, MD, who introduced me to the world of medicine, and to my boys Teddy, Duncan, and Brady, who are my inspiration.
Gerald E. Rodts, Jr, MD

Preface

This book is not about indications, and it is not about options. It is not a treatise on cervical spine surgery, and it is by no means comprehensive. What it represents is an organized, systematic compendium of techniques that the authors have adopted to treat cervical spine disease. Simply put, it is a "This is how *we* do it" atlas.

It represents an amalgam of the three authors' tricks of the trade, which we have developed over the years while treating patients with cervical spine disease. We continue to refine our techniques and view this work as a living document that will be updated and revised as newer technology is perfected and as we learn more about cervical spine disease. We emphasize that the procedures illustrated and described herein are the techniques and products that *we* prefer to use and have found useful and successful. There are many other fine products and techniques described by other learned spine surgeons that rival and may even surpass some of the ones we describe.

We credit the pioneers of cervical spine surgery, including Ralph Cloward, Wolfgang Caspar, Volker Sonntag, Alan Crockard, and others, who have blazed the trail before us. They have contributed to this volume indirectly by passing their wisdom and accumulated knowledge on to our generation through presentations, guidance, and academic integrity. It is evident in this work that the above masters have certainly played a role in influencing our education.

This work was written and illustrated so that chapters could either stand alone as isolated lessons on a particular technique or, if the reader desires, build on each other to serve as a learning continuum. The chapter illustrations are often sequenced so that the visual story can be told even without reading the figure legends.

While the focus of this book is primarily on degenerative disease of the cervical spine, the principles described can be applied to many traumatic and neoplastic diseases. A wise surgeon once said, "Often times when you are struggling in a case, it is because you do not have sufficient exposure." We strongly believe that adequate exposure and releasing techniques are critical to the success of any cervical operation and minimize postoperative complications. That is why we have dedicated a full chapter of this book to this important concept that serves as a springboard into the more advanced fusion techniques.

The first half of the book covers anterior cervical surgery from the top down, beginning with transoral techniques down to cervicothoracic junctional techniques. It also includes a chapter dedicated to special situations that require some additional nuances and tricks to remedy some of the more difficult cervical situations.

The second half of the book covers posterior approaches, instrumentation, and multiple options available to the surgeon for dealing with cervical disease from a posterior approach. It also addresses special, more unusual situations that require tailored techniques not often used by the average spine surgeon, yet nonetheless are familiar to a busy spine surgeon. A final section is devoted to cervical arthroplasty.

This book is intended first and foremost for spine surgeons who are looking to expand their repertoire of options to treat patients with spine disease. It was also written and illustrated for residents and fellows interested in spine surgery. It also will serve as a good resource for other health care professionals, such as physician assistants, nurses, and surgical assistants, so that they can better understand cervical spine surgery.

An enterprise of this magnitude cannot be undertaken without a dedicated team of individuals committed to the completion of the project. We would like to first thank our Medical Illustrator, Bill Winn, for his unwavering commitment and expertise in getting a project this size done.

Bill spent countless hours creating and recreating our multiple, minute corrections to make each figure anatomically, visually, and aesthetically authentic. The most unique aspect of this book is that the surgical procedures demonstrate examples with real, commonly-seen pathological conditions, rather than normal anatomical illustrations. Mr. Winn is a master of telling a story with pictures, and this book is a monument to his continuing drive for perfection.

There are many others who contributed to this book in their advice, technical support, and encouragement. We would like to specifically thank Rebecca Schmidt Gaertner, our editor, who had the patience to nurture this project and the perseverance to keep it moving forward.

We sincerely hope that the true beneficiaries of this book are our fellow physicians, who are dedicated to surgical excellence and our patients, who we hope, in some small way, may receive better care, endure less suffering, and realize quicker recovery.

Mark R. McLaughlin, MD
Regis W. Haid, Jr., MD
Gerald E. Rodts, Jr., MD

Foreword

The authors nicely discuss and illustrate the surgical techniques for operating on both the anterior and posterior cervical spine. The text offers excellent surgical drawings complemented by preoperative and postoperative diagnostic studies. A particular strength of this book is that most chapters include a section entitled "Common Pitfalls" to highlight typical technical stumbling blocks, and two chapters are devoted to unusual circumstances that surgeons might encounter when treating the posterior cervical spine (*Special Situation: Posterior*) and the anterior spine (*Special Situation: Anterior*). I found these two chapters to be especially useful. All chapters present step-by-step descriptions of specific surgical procedures, ranging from the transoral approach to posterior cervicothoracic fusion. The authors also thoroughly describe conventional techniques, such as posterior wiring, laminectomy, and keyhole foraminotomies. The text concludes with a chapter on future technologies for artificial discs, and they describe the step-by-step procedure for the placement of the Prestige cervical disc. Overall, I found this book to very nicely describe cervical surgical techniques. It also introduced me to terms such as "gardening" for removal of osteophytes and "West Virginia Measuring Stick." This book will be extremely helpful to residents, fellows, and young neurosurgeons learning or brushing up on various surgical techniques for the anterior and posterior cervical spine.

Volker K. H. Sonntag, MD
Phoenix, Arizona

Foreword

A surgical text worth having on your shelf has several critical characteristics. To be use*able*, it must be based in a consistent philosophy of education. To be worthwhile, it must be written by great surgeons. Finally, to be use*ful*, it must convey important information in an easy-to-assimilate fashion.

Drs. McLaughlin, Haid, and Rodts achieve all of these goals in the *Atlas of Cervical Spine Surgery*. Their goal is stated immediately in telling the reader what the text is and what it is not. It is clear from the first chapter that they deliver on their stated goal of "This is how *we* do it." Each chapter is based on the standard surgical technique and augmented with the authors' "pearls" and "pitfalls."

By "consistent philosophy of education," I mean several things. First, the chapter-by-chapter format and information content must be consistent. This has been accomplished in this text by focusing on drawings of key surgical maneuvers and by augmenting the drawings with limited description of the technique, along with important hints and warnings. But I mean more than that simple rote accomplishment. Great teachers have a unique combination of knowledge, humility, a thirst for continued self-learning, and the ability to inspire others. William Butler Yeats explained it as, "Education is not the filling of a pail, but the lighting of a fire." All three authors are well-known teachers who represent each of those traits.

What surgical text would be worth reading if it were not authored by great surgeons? We all know the phrase, "Good judgment comes from experience, which comes from poor judgment!" The authors' many years of experience are shared freely in this text. Their knowledge of anatomy and technical ability are well known to all and are reflected in their related "pearls." The "pitfalls" are intended to help us heed Ralph Waldo Emerson's warning, "Wise men learn by other men's mistakes, fools by their own."

Finally, one type of "useful" surgical text is one that gives the reader specific, easily understood, and rapidly accessible information on exactly how to safely and successfully complete common surgical procedures. This type of text is particularly useful for medical students and residents, and for those individuals, the "pearls" and "pitfalls' provide added value. Beyond that, however, the "pearls' and "pitfalls" are exactly what makes this text attractive to the more experienced surgeon. The "practicality" of this text, therefore, is compelling. Contrary to Petronius' statement in *The Satyricon* (circa 66 CE) (i.e., "I'm sure the reason such young nitwits are produced in our schools is because they have no contact with anything of any use in everyday life."), the readers of this text will use this information on a very practical level every day that they practice cervical spine surgery. The authors will produce no "nitwits" with this text.

Richard G. Fessler, MD
Chicago, Illinois

Contents

CHAPTER I

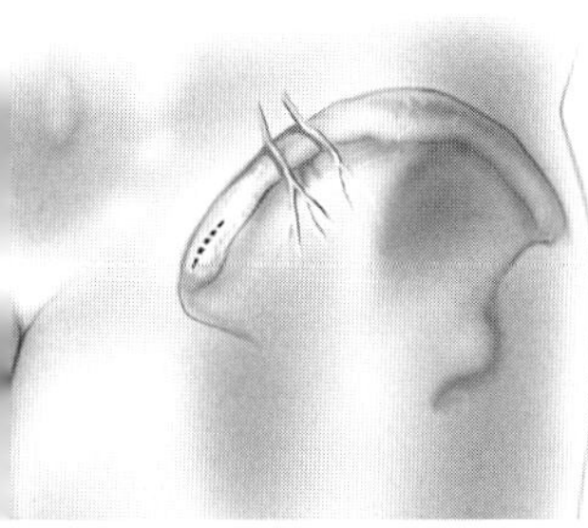

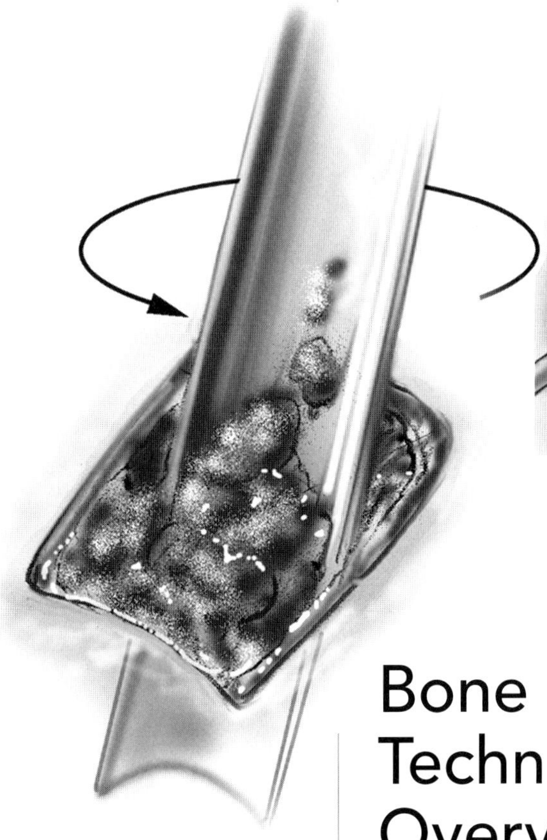

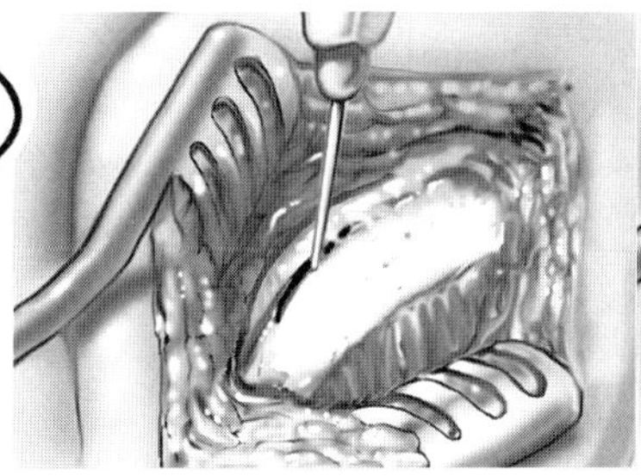

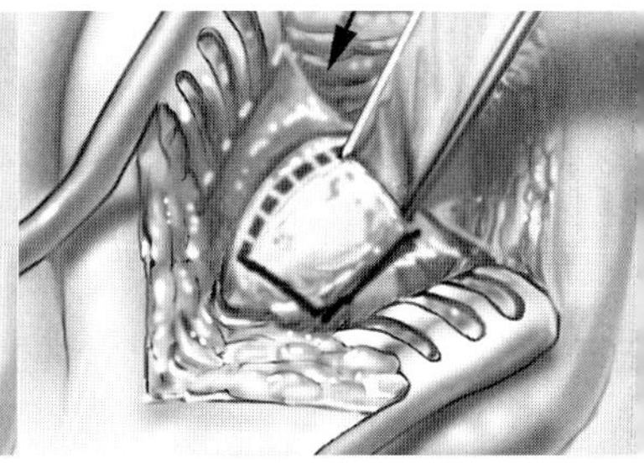

Bone Graft Techniques: Overview and Philosophy of Arthrodesis

BONE GRAFT TECHNIQUES

When performing any posterior fusion, our bias is that autologous graft or bone morphogenetic protein (BMP) should be used to augment the arthrodesis. Although local bone can be harvested from the spinous processes, it is primarily cortical bone with fewer cells and little bone morphogenetic protein. Our experience shows that the use of autologous graft increases the posterior fusion rate significantly. Conversely, with anterior approaches, we typically use allograft bone for arthrodesis because the fusion rates are extremely high regardless of the type of bone used. In patients with significant risk factors for pseudoarthrosis, such as long-term smoking history or failed prior fusions, we may use autologous iliac crest graft anteriorly or BMP as well.

Autologous rib graft is also an excellent source of "type A" bone that can be used for posterior procedures to augment arthrodesis. These grafts are useful in occipital-cervical fusion because the bone can be split with an oscillating saw and placed as an onlay over a morselized graft bed. The curvature of the rib is well suited for the occipital-cervical junction. This chapter discusses the following three approaches to harvesting autograft bone:

- Posterior/Superior Iliac Crest Graft
- Anterior Autologous Graft Technique
- Rib Graft.

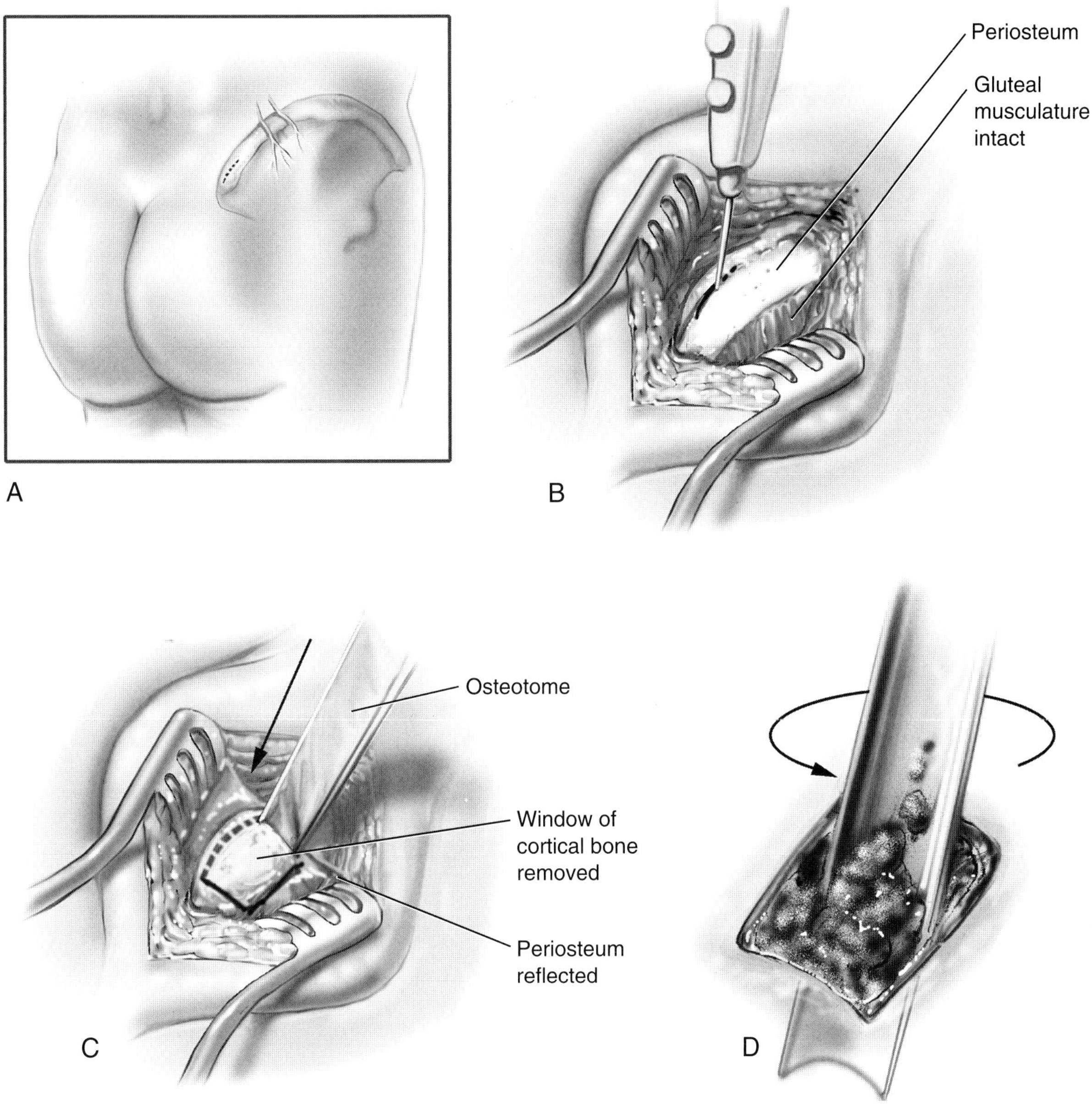

Posterior/Superior Iliac Crest Graft (Figures 1-1, 1-2, and 1-3)

Figure 1-1, A–D. **A,** The posterior/superior iliac spine is identified by palpation and prepared as a separate surgical region for any posterior cervical procedure. An incision line approximately 2 to 3 cm in length is made over the posterior/superior iliac spine well medial to the superior cluneal nerves. A linear incision centered over the osseous ridge will still allow harvest of approximately 30 cc of morselized autologous graft. **B,** The incision is carried down to the roof of the posterior/superior iliac spine. Using a subperiosteal dissection, the cortical bone overlying the iliac wing is dissected using monopolar cautery and an elevator. Since only the superior cortex needs to be exposed, great care is exercised in preserving the gluteal musculature. Minimal gluteal dissection decreases postoperative graft site pain. **C,** After adequate exposure of the posterior/superior iliac spine, an osteotome is used to chisel a square window of cortical bone off the iliac wing. By unroofing the posterior/superior iliac spine, the surgeon gains access to the cancellous bone underneath without significant gluteal musculature disruption. We credit spine surgeon pioneer Dr. Ralph Cloward with this *puka*-style harvest. (Clowerd practiced in Hawaii and adopted *puka*—the Hawaiian word for "small hole"—to describe this technique.) **D,** Using a curved bone gouge, the morselized bone is removed from the iliac crest. This is best achieved by placing the bone gouge within the cancellous bone and rotating the gouge in a circular fashion to remove all of the underlying cancellous bone.

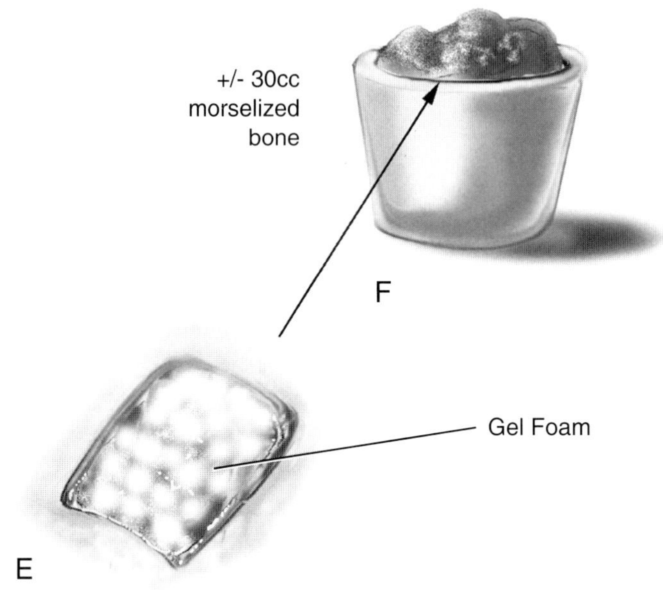

Figure 1-1, E and F. By using this rotating technique, a large amount of morselized autologous iliac crest graft can be harvested without exposing or disrupting a large cortical surface of the iliac crest. Approximately 30 cc of morselized bone graft can be harvested using this technique. Once the bone graft has been harvested, the wound is irrigated with antibiotic irrigation and packed with cellulose matrix (Gel Foam) or sealed with bone wax. The fascia and subcutaneous tissues are closed in a watertight fashion with interrupted absorbable sutures.

Figure 1-2, A–E. For longer segmental fusions, more bone is typically required, and therefore a larger exposure of the iliac crest is warranted. A larger portion of the iliac crest is cut with an osteotome, and the cancellous bone is harvested with curettes and gouges. The cortical bone removed from the posterior iliac crest wing can be cut into strips for the onlay fusion. The disadvantage of this technique is that the detachment of the gluteal musculature increases postoperative graft site pain.

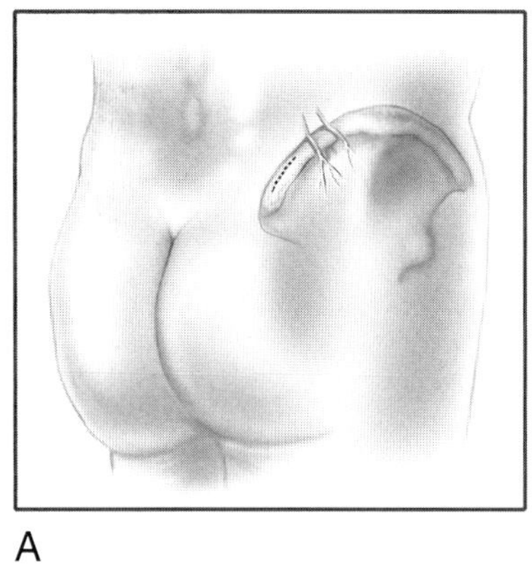

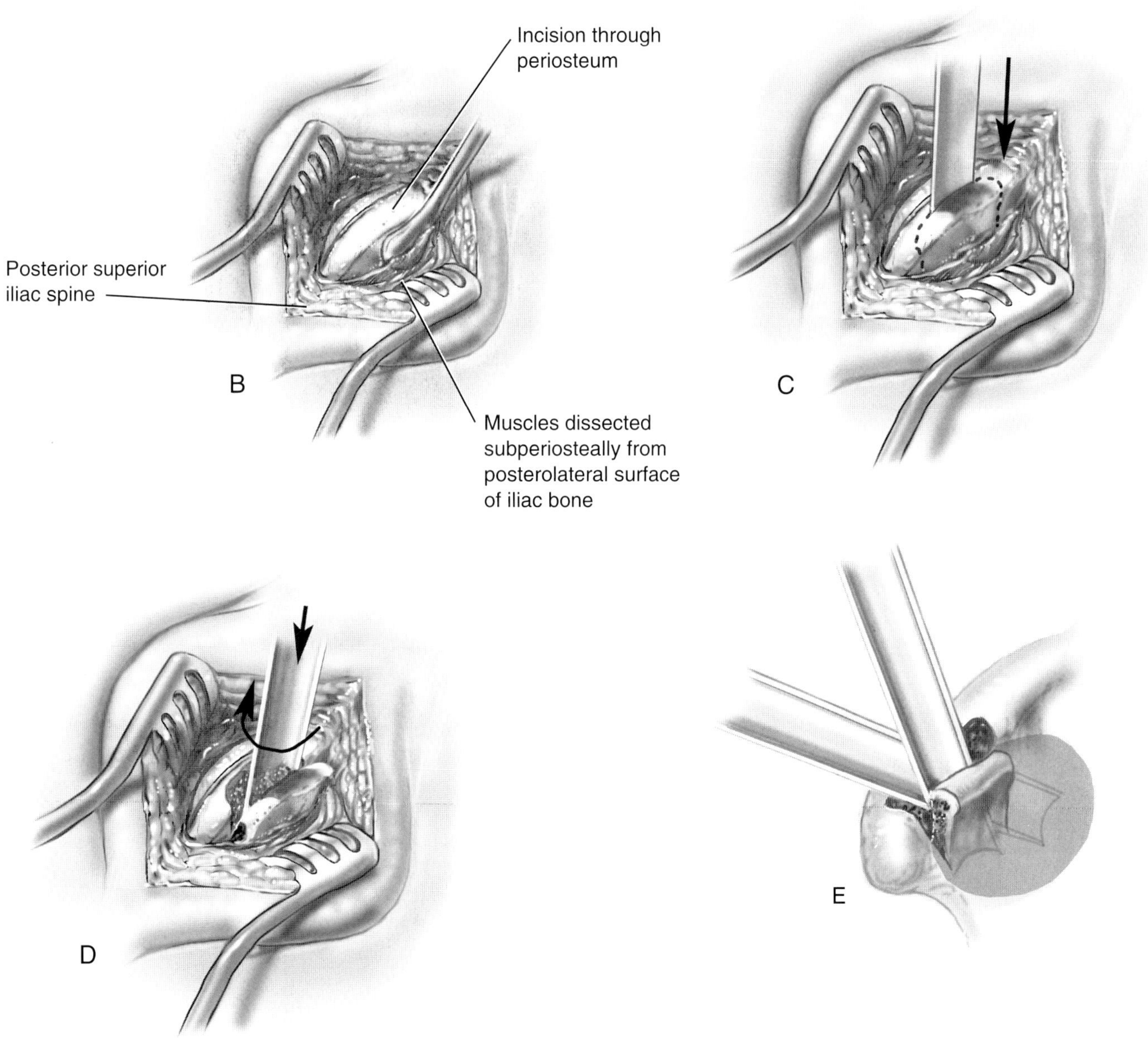

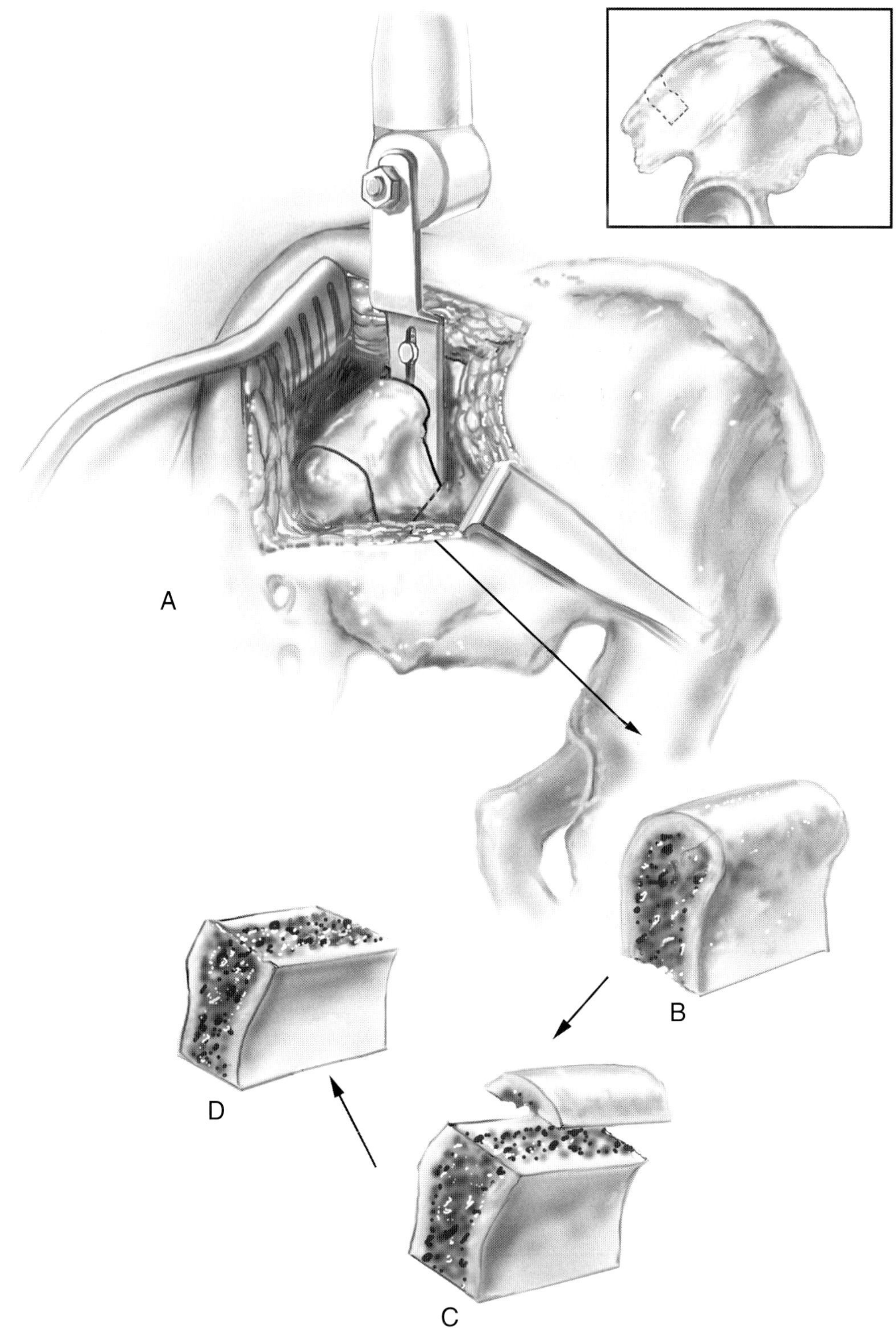

Figure 1-3, A–F. Autologous graft for C1-C2 fusion. The ideal region for this graft is located more lateral on the iliac wing, where the contour more closely approximates the curve of the C1 posterior rim. The tricortical graft is harvested with an oscillating saw, and the rostral cortical margin is then removed to create a bicortical graft. The two cortices will interface the inferior rim of C1 and the superior rim of C2. When using a Sonntag cable technique, the graft must be at least 4 to 5 cm in length so it can be incorporated into the cable construct. For an interlaminar clamp technique, the graft width must be shorter because the clamps attach lateral to the graft. The surgeon needs to ensure the height of the graft is adequate for optimal bone graft-spine contact. Therefore, we try to oversize the initial bone harvest and then customize the graft to the optimal size. Remaining trimmed bone is then morselized and placed in the lateral gutter.

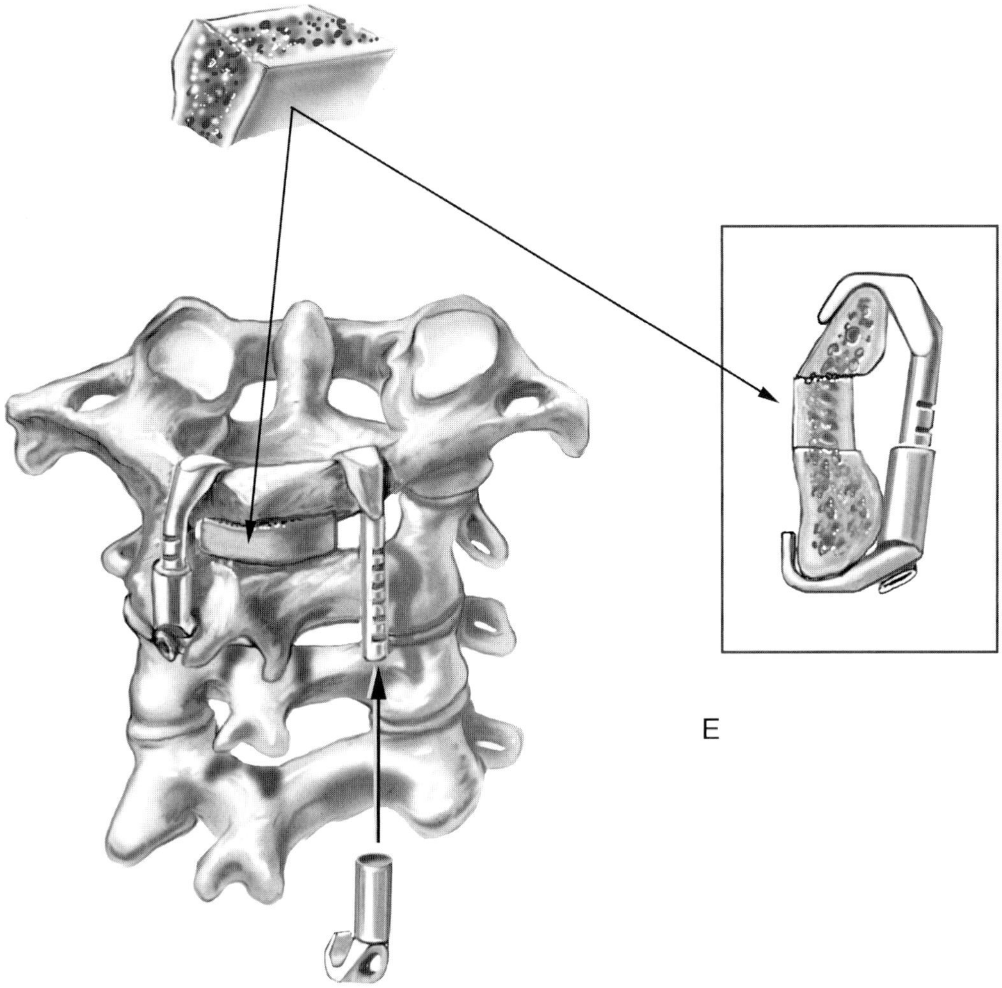

E

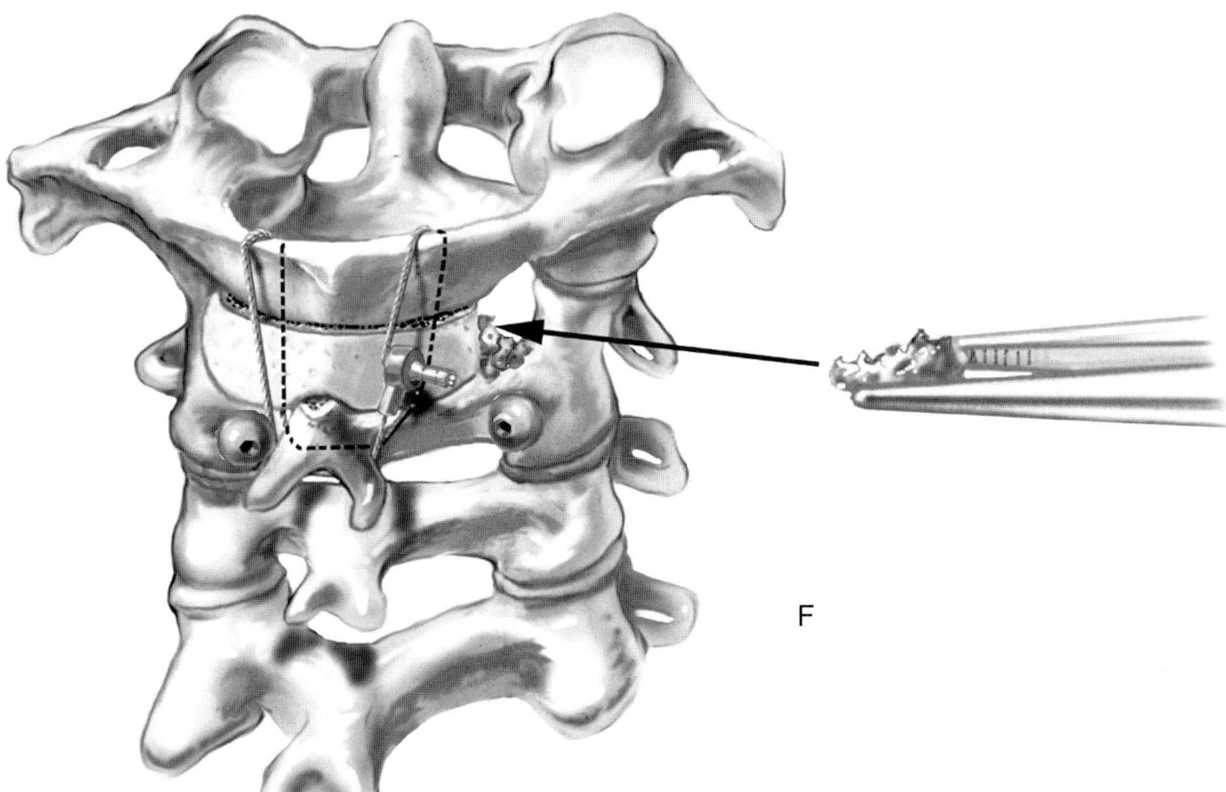

F

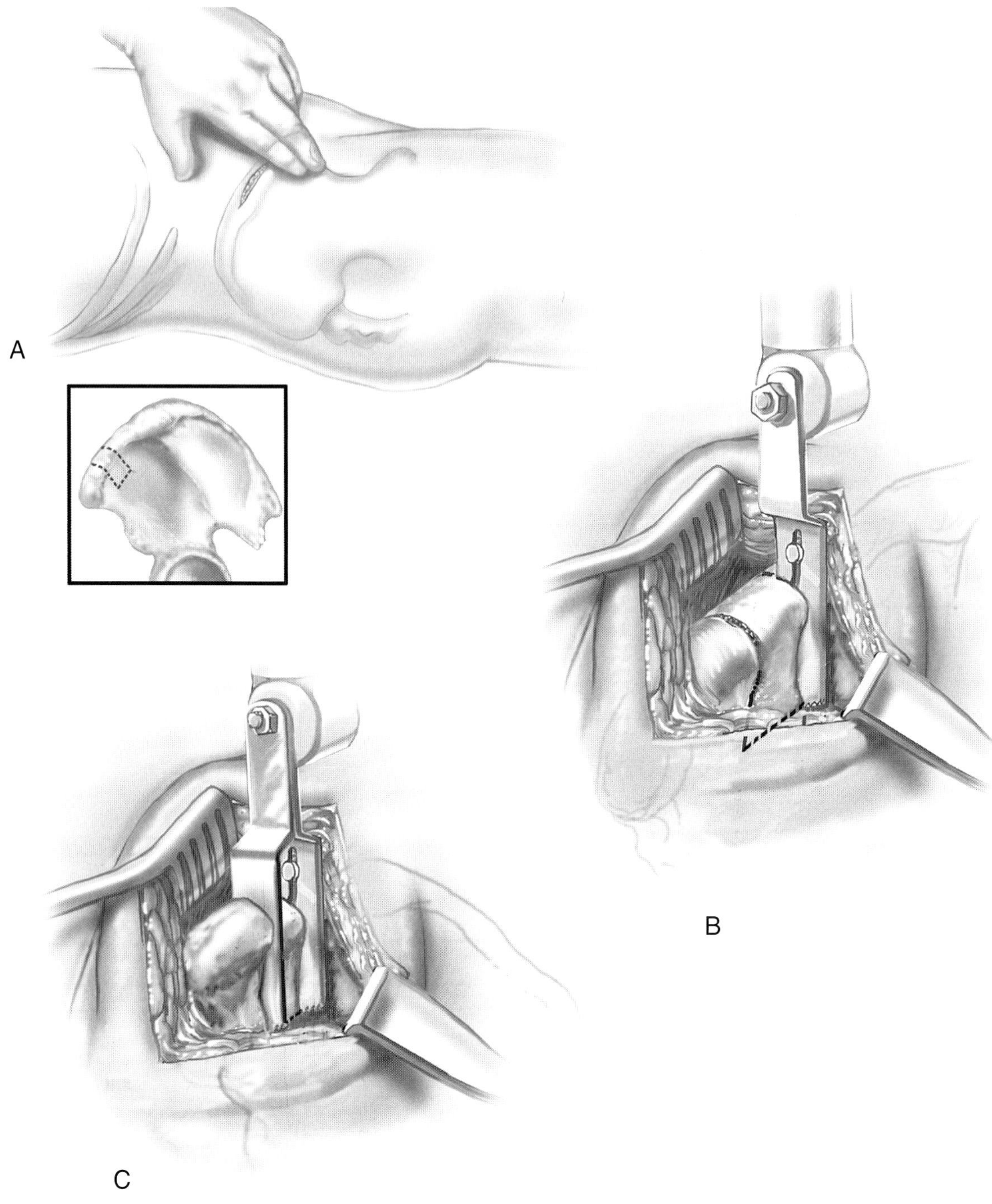

Anterior Autologous Graft Technique (Figure 1-4, A–G)

Figure 1-4, A–C. A, With the patient in a supine position, the anterior/superior iliac spine is palpated and an incision is marked two fingerbreadths laterally to the anterior/superior iliac spine. By placing this incision two fingerbreadths laterally, the lateral femoral cutaneous nerve is avoided. Typically it runs medially to this region, and the insertion of the sartorius is adequately preserved to avoid an avulsion fracture of the anterior/superior iliac spine. In patients from whom a single tricortical graft is harvested for anterior cervical discectomy and fusion, the 2- to 3-cm incision is used. When a corpectomy is performed and a larger graft site is required, the incision can be extended to obtain a larger autologous graft. **B,** After exposure is obtained in a subperiosteal fashion, retractors are placed, and the interspace to be fused is measured with a caliper. **C,** This measurement is then used for the chosen width of the double-bladed oscillating saw (i.e., 8 to 10 cm). We prefer this technique because it ensures a properly sized graft and a customized fit for the graft into the interspace. In cases of corpectomy, or when a longer tricortical graft is needed, a single-blade oscillating saw is used to make two separate cuts of the desired length.

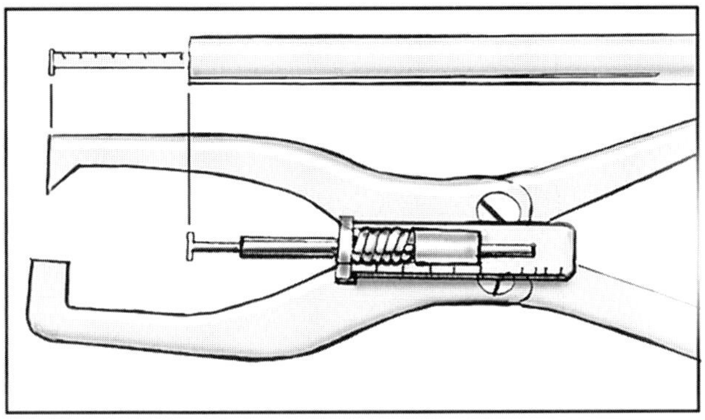

D

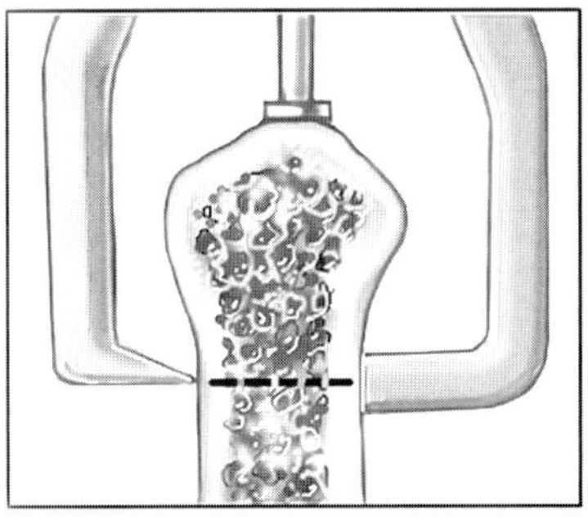

E

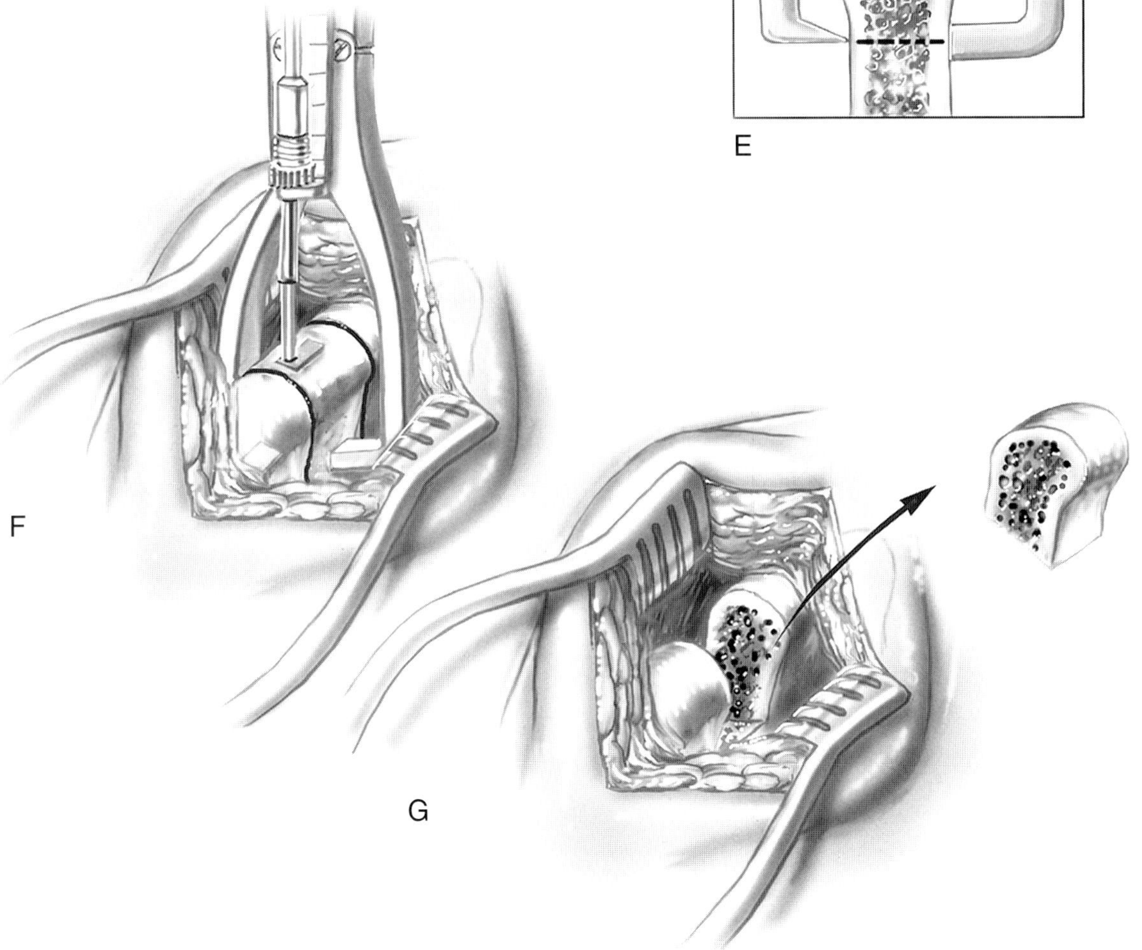

F

G

Figure 1-4, D–G. For a single-level disc, a "bone chomper" (Aesculap, Germany) is used to make the bottom cut deep into the iliac crest. We prefer this instrument because, again, it ensures a customized graft to the premeasured intervertebral space. This instrument also has a caliper that can preset the desired depth of the graft. The depth of the graft is determined from measurement of the interspace and is also measured from the intervertebral space and set on the instrument before the graft is cut. Care should be taken to ensure there is no fascial defect. Bone wax is used to stop bone bleeding, and cellulose matrix is placed into the defect.

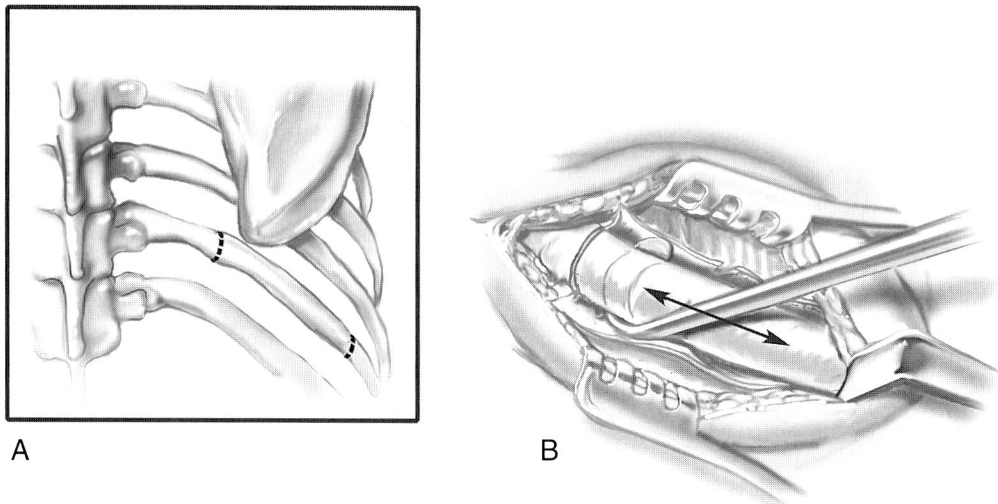

A B

Rib Graft (Figure 1-5)

Rib serves as an excellent source of grafting material. Although weak in structure, its propensity for fusion is excellent. Rib is routinely our material of choice for pediatric occipital-cervical fusions as well. It can also serve as a source of structural graft in a posterior cervical cerclage technique, although our preference is a screw rod technique.

Figure 1-5, A. When the patient is placed in a prone position, a region below the scapula is carefully prepared for rib graft harvest. Usually, the rib below the scapula is the T8 rib and serves as an excellent source of autograft bone. This rib is palpated, and a linear incision line is made paralleling the rib contour approximately 5 cm in length. A significantly longer section of rib may be harvested with skin retraction using an Army-Navy retractor.

Figure 1-5, B. After the incision is made and carried down directly to the periosteum of the rib, retractors are placed using the Alexander periosteal dissector as well as a "pigtail" (Doyen) periosteal dissector. The rib is dissected free from its neurovascular bundle. Although the length of the incision is only approximately 5 cm, a significant portion of the rib lateral to the incision can be dissected to obtain more bone graft without making a longer incision. The neurovascular bundle lies at the inferior portion of the rib, and care should be maintained to preserve this structure.

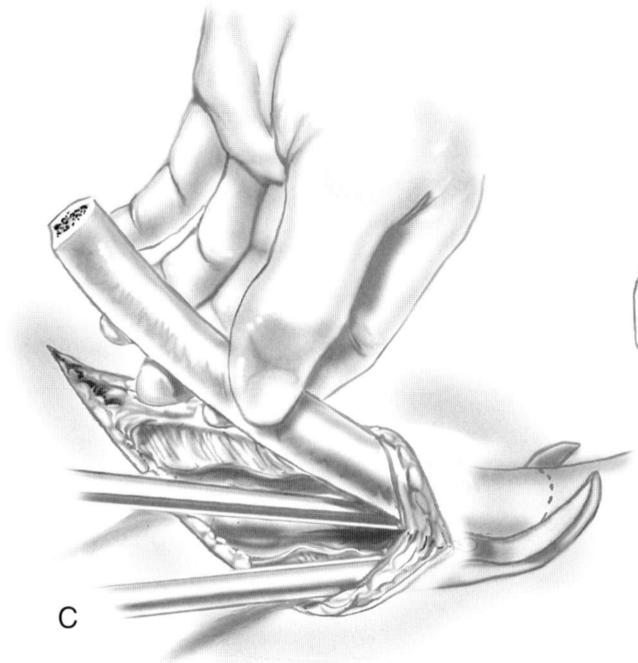

C

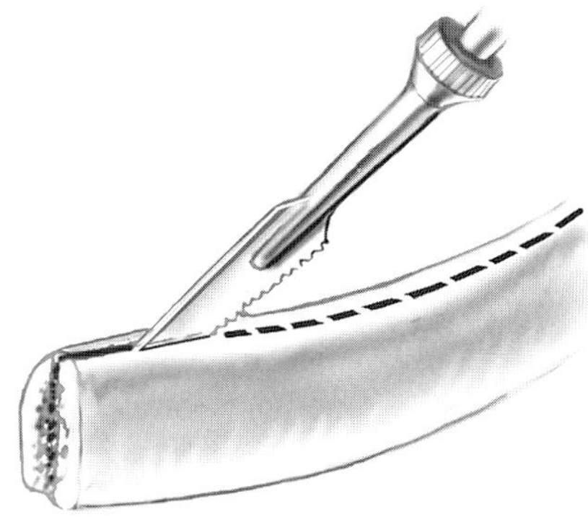

D

Figure 1-5, C. Once the rib has been dissected from intercostal musculature and the neurovascular bundle, a guillotine is used to cut the rib as distal as possible under the incision line. The rib is then removed from the operative bed, and the bone edges are waxed. The fascial layer is then closed with interrupted O-Vicryl sutures, and subcutaneous tissues are approximated with interrupted sutures as well. It is important to note that this technique involves a small chance of pneumothorax. We routinely obtain chest x-rays in the recovery room to verify no pneumothorax is present.

Figure 1-5, D. After the rib is harvested, a reciprocating saw is used to create a split-thickness bone graft. A portion of graft that has cancellous bone on the convex surface is ready for an onlay or wire fusion in the posterior cervical or occipital-cervical region. The portion of the graft with cancellous bone on the concavity is then forced into a greenstick fracture to mirror its counterpart. These grafts then can be augmented with autologous iliac crest in the posterior cervical region or wired with either a facet wiring technique or an interspinous wiring technique. The rib can be used whole or can be split to extend graft matter. The natural contour of the rib often approximates the cervical lordosis.

COMMON PITFALLS

- When choosing a bone graft, it is important to consider the function of the graft. If one only needs morselized bone to augment a posterior fusion, then the posterior/superior iliac crest graft–type exposure is best suited for bone graft harvesting. It is important not to dissect the gluteal or gluteus musculature from the iliac wing because this usually is associated with increased postoperative pain. Only the posterior/superior iliac spine needs to be dissected to allow access to harvest morselized bone.
- It is important to perform an upright chest x-ray in the recovery room after harvesting autologous rib graft to verify there is no pneumothorax related to an inadvertent violation of the pleura during harvest.

CHAPTER II

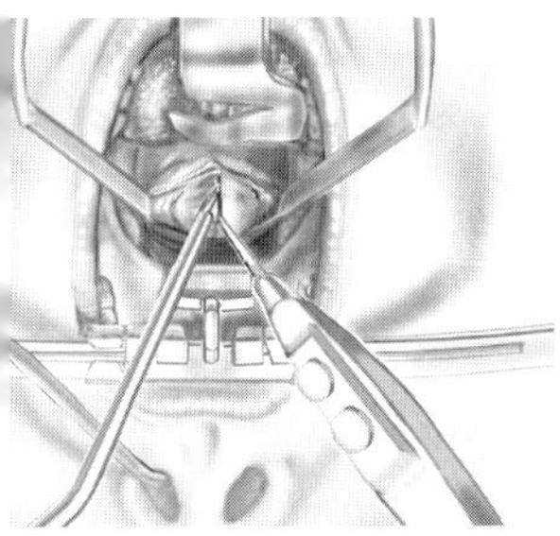

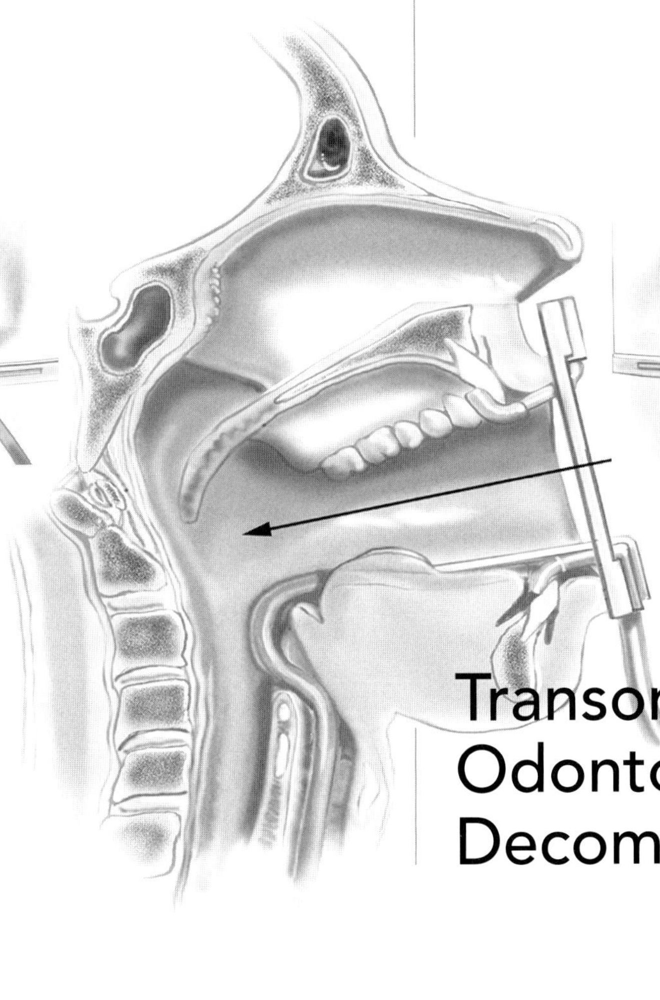

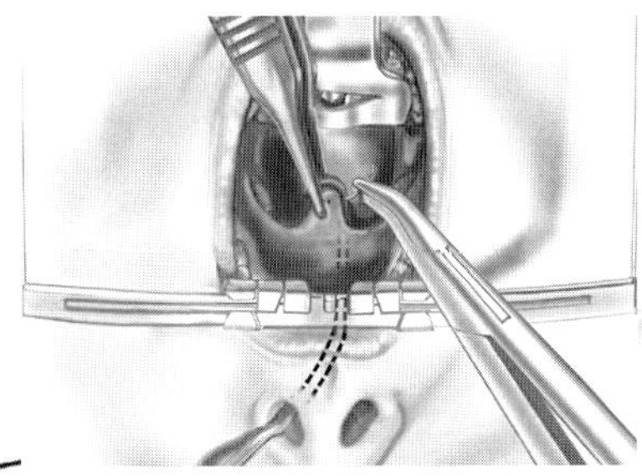

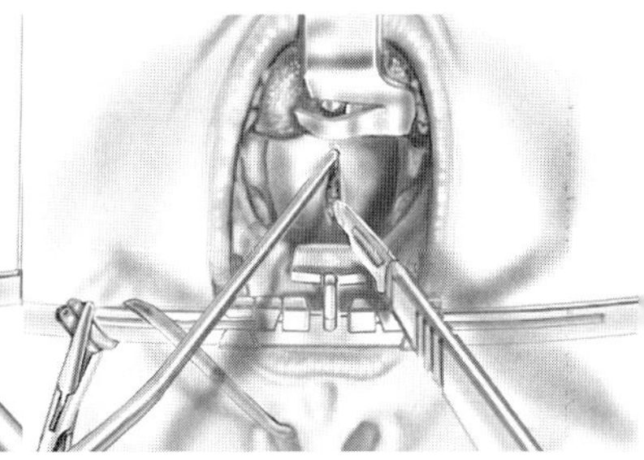

Transoral Odontoid Decompression

When considering a patient as a candidate for a transoral decompression, it is important to include an examination of dentition and jaw opening (particularly in rheumatoid patients whose jaw excursion may be limited). A good rule of thumb is a minimal jaw excursion of two fingerbreadths. Some patients with poor mandibular excursion may require a transmaxillary or transmandibular approach. In properly selected patients with good retractor placement, the surgeon can usually have access from the inferior clivus down to approximately the C2–C3 interspace.

Oral hygiene should be optimized preoperatively; we have had one patient develop an epidural abscess that was presumed to be related to extremely poor dentition. Computed tomography (CT) scans should be reviewed with careful attention to any rotatory component of C1–C2. If there is rotation, the position of the vertebral artery may be slightly more midline, putting this structure more at risk.

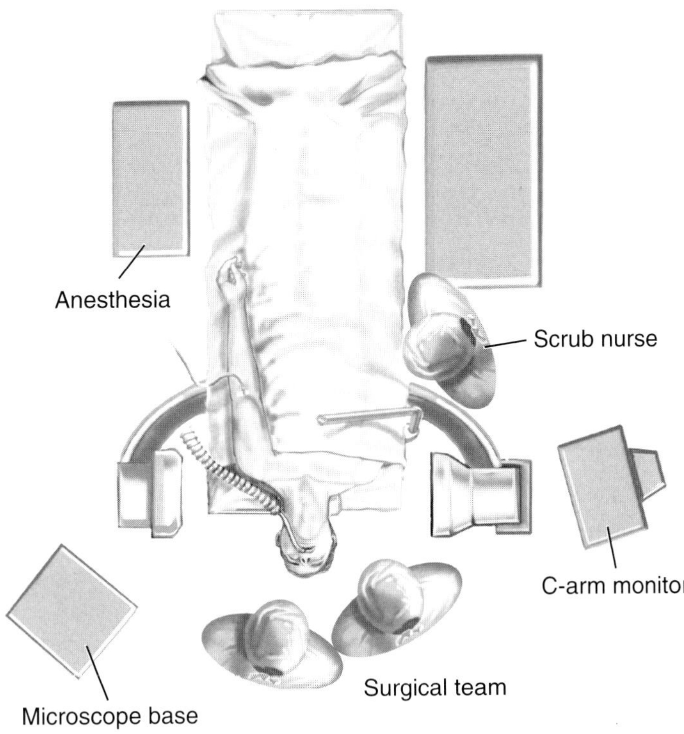

OPERATING ROOM SETUP

Figure 2-1. The setup and patient positioning for this operation are critical in maintaining a flow. The patient should be extended and positioned awake before induction of anesthesia and intubation. This awake hyperextension ensures optimal visualization and permits neurological assessment prior to anesthesia. It is critical that the patient's head be kept in a neutral (nonrotated position). We have found that tracheostomy is rarely necessary in patients requiring transoral approaches. Patients are kept intubated for approximately 3 days; extubation is then performed with the patient in the intensive care unit after airway patency is verified by deflating the endotracheal tube cuff. Because patients are intubated for 3 days and their diet after extubation is only slowly advanced, we place a low-profile feeding tube under direct vision in the operating room after closure of the mucosa. This tube is sutured in place and used until adequate p.o. intake is verified by calorie counts. Nutrition in the early postoperative period is critical for wound healing, and we aggressively advance tube feeds on the first day after surgery. High-dose penicillin or clindamycin is administered in the perioperative setting and continued for 5 days postoperatively.

Although spinal cord monitoring is sometimes used, we prefer awake positioning to monitor the patient's neurological status. Each piece of equipment is placed to allow the surgeon the most comfortable position for working within a limited surgical field. The placement of the C-arm, anesthesia, monitor, and scrub team allows the surgeon to easily access instruments and easily view any point of the operation on fluoroscopy. Usually, the microscope is kept at the patient's left side, out of the field until adequate exposure is obtained. The C-arm is placed perpendicular to the patient for the lateral view and is tilted under the table to allow the surgeon more leg room. The fluoroscopy monitor is placed in front of the surgeon and to his or her right so that any changes to depth or bone removal can be visualized in real time with fluoroscopic guidance. Other methods of computerized spinal navigation can also be used.

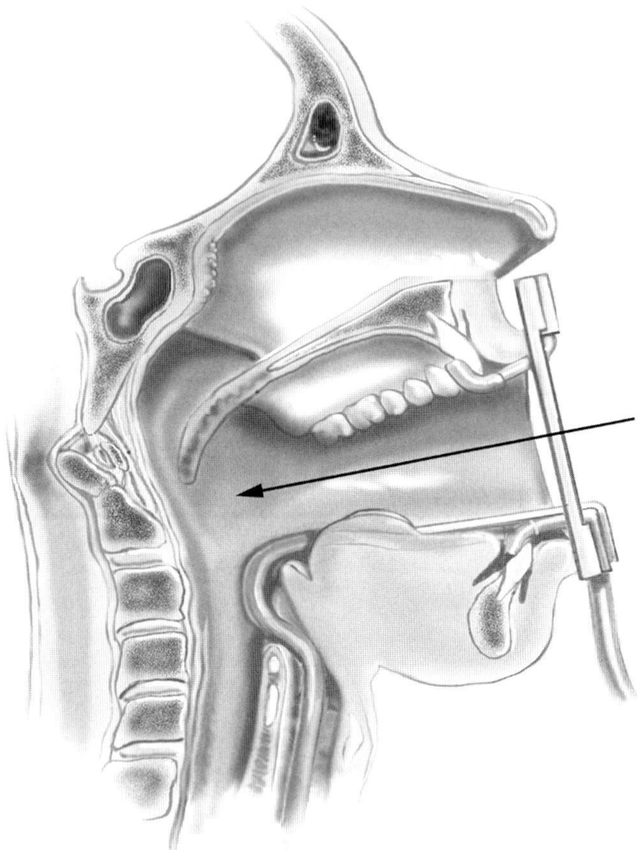

Figure 2-2. We routinely use the Spetzler-Sonntag (Aesculap, Germany) retractor to hold open the mouth. We also use the Crockard (Codman) self-retaining retractor to retract the mucosal and pharyngeal constrictor muscles. Once the retractor is placed, the uvula is mobilized cephalad to expose the upper craniocervical junction. The uvula can be retracted superiorly by placing a red rubber catheter through the nose and down into the oropharynx. Then, using a suture, the uvula is sewn to the tip of the tubing, and the tubing is gently pulled through the nose. This will retract the uvula superiorly and expose a significant portion of the upper C1 and clival region. Although a second soft palate retractor is placed, the catheter holds secretions in place.

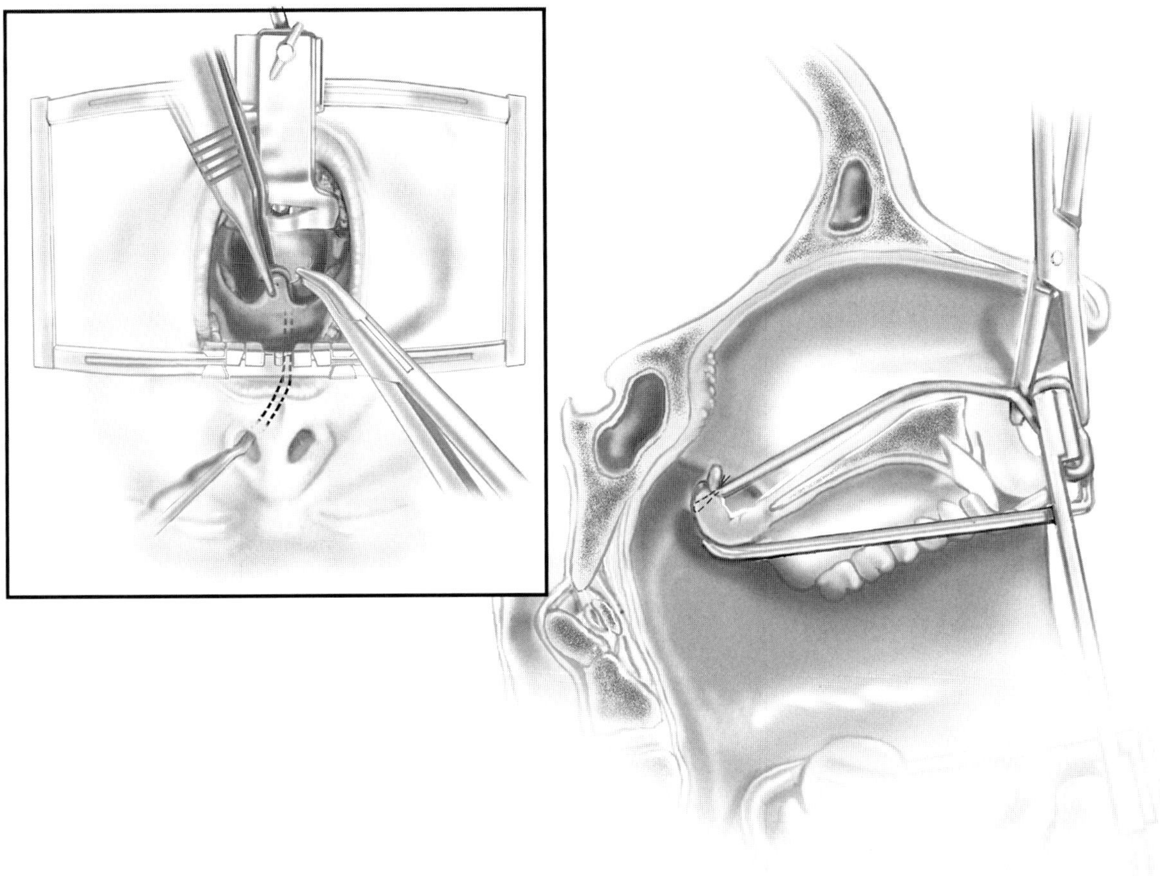

Figure 2-3. This lateral view demonstrates the additional exposure when the uvula is retracted with the proximal tubing sewn to the uvula, and the distal tubing is clamped to the retractor (see *inset*). The additional soft palate retractor has also been placed. Once the retractors have been placed and the uvula is retracted, a clear view to the C2, C1, and inferior clivus is possible.

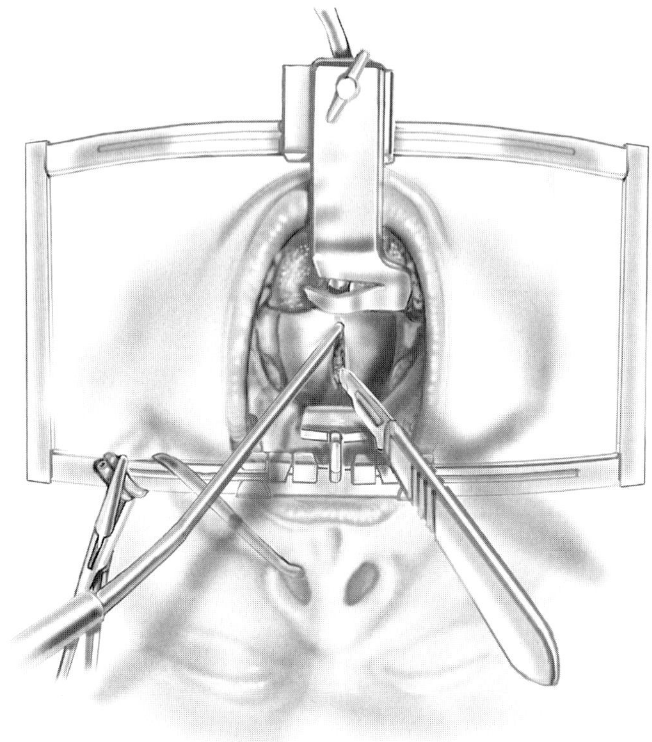

Figure 2-4. Before the incision, the anterior tubercle of C1 can be palpated. The C-arm imaging may confirm the appropriate location of the incision. After the mucosa has been infiltrated with local anesthesia and epinephrine, a midline incision is made over C2 and the anterior tubercle of C1. Careful attention is paid to make a full-thickness cut through the mucosa. Once this incision is made, all efforts are made not to manipulate the superficial mucosa to preserve its integrity for closure. The mucosa is then gently retracted with suction, and the dissection is carried out laterally with the monopolar cautery. When placing the retractor, it is important to keep in mind that the mucosal incision will lengthen as the retractor is dialed open. Therefore, a slightly smaller incision than necessary is made first; then the remainder of the opening enlarges in a rostral caudal direction as the retractor is placed.

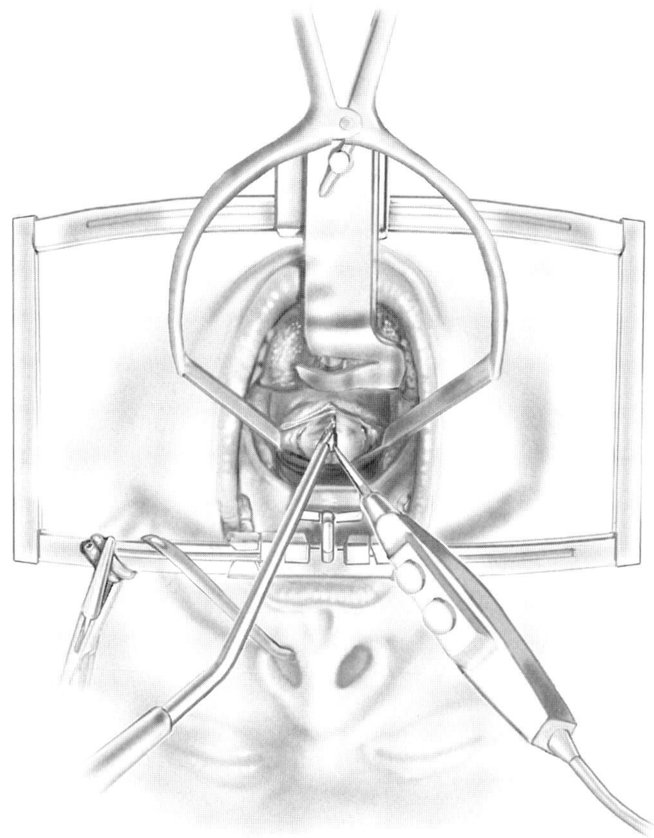

Figure 2-5. The initial subperiosteal dissection should occur along C1 approximately 1 cm from each side of the midline. An insulated monopolar is used to cauterize the C1 bone. The inferior dissection typically requires about 7.5 mm on each side lateral to the midline over the C2 body. This dissection will afford adequate exposure of the dens. Once the subperiosteal dissection has been carried out laterally, a Crockard self-retaining retractor is placed to retract the tissues laterally. We have found this retractor to be extremely helpful because it is easy to seat and holds the tissues well. Once this retractor is placed, the surgeon should have an excellent view of the anterior tubercle of C1, the medial portion of the C1 ring bilaterally, and the superior portion of C2. Retraction is increased as the dissection is carried laterally.

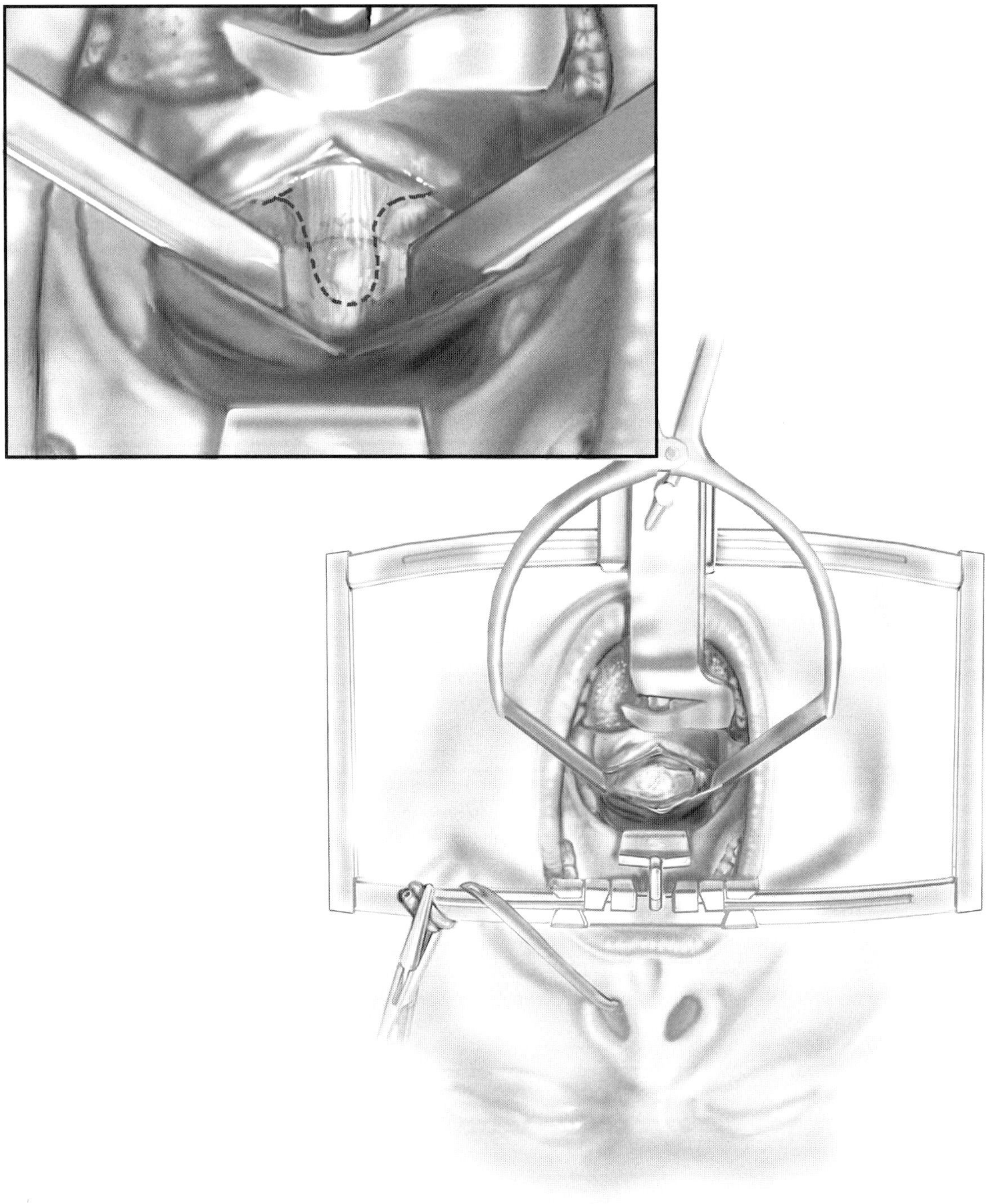

Figure 2-6. View of the operative field demonstrating the relationship of C1 and C2. **Inset**, Magnified view.

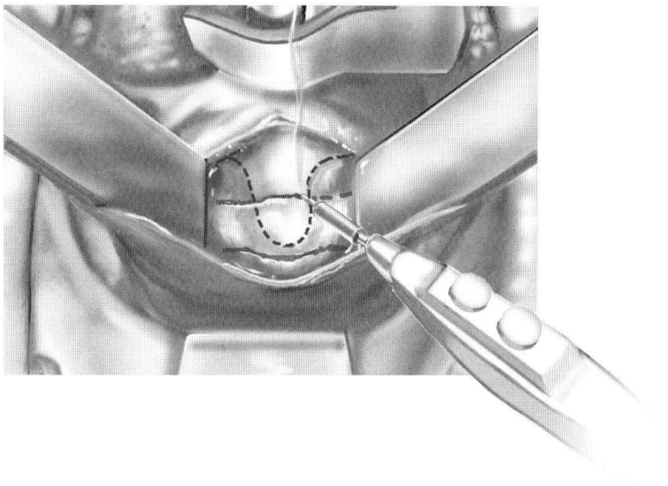

Figure 2-7. The ligamentous structures are then carefully dissected from the C1 ring. The superior dissection will clear the superior portion of the C1 ring, and the inferior dissection of the C1 ring will help the surgeon visualize the shoulders of the dens.

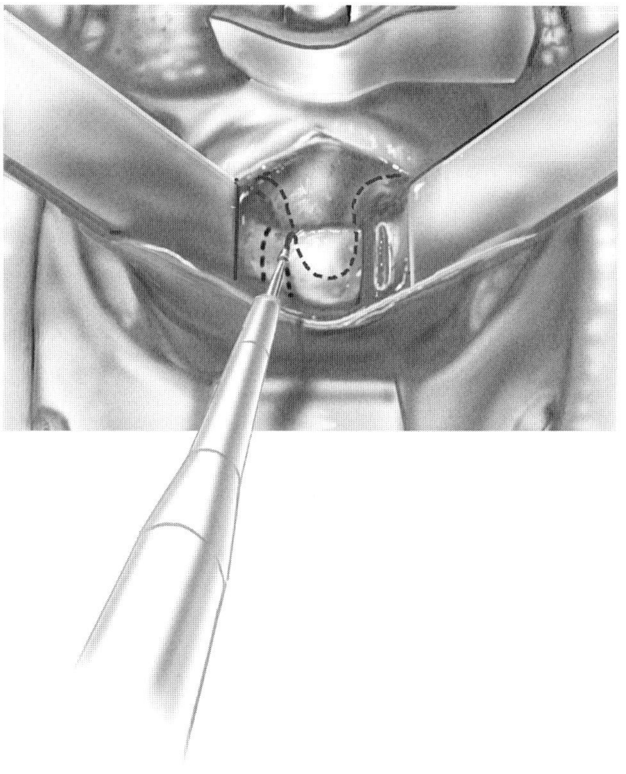

Figure 2-8. Once the bony exposure has been obtained, a high-speed drill (Midas Rex) is used with a small matchstick-tip bit to drill a trough on the lateral portions of the C1 ring for its removal. This tubercle can also be removed with a needle-nose rongeur much the same way. A common mistake is to not perform a wide removal of the anterior C1 ring; wide removal is critical for visualization of the shoulders of the dens, which provides the surgeon with a helpful anatomical landmark.

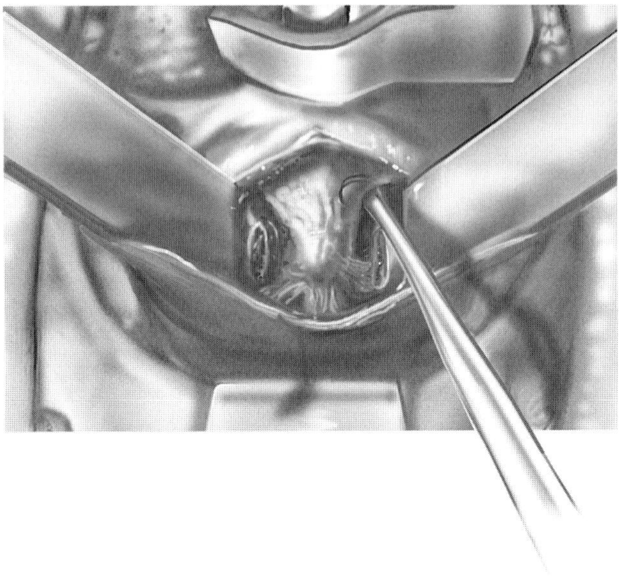

Figure 2-9. Identify the shoulders of the dens. Once the C1 ring has been removed, the dens can clearly be identified. Using a small, forward-angled curette, the dens is circumferentially dissected free from the alar and apical ligaments.

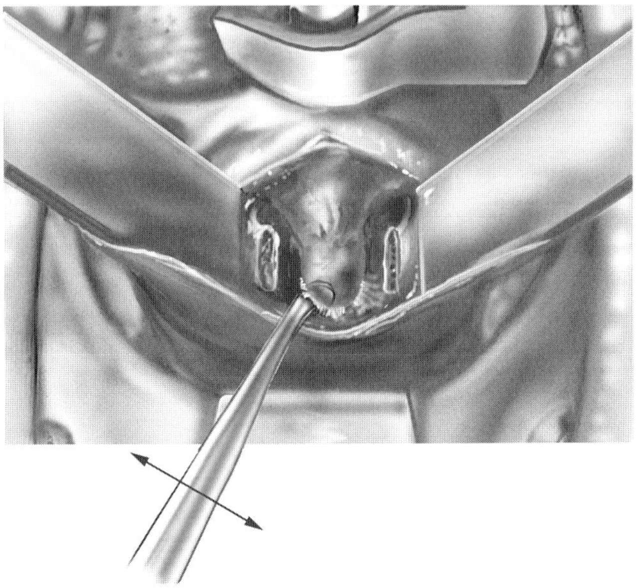

Figure 2-10. Using this forward-angled curette, the shoulders of the dens is dissected free. Once all the ligaments have been dissected off the dens, the curette can be advanced posterior to the dens, and the dens can sometimes be mobilized. Gently lift the dorsal side of the odontoid to verify that the curette is completely around the dens. It is critical to do this soft tissue dissection circumferentially around the dens before drilling (see *arrows*). If attachments are left on the dens, drilling may disarticulate the cortex from the base of C2. Any remaining cortex that is still attached to these ligaments is then difficult to remove without significant manipulation.

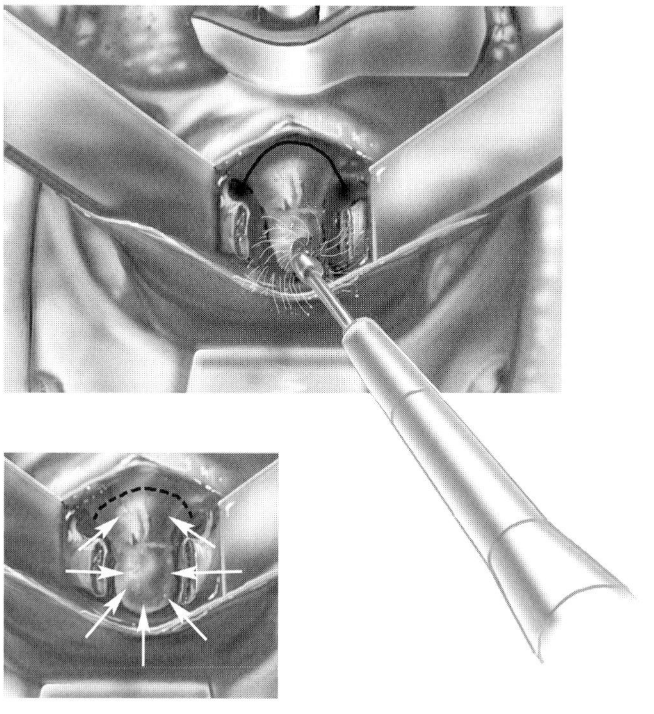

Figure 2-11. Once the dens has been completely freed of its ligamentous structures, drilling can be initiated from a lateral-to-medial and rostral-to-caudal direction. A high-speed drill is used to drill from the rostral tip of the odontoid caudally to the base. It is important to drill from the tip down instead of transecting the dens at the base. This is critical because, invariably, some of the posterior ligaments are still attached to the underside of the dens. If one transects the base of the dens, typically the fragment becomes mobile, making it extremely difficult to remove the remainder of the bone. Rather, we prefer to drill from the tip of the dens down, not allowing for a free fragment to become loose (i.e., "Attack from the perimeter." See *inset*.).

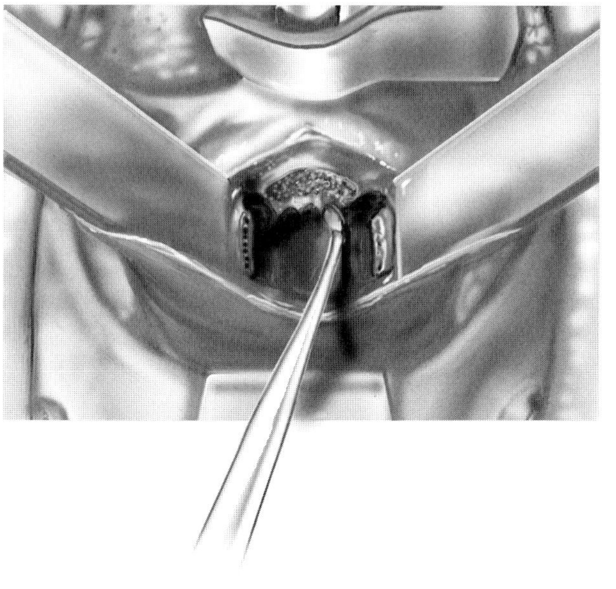

Figure 2-12. Once the major portion of the dens has been drilled, there is a thin eggshell cortical mantle present at the posterior aspect of the dens. Curved-angle curettes are used to remove this final fragment. We describe this as an "eggshell technique."

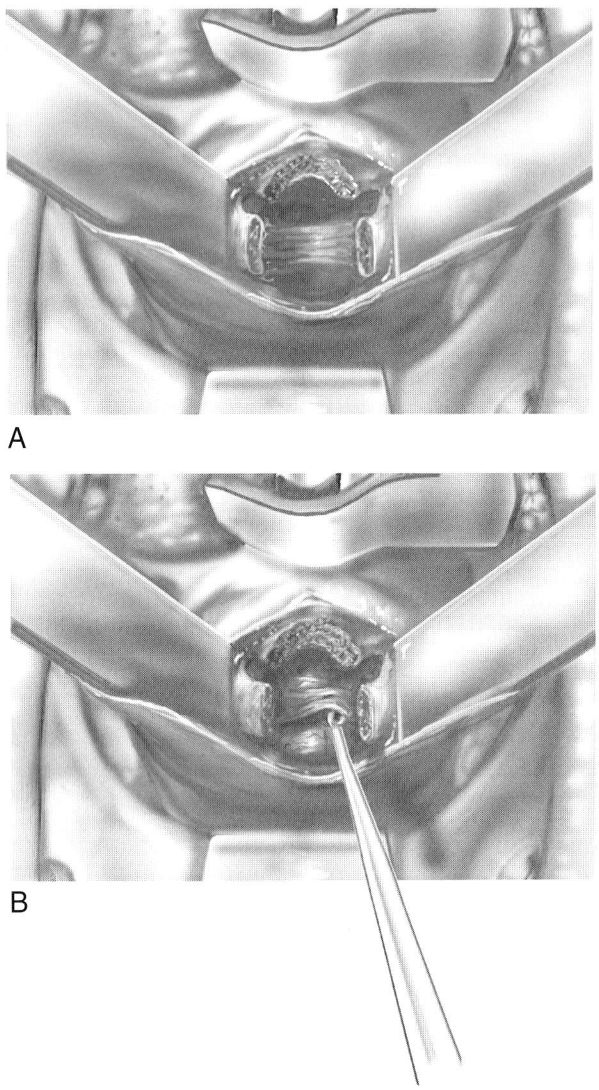

Figure 2-13. Once the dens has been removed **(A)**, the cruciate ligament is identified **(B)**. It is important to remove more of the rostral C2 body than what is initially thought necessary. We have found inadequate resection of the rostral C2 body to be a common problem that can leave the patient with residual cord compression after the odontoidectomy.

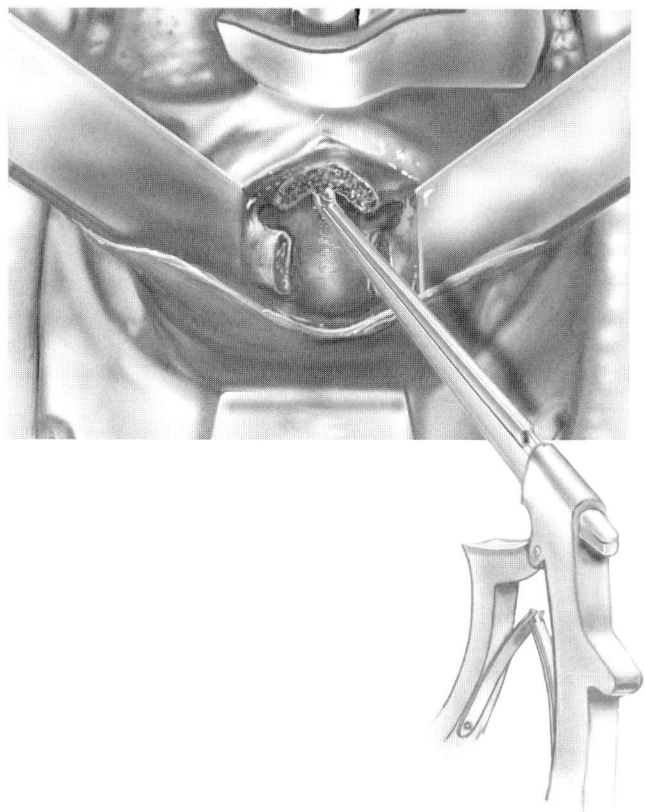

Figure 2-14. With the ligament removed and the dura exposed, the surgeon must determine the amount of soft tissue that should be removed. Sometimes considerable pannus removal should be considered. Depending on the level of compression behind the C2 body, a Kerrison rongeur might then be used to undercut this area. Our early experience was that we did not remove as much as was perceived during the operation. In the majority of these patients, compression is caused by bony compression. If there is a significant soft tissue pannus, this is debulked with a curette and Kerrison rongeur. We do think, however, that the high risk associated with a cerebrospinal fluid leak might outweigh any significant benefit from exposing the dura. Therefore, sometimes we elect to leave the ligament intact and just perform a bony decompression.

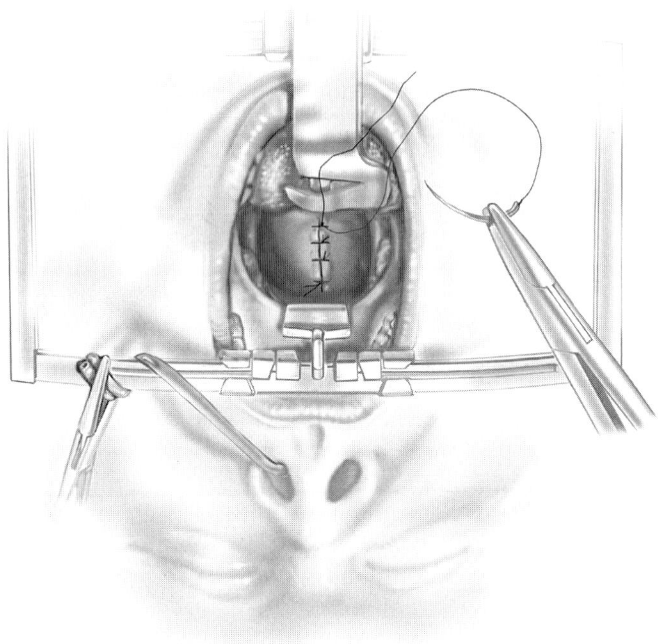

Figure 2-15. Closure. Once the decompression is complete, the wound is irrigated with small amounts of antibiotics. We do not use bone wax to stop bone bleeding because in this contaminated wound, we believe its use carries a high risk for infection. Once hemostasis is obtained, the mucosa is closed in a single layer with interrupted 3–0 chromic sutures that incorporate multiple layers of tissue.

COMMON PITFALLS

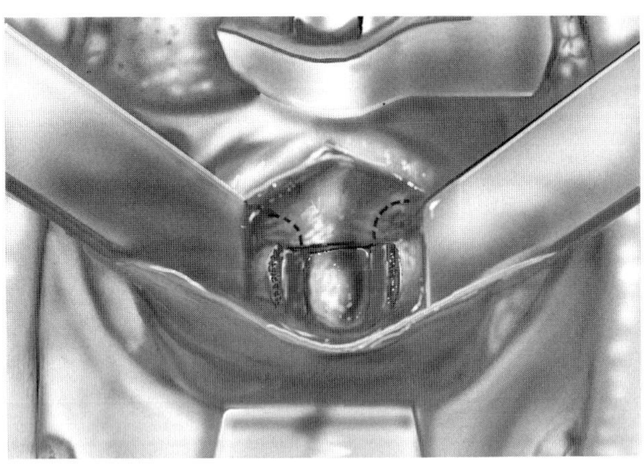

Figure 2-16. Suboptimal exposure and removal of the C1 ring can limit the odontoid resection. It is important to dissect at least 7.5 mm lateral to the anterior tubercle to properly visualize the true lateral walls of the dens. This will allow for adequate arch removal. If the arch is not removed to this lateral extent, it will be difficult to identify the shoulders of the dens and, subsequently, to remove it.

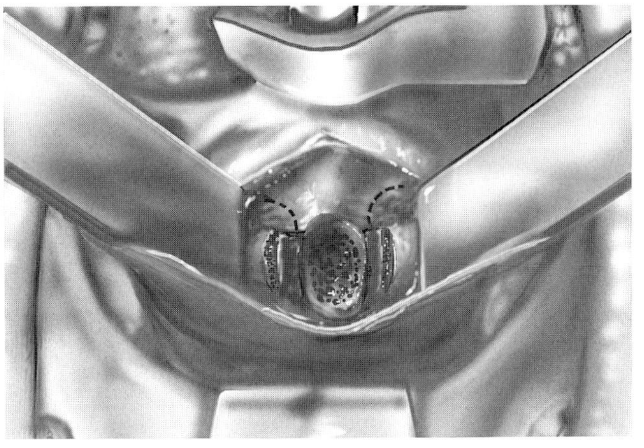

Figure 2-17. Some surgeons have used a "tumor-debulking" technique to remove the odontoid. This consists of drilling of the central portion of the odontoid and leaving the lateral, ventral, and superior vertical rim intact. By doing this, the cortical rim fragments can then be fractured centrally to decompress the brain stem. The difficulty with this technique is that there are still extensive ligamentous attachments to the cortical mantle ventrally and superiorly. When using this "tumor-debulking" technique, it is much more difficult to remove these fragments, and an inordinate amount of time is added to the process. By drilling from the rostral tip and in a lateral-to-medial fashion, it is easier to remove the odontoid (i.e., "Attack from the perimeter.").

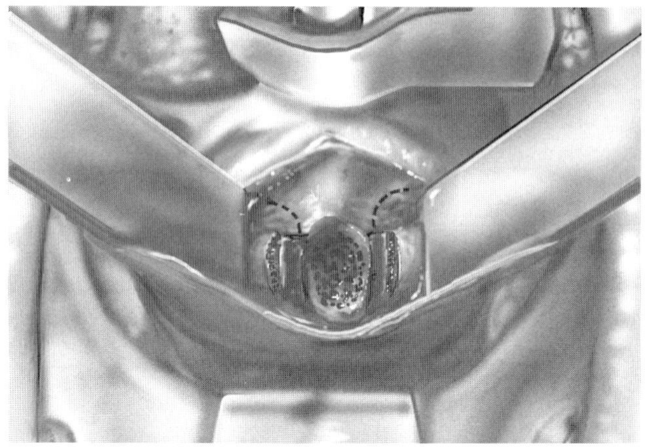

Figure 2-18. Suboptimal resection of the ventral compression is a common difficulty with this operation. Several times early on in our experience, we reviewed postoperative studies that demonstrated some residual ventral compression due to suboptimal decompression. The amount of compression must be determined preoperatively with CT and magnetic resonance imaging (MRI). The surgeon must have a good understanding of how much of the C2 body must be resected to provide adequate decompression. This is usually best visualized on the CT scan. Resection can vary from simply removing the very tip of the dens to removing the complete C2 body. Decompression is achieved using a Kerrison rongeur and a high-speed drill. To gauge the amount of bony removal and decompression, the surgeon can deliver a small dole of iohexol contrast into the decompression bed and check a lateral fluoroscopic view. This radiographic image can help the surgeon in assessing the amount of C2 bone removal.

CHAPTER III

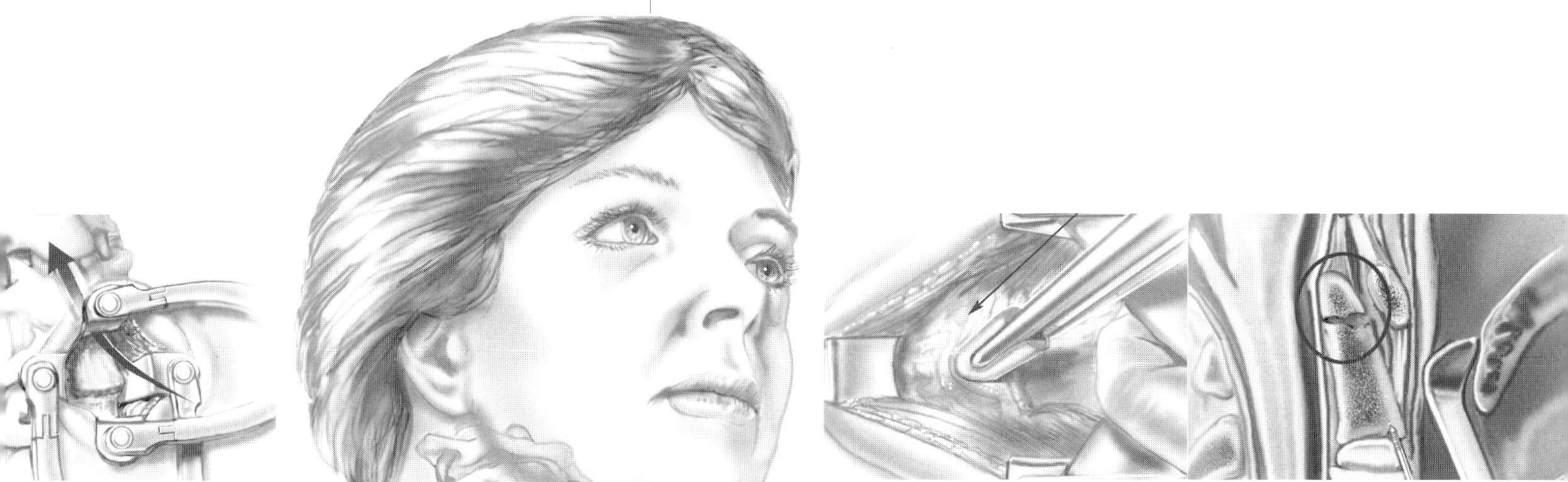
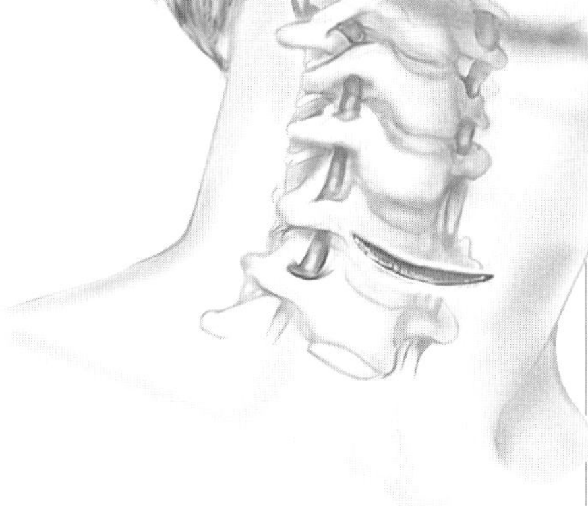

Anterior Odontoid Screw Fixation

With regard to anterior odontoid screw fixation, important points to consider are the patient's body habitus, the direction of the fracture line, and the amount of displacement. Patients with short necks or barrel chests may not be good candidates for this procedure because screw trajectory may not be optimal for fracture fixation. Patients and their families need to be informed during consent that anatomical variables may prevent screw placement and as a result may require either an alternate posterior C1–C2 approach or halo fixation instead of anterior screw fixation.

Oblique fractures or fractures in the coronal plane may not be amenable to screw fixation because the course of the screw may project along the fracture line.

Lastly, displaced nonreducible fractures do not provide optimal conditions for anterior screw fixation. It has been our experience that posteriorly displaced fractures can be gently reduced under fluoroscopic guidance with anterior translation of the head. Anterior fractures can be reduced after intubation by placing a finger in the patient's mouth and gently pushing posteriorly on the C1 arch under fluoroscopic guidance. If the fracture is reduced, anterior fixation can be achieved. If the fracture is not reducible, alternate forms of fixation must be considered.

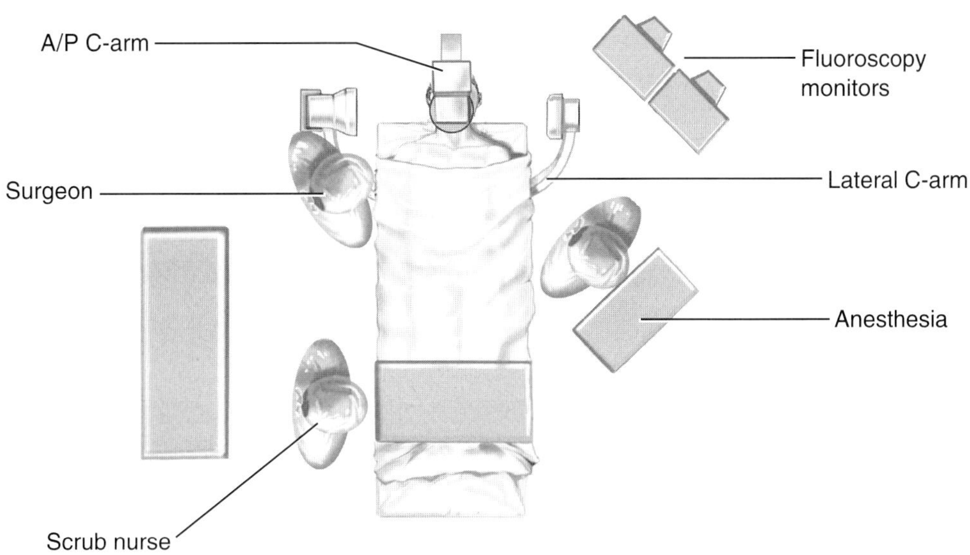

Figure 3-1. This schematic of the operating room setup demonstrates a right-handed surgeon in position with biplanar fluoroscopy. We have found that this setup allows the surgeon to view both fluoroscopy monitors and work unimpeded for screw placement. Reduction of the fracture and adequate biplanar fluoroscopic visualization of the C1–C2 complex is critical and must be optimized before the incision. If there is not adequate visualization of these structures or if there is inadequate reduction, this procedure cannot be performed, and alternate therapies such as posterior C1–C2 screw fixation or halo immobilization must be considered. This technique can be difficult to perform with barrel-chested patients. (Sometimes anterior translation of the head toward the ceiling can overcome this problem.)

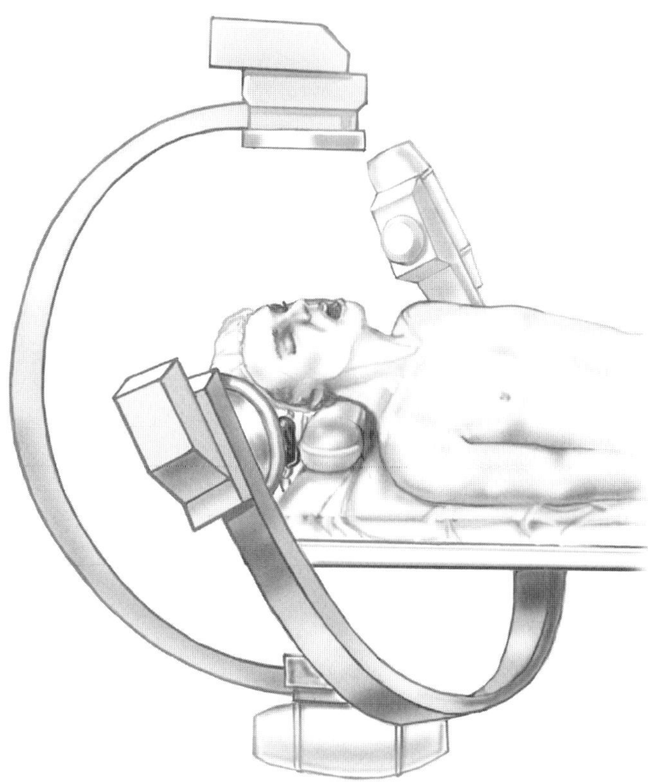

Figure 3-2. When positioning both fluoroscopic machines, it is important to first place the lateral one with the gantry tilted under the bed. This will allow the anterior/posterior fluoroscopic machine to be moved into position without difficulty. A radiolucent bite block is placed to open the patient's mouth, ensuring adequate visualization of C2. Rolled gauze can be used as an alternative.

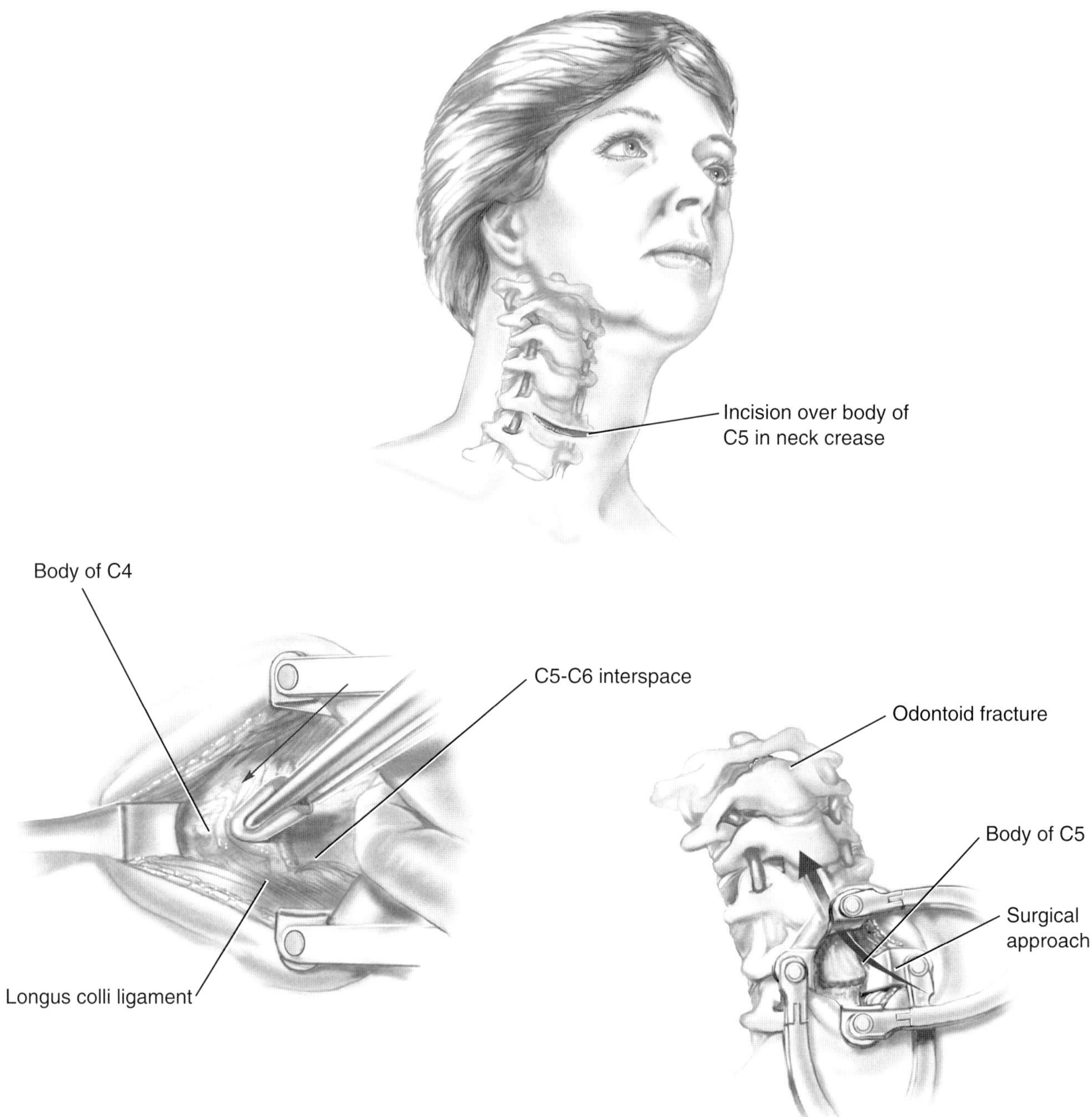

Figure 3-3. The incision is made at approximately the C5–C6 skin level. We typically use a standard transverse incision and an anterior cervical discectomy approach. Once the prevertebral fascia has been identified, a medial-to-lateral Caspar retractor system may be placed, and blunt dissection is performed superiorly with Kittner dissectors up to the C2–C3 disc space. As dissection occurs superiorly, the level should be intermittently checked using lateral fluoroscopy. The majority of this procedure is performed blindly until the C2–C3 interspace is identified on fluoroscopic image. We rarely use the two-bladed rostral-caudal retractor. A single cephalad retractor is placed.

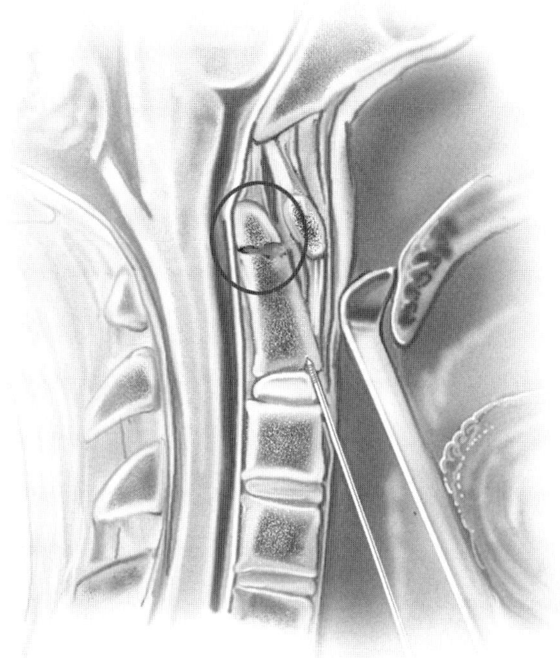

Figure 3-4. Once the C2–C3 interspace is identified, a retractor is placed to expose the pertinent anatomy. Retractor systems include the UCSS (Universal Cannulated Screw System, Medtronic Sofamor Danek) and the Apfelbaum retractor system (Aesculap).

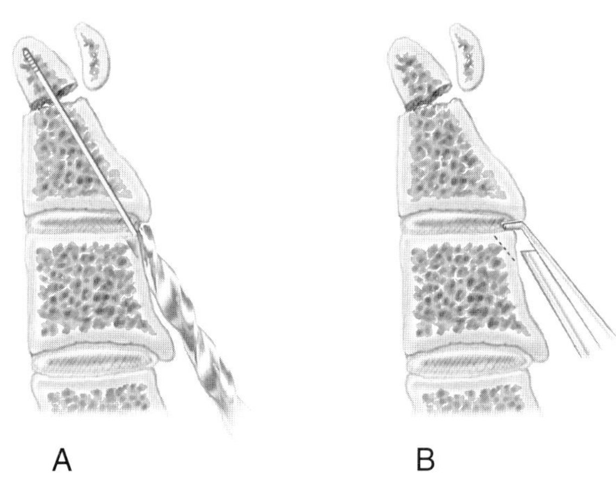

Figure 3-5, A and B. A K-wire is placed under the C2 anterior lip in the midline. The midline is assessed by anteroposterior fluoroscopic imaging. Sometimes a surgeon must remove a portion of the superior anterior surface of C3 to get a more optimal trajectory. This can be achieved with an Apfelbaum hand drill slid over the K-wire or a Kerrison rongeur held upside down. By removing this portion of bone, the surgeon can dock the cannulated drill and screw system and ensure an adequate trajectory to incorporate the dens fracture.

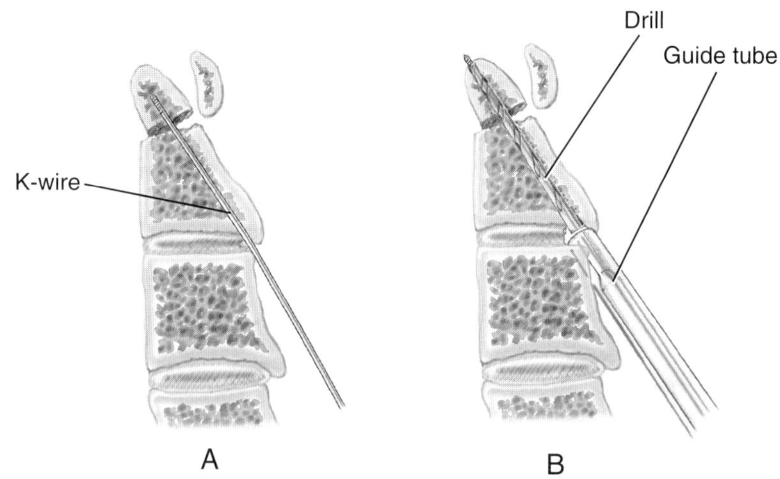

Figure 3-6, A. Once the trough is created, a K-wire is inserted using a mini driver drill. Under direct biplanar fluoroscopic guidance, the K-wire is advanced through the fracture site into the fragment.

Figure 3-6, B. Once the K-wire is in an adequate position, a drill guide is placed over the K-wire, and the drill bit is drilled over the K-wire. Care should be taken not to advance the K-wire when drilling. The drill is completed through the distal segment of the fracture incorporating the distal cortex. We prefer using the UCSS for screw placement.

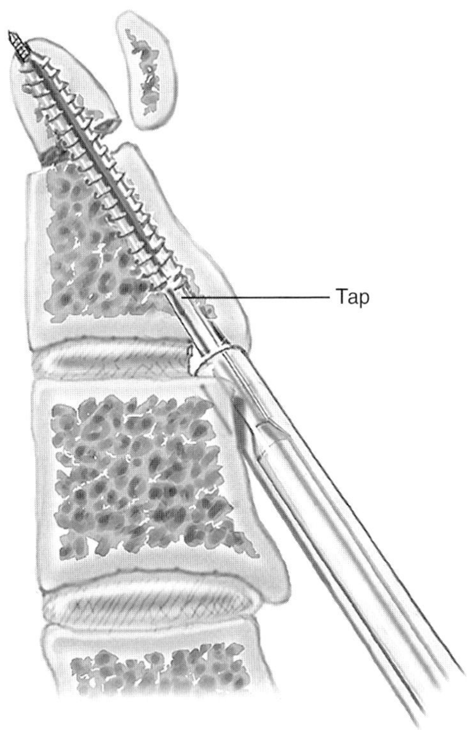

Figure 3-7. After drilling is complete, the channel is tapped over the K-wire, avoiding advancement of the K-wire. The lag screw is then placed. One must account for the few millimeters of lag distance when selecting screw length.

Box 3-1 Choice of Screw

Measure 38 mm, use 36 mm screw
Measure 40 mm, use 38 mm screw
Measure 42 mm, use 40 mm screw

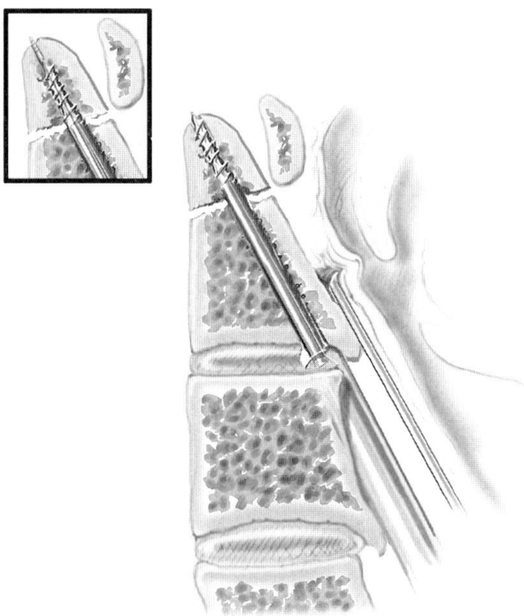

A

Figure 3-8, A. As the lag screw crosses the fracture line, the K-wire is removed to avoid bending of the wire to the screw.

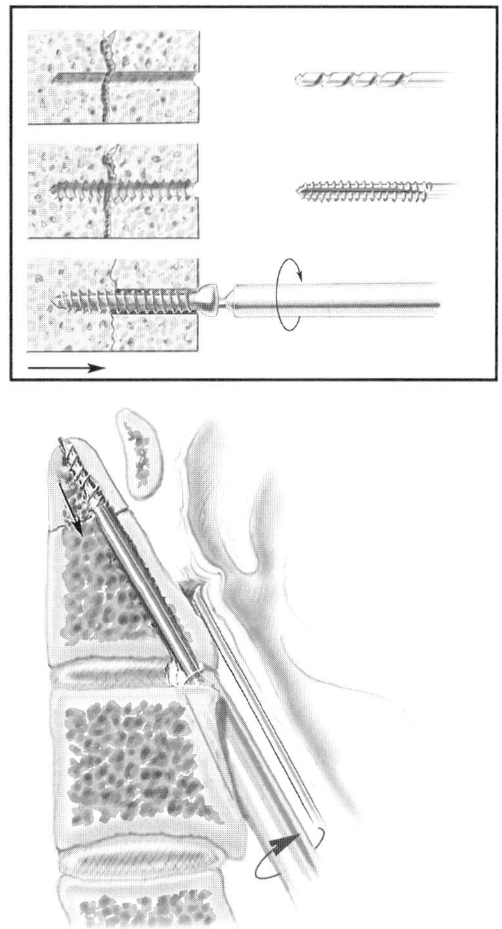

B

Figure 3-8, B. The final lag effect occurs at the last turn of the screwdriver. Occasionally, the fragment will not lag completely. If the lag screw is not available, the larger drill bit can be used to overdrill the proximal segment. (gliding hole). Then a fully threaded screw can be used; this will still achieve a lag effect on the tapped region (see *inset*).

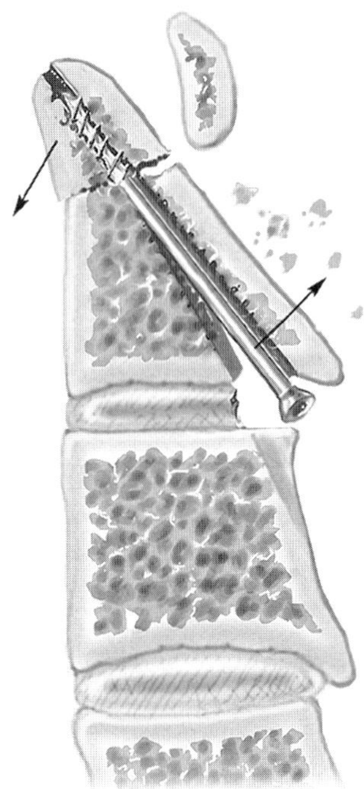

COMMON PITFALLS

It is on option premeasure screw length based on preoperative computed tomography (CT) scanning to obtain the optimal lag purchase. Even though these measurements are helpful, the surgeon must ultimately judge the screw length during intraoperative fluoroscopy. Patients and their families must be counseled preoperatively regarding the possibility that odontoid fixation cannot be performed due to body habitus or an inability to obtain adequate reduction. As a result, alternative posterior C1–C2 fixation may need to be performed.

Figure 3-9. If the screw is placed too far anteriorly, it may fracture through the anterior face of the C2 body. Preoperatively, a thin-section CT scan with sagittal and coronal reconstructions should be obtained, and careful attention to the orientation of the fracture is critical. If a coronal fracture is present, the patient's anatomy may not be amenable to direct screw fixation.

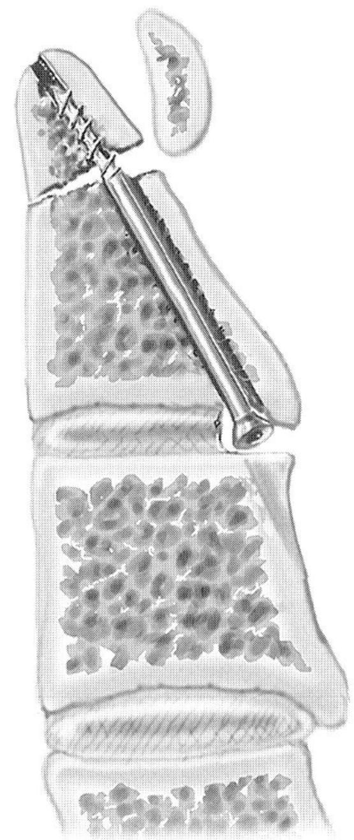

Figure 3-10. Screw threads are proximal to the fracture line, which can prevent any desired lag effects of the screw.

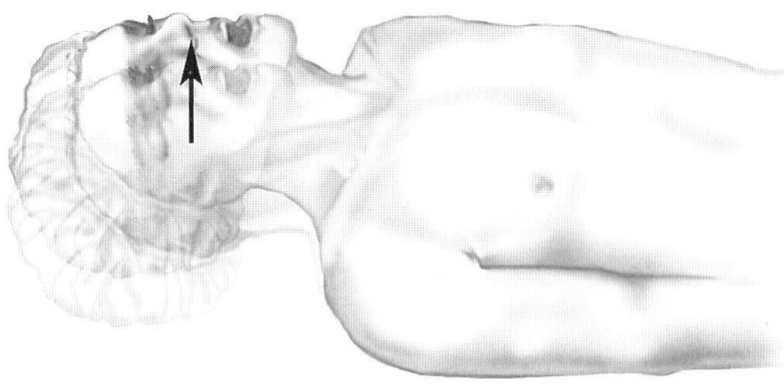

POSTOPERATIVE RESULTS

Figure 3-11. Anterior translation of the head can help achieve adequate reduction. Reduction can also be achieved for anteriorly displaced fractures by gentle finger pressure through the mouth of an anesthetized patient. This reduction technique should be performed under direct fluoroscopic guidance.

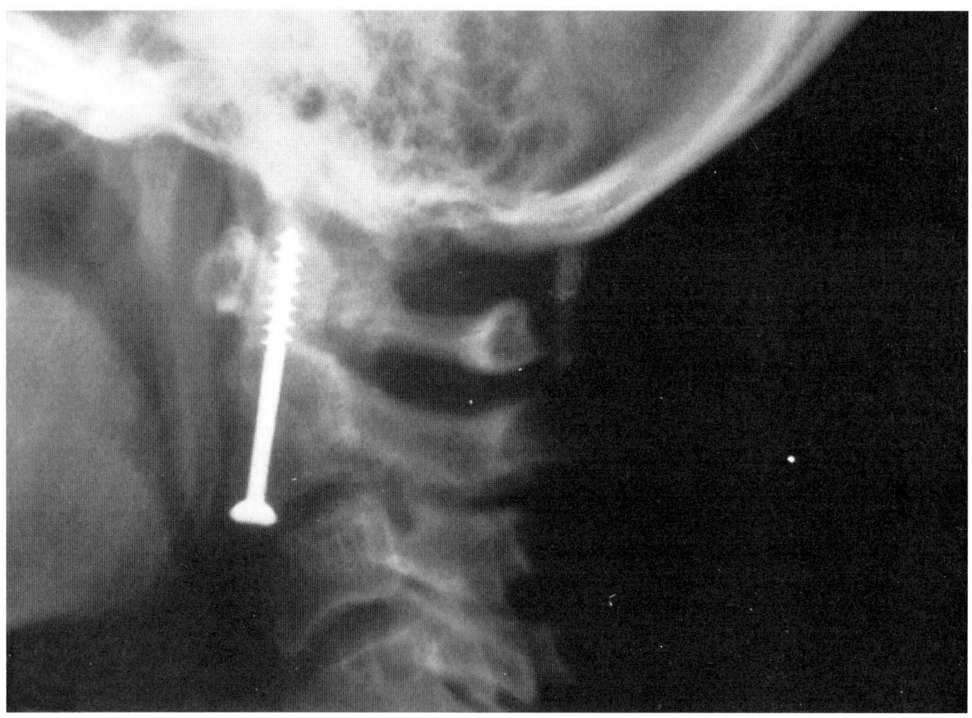

Figure 3-12. Lateral cervical spine x-ray demonstrating anterior odontoid screw fixation. Note the lag portion of the screw sits only within the dens portion of the fracture. This allows for the lag effect to "pull" the fracture down.

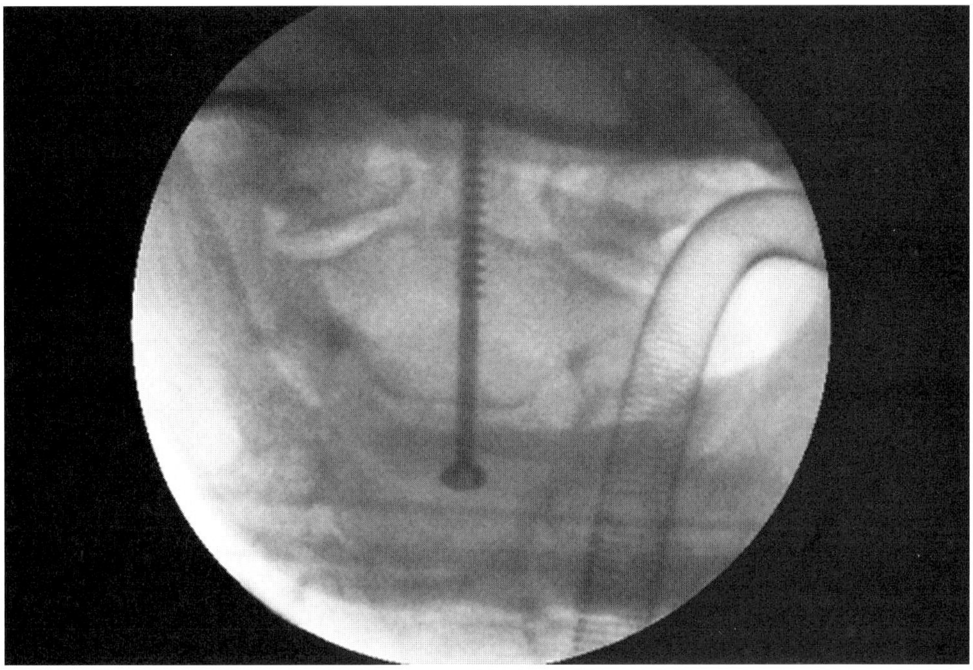

Figure 3-13. The anteroposterior view of this patient demonstrates the common pitfalls of screw choice—the screw is too long and may be prominent on the anterior aspect of C3. In addition, the lag portion of the screw is too long, thus eliminating the lag effect of the screw.

CHAPTER IV

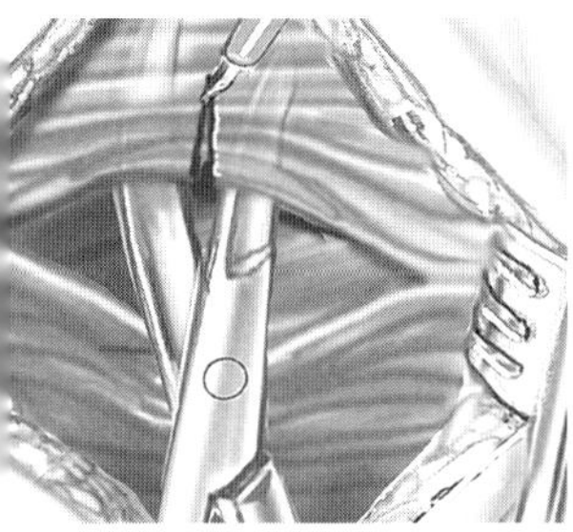
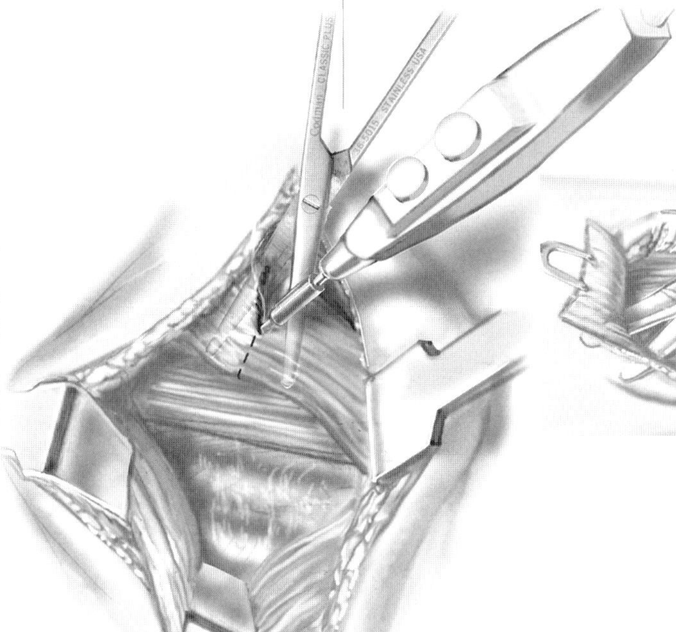
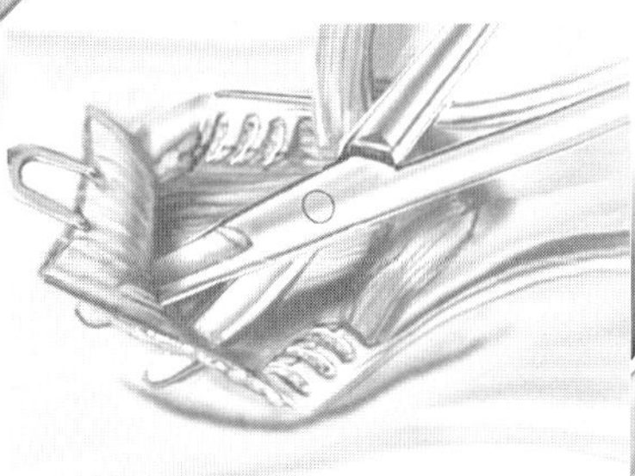
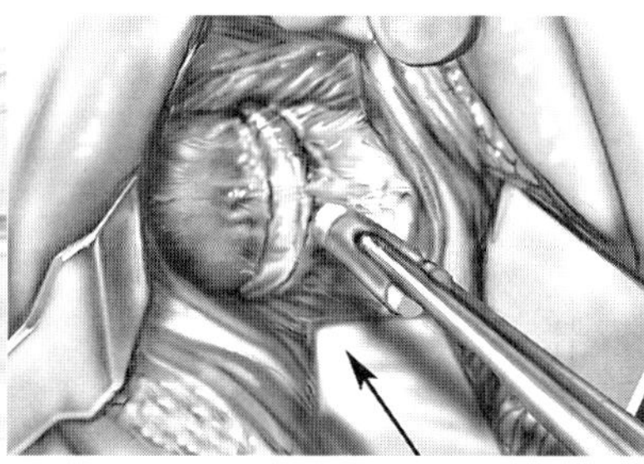

Anterior Cervical Approaches: Exposure and Releasing Techniques

This chapter is a springboard for exposures of the anterior cervical spine. The main emphasis on the anterior dissection is that a well-dissected, relaxing-type exposure is less traumatic to the cervical musculature and reduces postoperative soft tissue swelling. We have found that division of the omohyoid muscle allows for a wider dissection with less tension and does not result in any demonstrable disability related to division of this muscle. Although we do not routinely reapproximate the muscle with sutures, this can be achieved easily if a surgeon wishes to do so. With the exception of sharp dissection to undermine the platysma and the opening of the investing sheath of the sternocleidomastoid, the majority of the remaining dissection is performed bluntly with a Kittner and finger dissection.

Any large anterior jugular vein that courses through the field that might obscure or lessen exposure should be tied off and divided to optimize exposure. Single- or double-level exposures can be achieved with a transverse incision. An exposure of three or more levels may require a vertical incision along the medial border of the sternocleidomastoid.

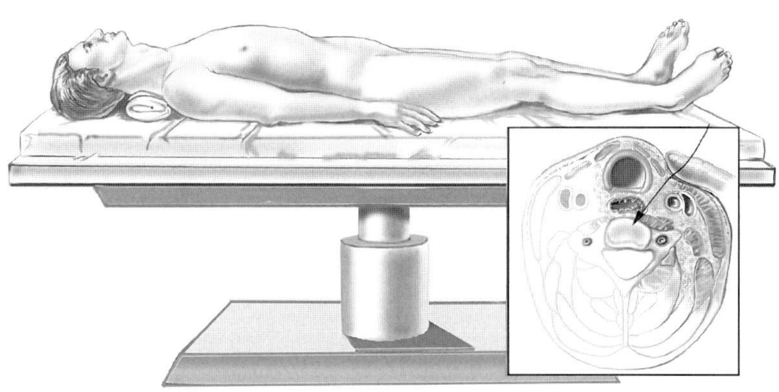

Figure 4-1. The patient is positioned in the supine position on an electric table with a 1-L IV bag wrapped in a towel supporting the cervical region to enhance lordosis. All appropriate pressure points are padded, including the ulnar nerves bilaterally and the heels. Some prefer to use a doughnut to stabilize the head. However, we have found that the doughnut can reduce the cervical lordosis established by the IV bag. It has been our preference to leave the head gently extended and resting on the bed. In patients with severe cervical stenosis or large disc herniations causing significant spinal canal narrowing, a cervical extension test may be performed before intubation and positioning before anesthetic induction.

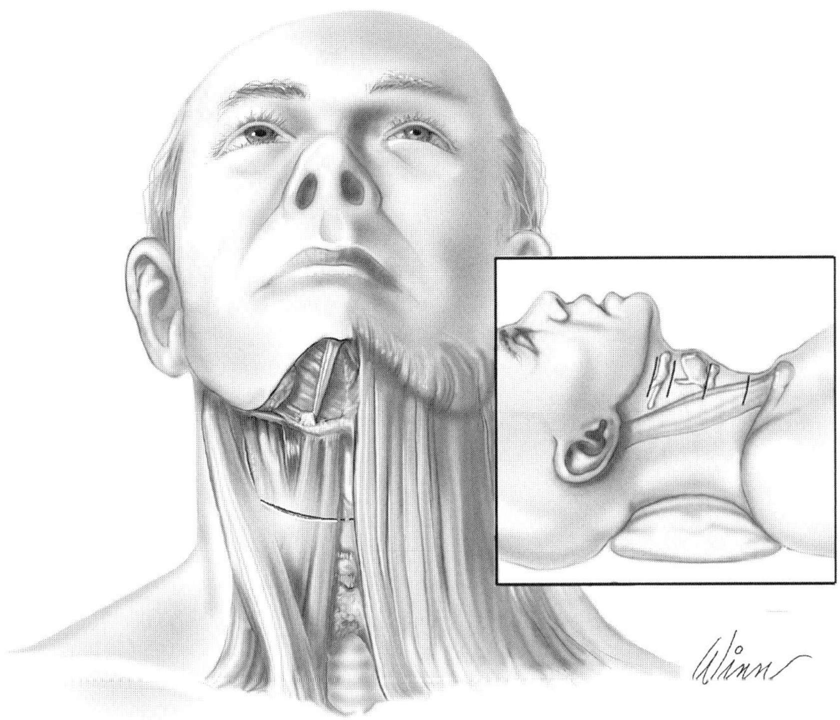

Figure 4-2. This general overview of the cervical musculature demonstrates a typical transverse incision for a routine anterior cervical discectomy and planned route of approach (see *inset*). This incision begins at the midline and extends laterally along the skin crease to the medial border of the sternocleidomastoid muscle. The level of the incision is determined by palpation of external and internal bony landmarks. Using gentle finger pressure medially, one can palpate the C6 tubercle (Chassaignac's tubercle) to get a better idea of what level is appropriate for placement of the incision. Also, the cricothyroid membrane is typically at the C5–C6 interspace, and this landmark is reliable in helping the surgeon choose the proper incision level (see Figure 4-1 inset). In older adults, we caution against vigorous palpation of the C6 tubercle because patients may have concomitant vascular disease in the carotid region, and atherosclerotic plaques may be disrupted and cause embolic events.

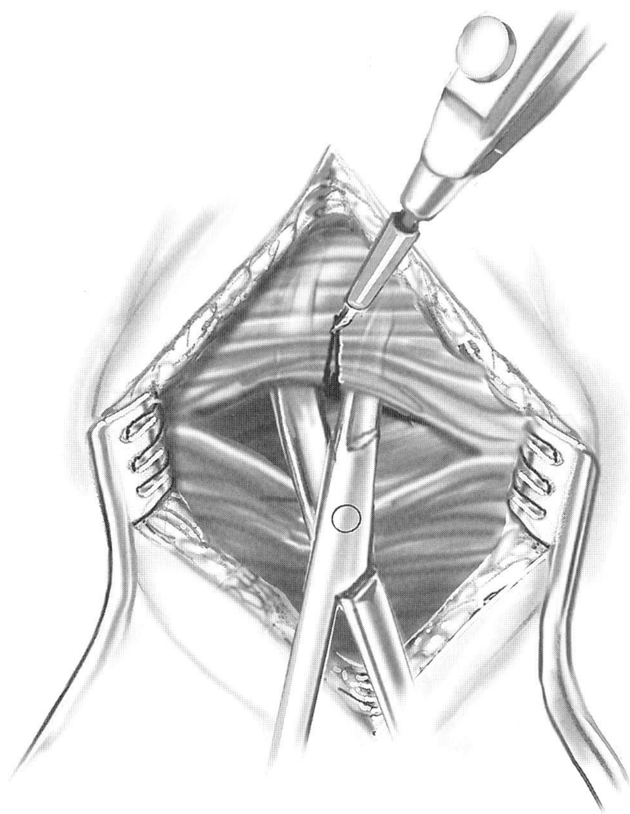

A

Figure 4-3, A–C. **A,** A transverse incision is made down to and through the subcutaneous tissues and fat. The platysma muscle is identified and elevated. Using Metzenbaum scissors, the platysma is opened, undermined, and transected with monopolar cautery. **B,** After the platysma is transected, we perform an extensive releasing technique by undermining the platysma superiorly and inferiorly. This is especially useful once the retractor blades are placed. If an inadequate platysma release is performed, when the medial lateral retractor is placed deeply, upper tissue layers will become taut and difficult to retract in a rostral-caudal direction. **C,** Once the platysma has been undermined, the omohyoid muscle is identified. The omohyoid muscle can typically be identified at the C5–C6 level and is crossing in an oblique fashion almost perpendicular to the sternocleidomastoid. We have found the division of the omohyoid to be very useful in gaining extensive exposure to the anterior cervical region. At the completion of the procedure, we do not reapproximate this muscle and have had no postoperative problems with this technique.

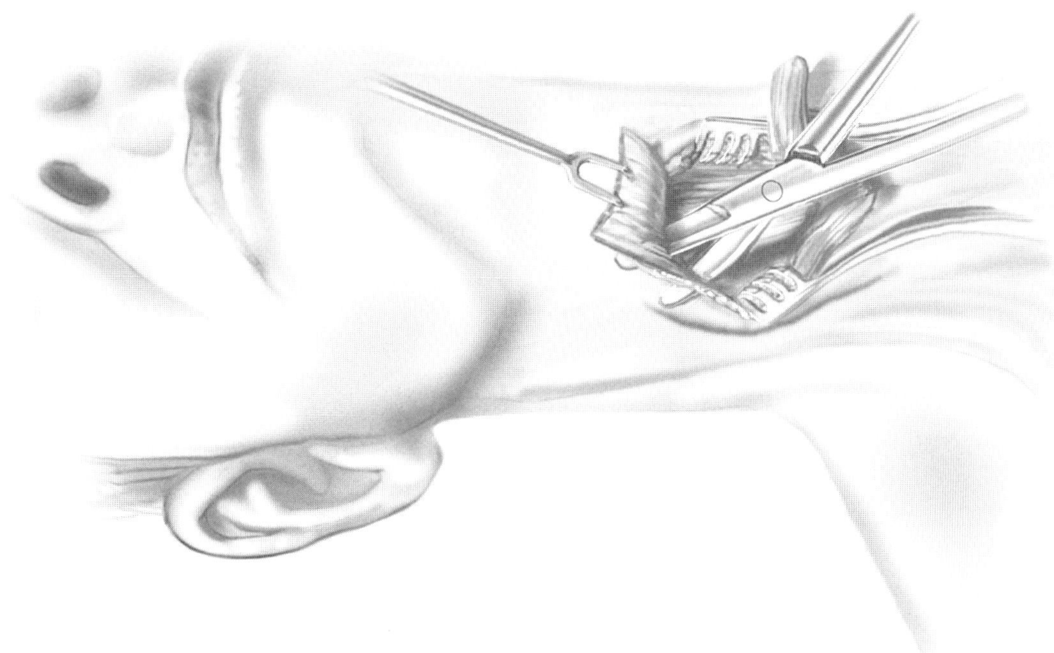

B

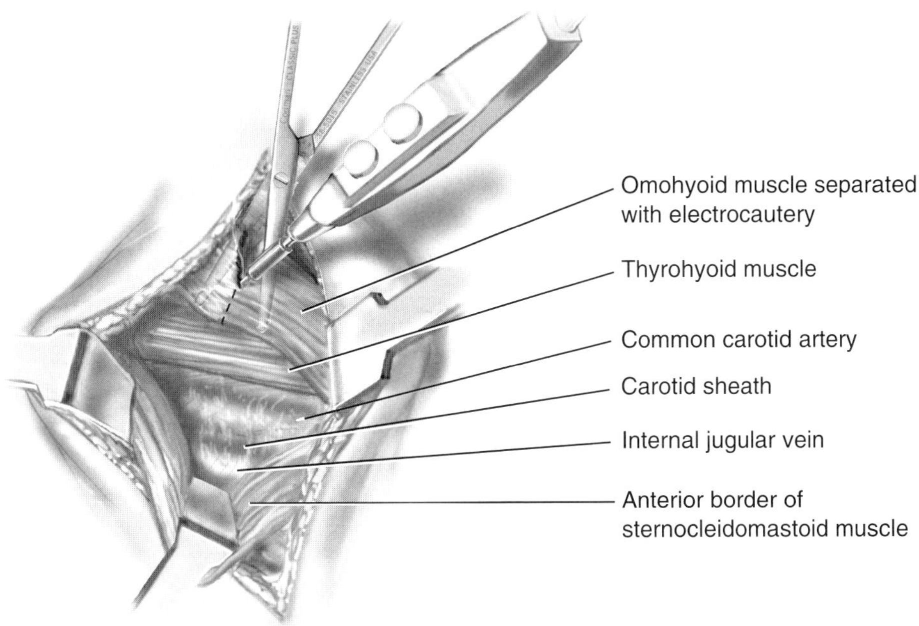
Omohyoid muscle separated with electrocautery
Thyrohyoid muscle
Common carotid artery
Carotid sheath
Internal jugular vein
Anterior border of sternocleidomastoid muscle

C

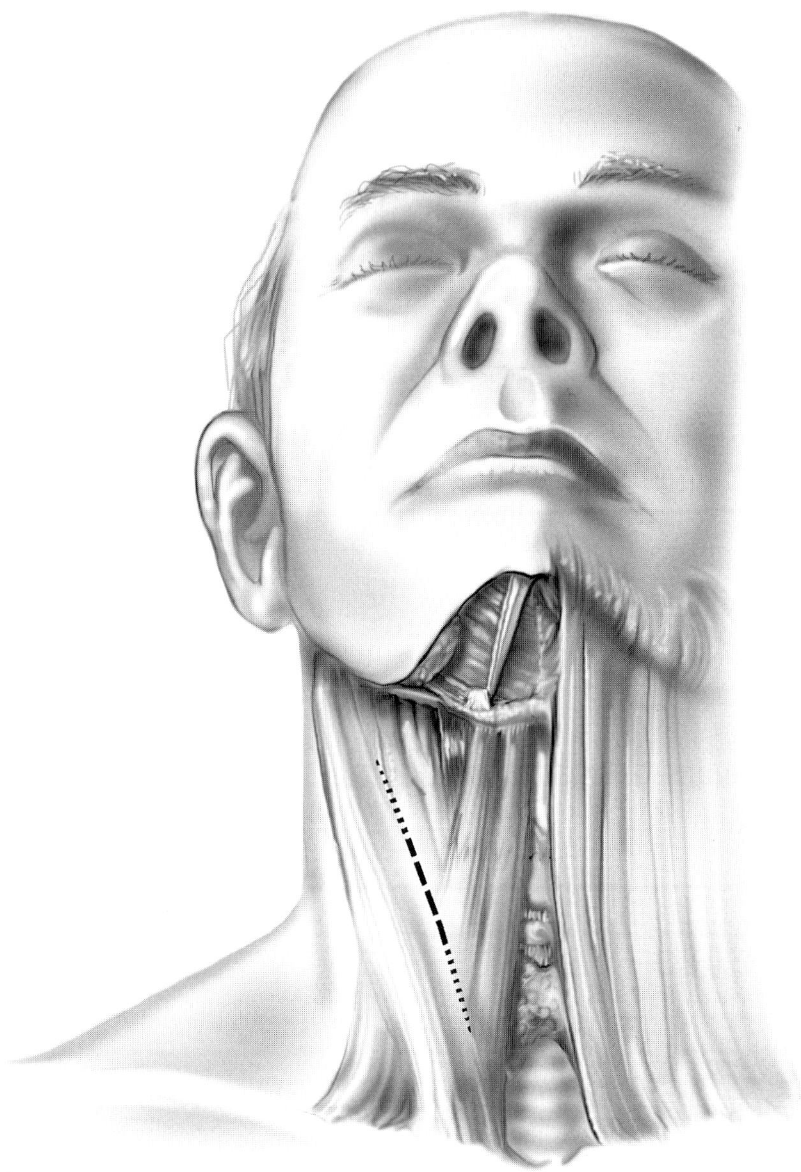

A

Figure 4-4, A–C. **A,** For multilevel exposures, a longitudinal incision along the medial border of the sternocleidomastoid can be used. We reserve this incision for multilevel discectomy of more than two motion segments or for any multilevel vertebrectomy. **B,** With the longitudinal incision, the platysma does not need significant undermining to obtain adequate exposure. The longitudinal incision provides wide access to the anterior cervical region. **C,** The dissection is carried down through the avascular plane between the sternocleidomastoid and carotid sheath laterally and the trachea and esophagus medially. Using a combination of blunt and sharp dissection, the prevertebral fascia is exposed.

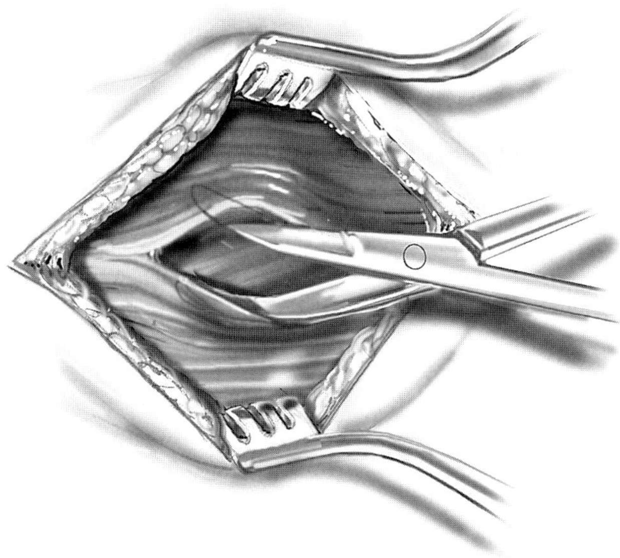

B

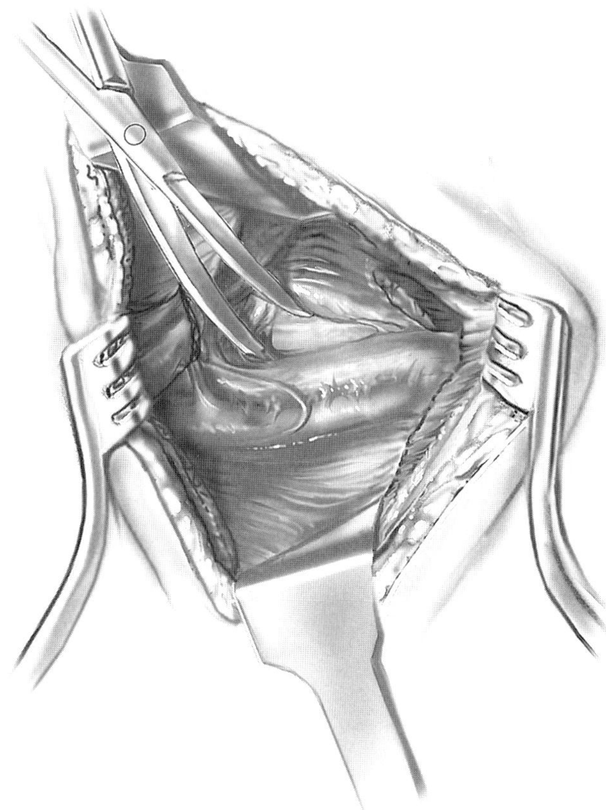

C

Figure 4-4, B–C. *Continued.*

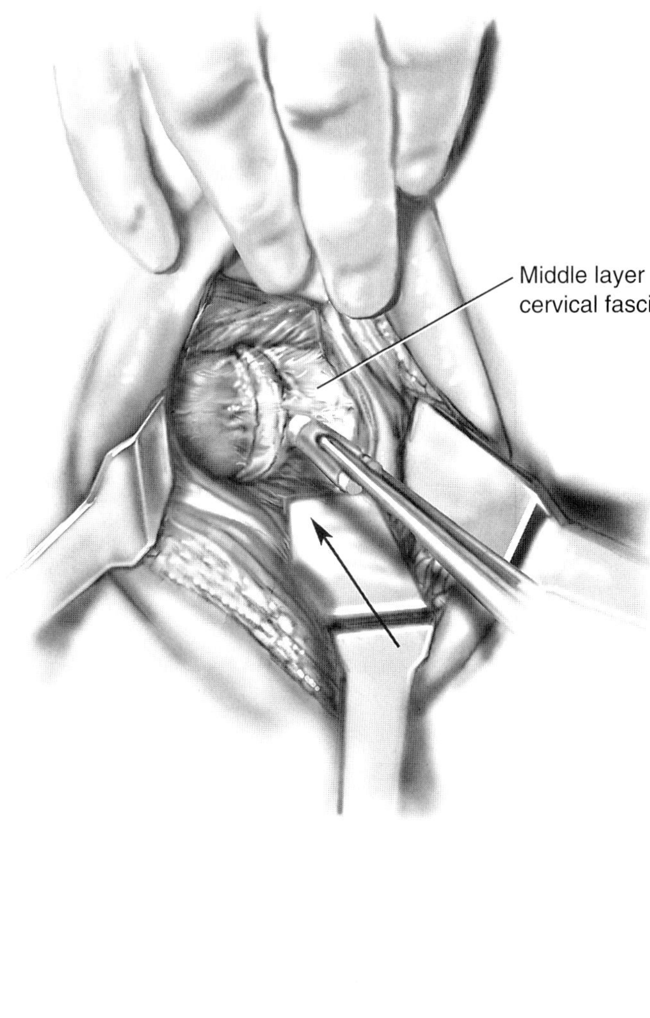

Figure 4-5. Once the prevertebral fascia is identified, a Kittner dissector is used to open the area.

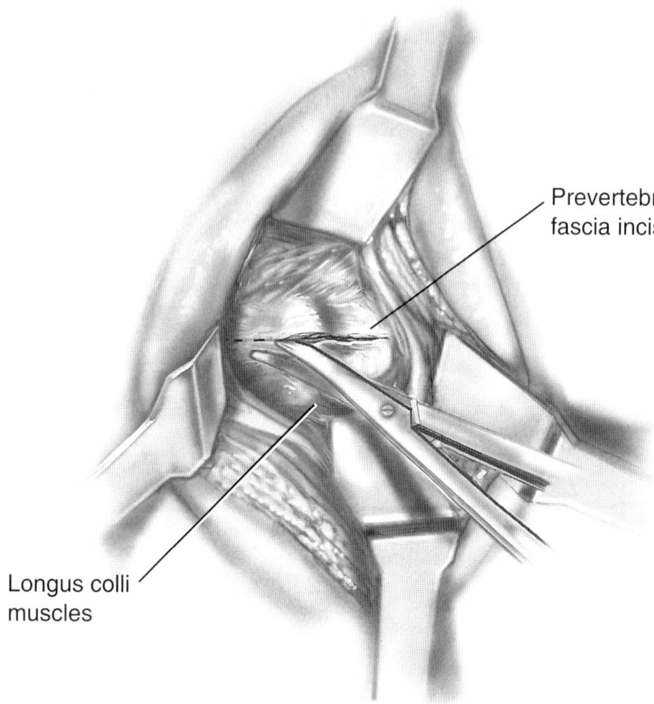

A

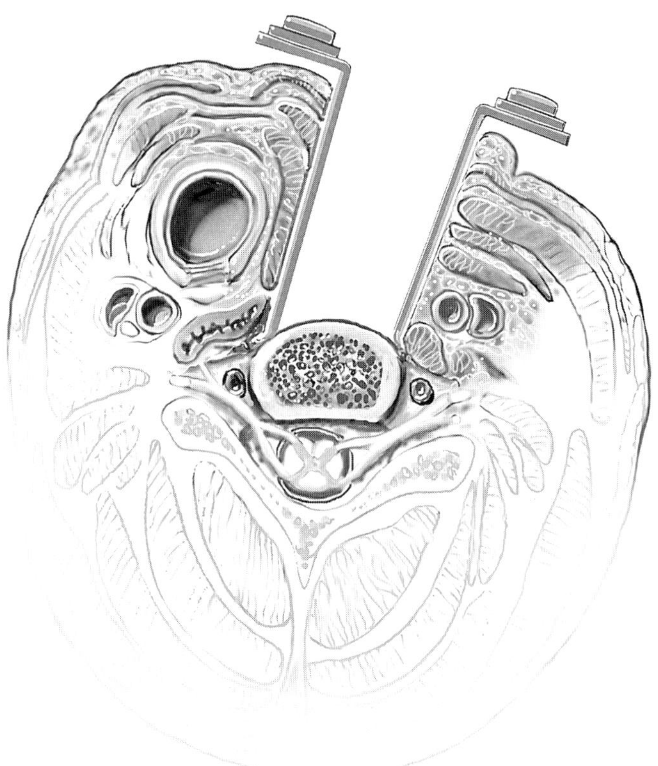

B

Figure 4-6, A and B. **A,** If necessary, the prevertebral fascia is opened sharply. A monopolar cautery is utilized to dissect the longus colli muscles laterally. The longus colli muscles are released from the medial attachments and are dissected in a subperiosteal fashion. They can usually be retracted during this dissection with a Fraser tip suction. The interspace is then identified, the needle is placed into disc space (or a Caspar distraction pin is placed into a vertebral body), and a localizing x-ray is taken. **B,** The Caspar retractor system is then placed in the medial lateral direction with the trachea and esophagus medially and the carotid sheath laterally.

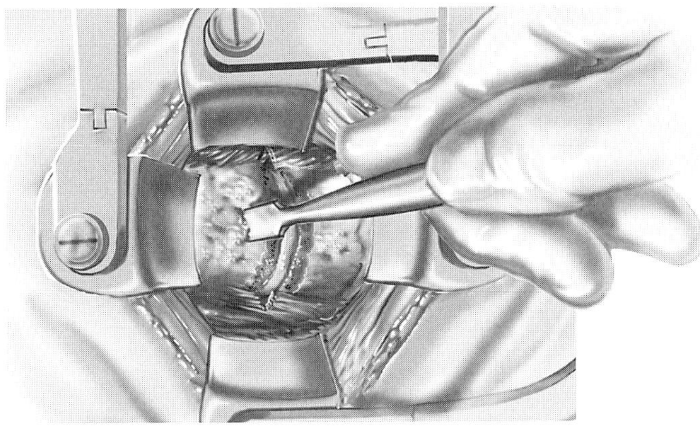

Figure 4-7. Once the appropriate level has been identified, the longus colli dissection is carried laterally to identify the uncovertebral joints bilaterally. If a quarter-inch key elevator is used, soft tissues can be dissected away from the cortical surface, and the osteophytes can be identified. The key elevator is very helpful in exposing bone surface area so that the surgeon can identify the shape of the vertebral body.

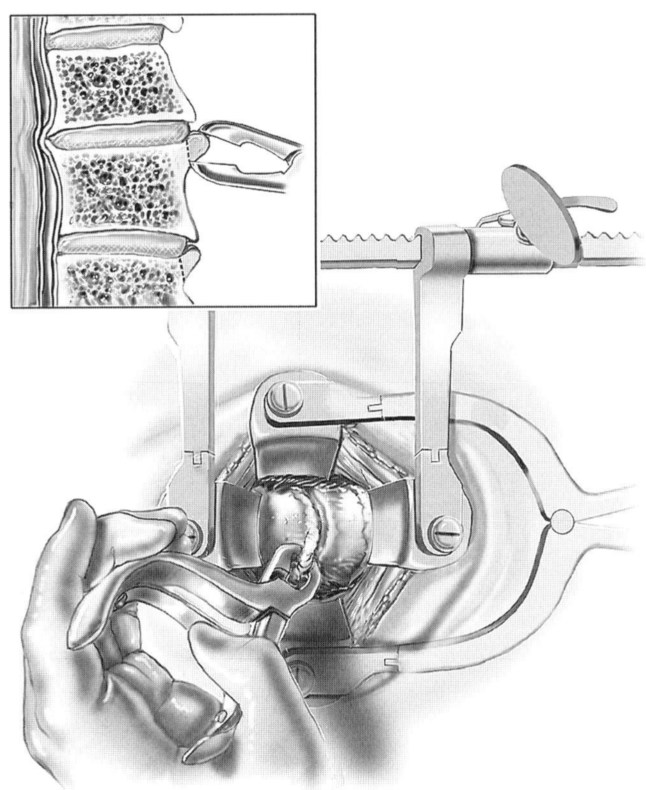

Figure 4-8. All osteophytes are removed with a Cushing rongeur to ensure a flat surface of bone that ultimately will facilitate plate fixation. This technique, called *gardening*, helps the surgeon to identify the disc space and to begin the preparation of the cortical surfaces for placement of a cervical plate (see *inset*). The removal of osteophytes facilitates exposure of the uncovertebral joints, thereby helping the surgeon to identify proper lateral exposure and thus the midline. It also allows for a cervical plate to lay flush against the anterior surface of the spine.

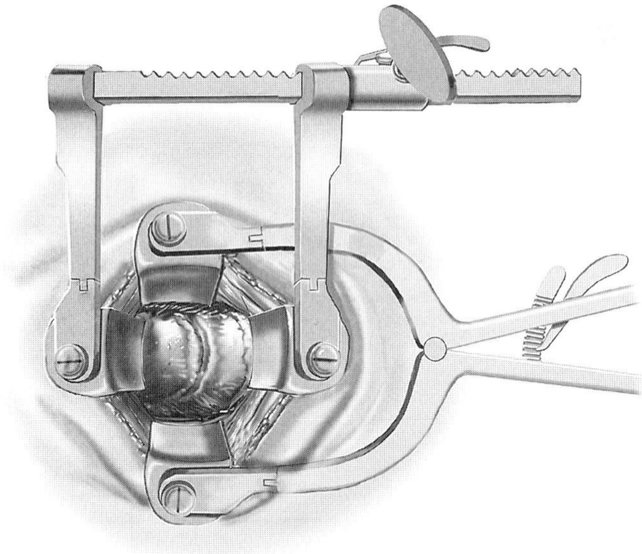

Figure 4-9. The correct level is identified, adequate tissue release is performed, and all osteophytes are removed from the diseased segment. The fixed retractor system is then placed. We typically use the toothed Caspar retractor blades in the medial-to-lateral direction and blunt retractor blades in the rostrocaudal direction.

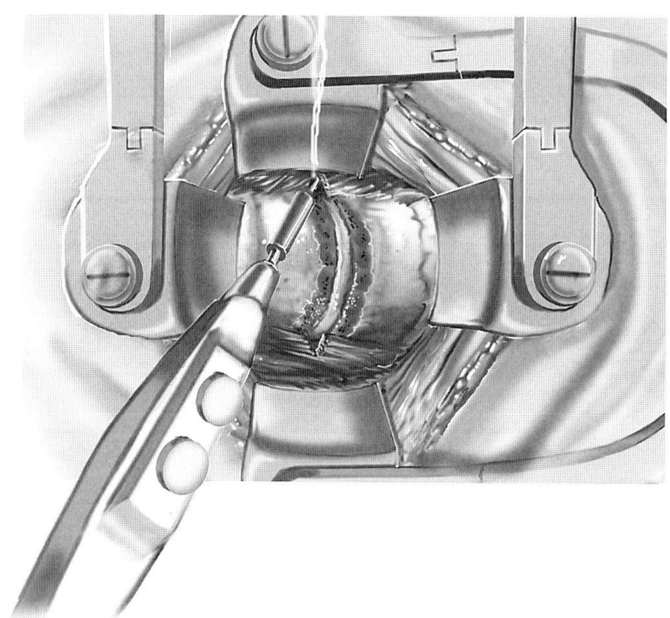

Figure 4-10. Once the medial lateral retractor blades have been placed and anchored into the longus colli muscle, the rostrocaudal retractor system is placed into position, centering the diseased segment within the operative field. This exposure is typical for a C5–C6 anterior cervical anterior discectomy and fusion and will allow the surgeon adequate room to place the distraction pins, perform the discectomy, place the graft, and fix a plate if desired. The lateral uncinate region is cleaned of the longus colli with monopolar cautery. If an artificial disc is placed, a slightly larger exposure may be necessary. We have found it helpful to obtain a lateral exposure at the disc level to provide optimal foraminal decompression.

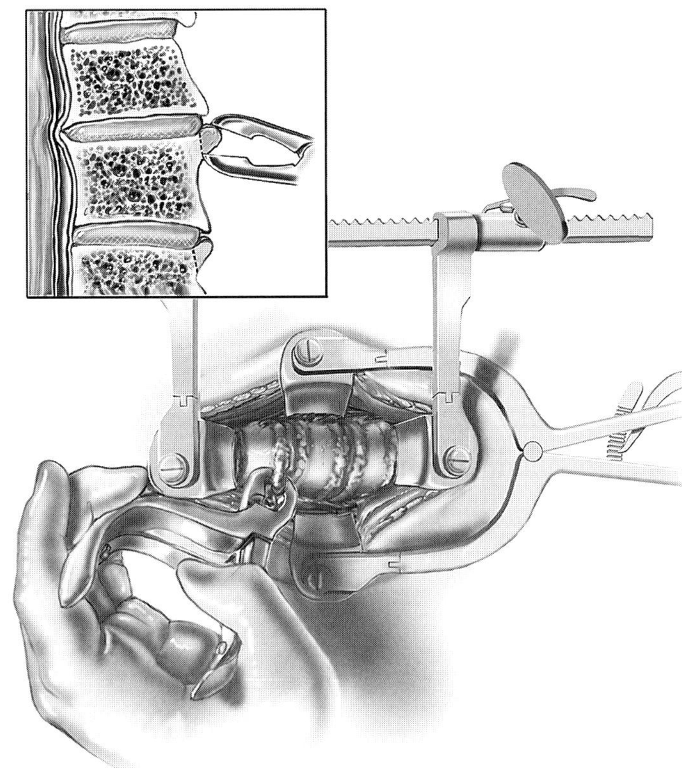

Figure 4-11. In the long segment exposures, once the retractor blades have been placed, gardening of the osteophytes can continue to provide adequate exposure and prepare cortical surfaces for future plating.

COMMON PITFALLS

The most common pitfalls of anterior cervical exposure include the following:

- Inadequate release of the soft tissues and suboptimal gardening of anterior osteophytes. Our bias is that the dissection to expose the affected part of the spine must adequately release all tissues above and below the level of surgery. There should be no tension on the midline structures when the retractors are placed. Excessive tension will result in soft tissue swelling and subsequent airway edema postoperatively.
- Gardening of all osteophytes is absolutely critical for optimal bone plate interface and screw purchase. If the osteophytes are not completely removed to leave a level surface for the plate, stress risers will cause the plate to be compromised and rock when the screws are tightened.

CHAPTER V

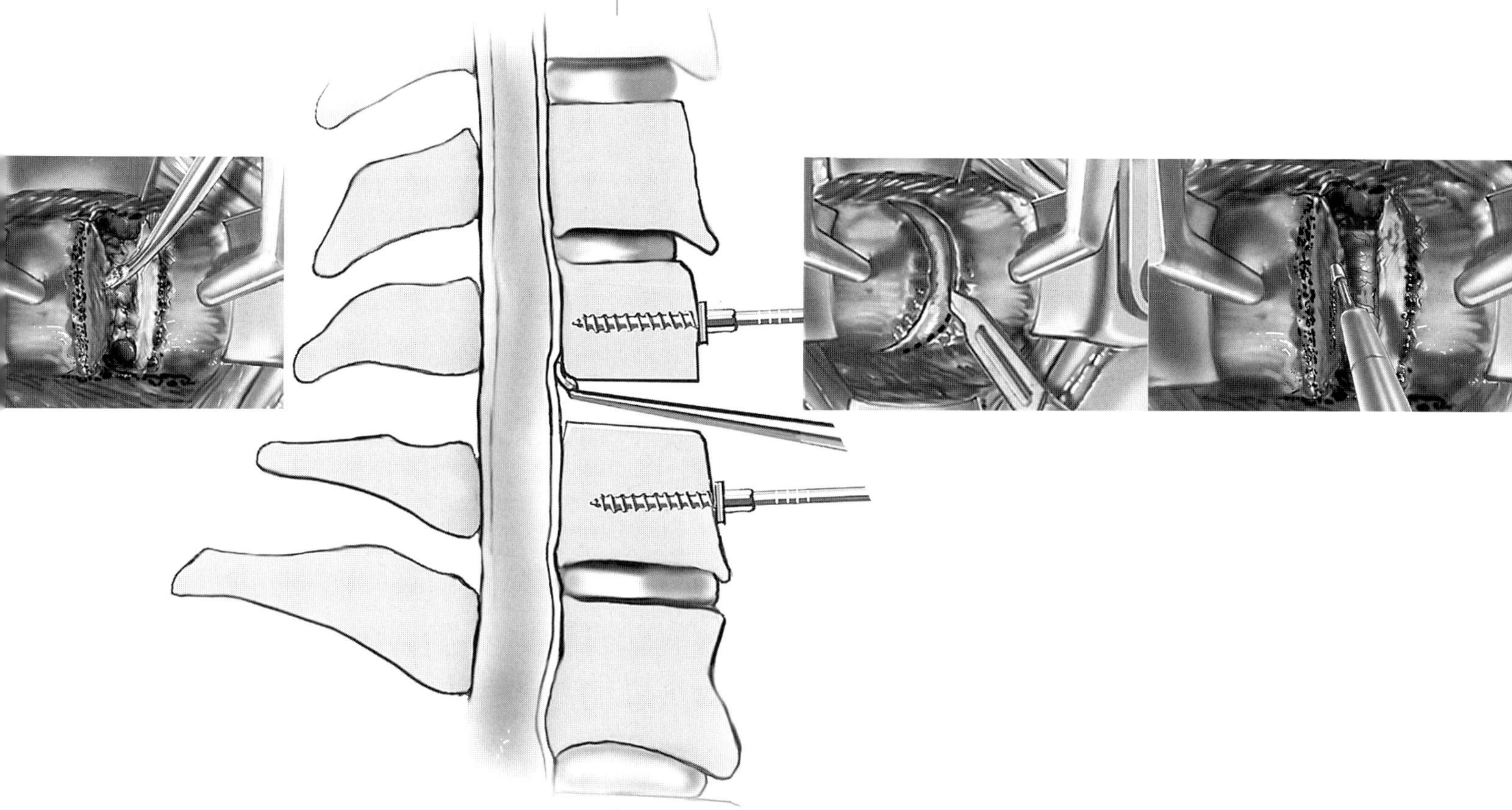

Single-Level Discectomy

Anterior cervical discectomy and fusion is a highly effective method for treating patients with cervical radiculopathy unresponsive to conservative measures and cervical myelopathy. Although a posterior keyhole foraminotomy is sometimes an option for soft disc herniations, we prefer the anterior approach for any central disc herniations and for hard disc/osteophyte compression.

This procedure is widely used with many variations, but we have found the Smith-Robinson fusion technique combined with direct decompression to be the most effective approach to anterior cervical discectomy and fusion. Gardening, or preparation of a smooth anterior vertebral body plane, is important in identifying the midline, allowing for proper distraction pin placement and good bone plate interface if a plate is to be used. Careful restoration of lordosis with diverging distraction pins and meticulous end plate preparation are keys to the success of this operation.

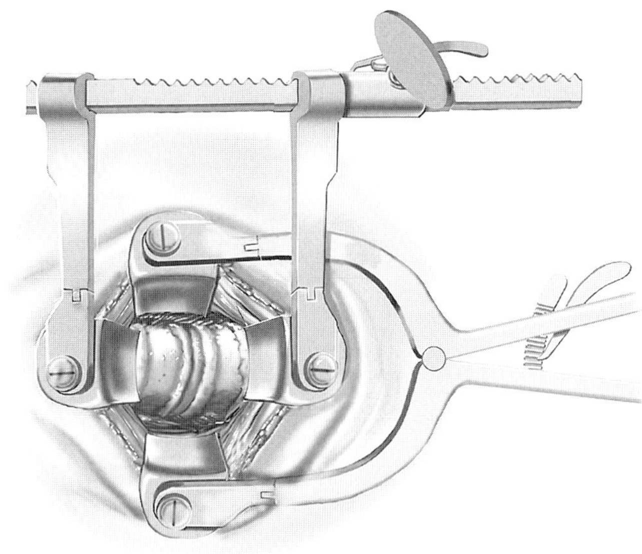

Figure 5-1. The Caspar retractor system provides excellent retraction and exposure. We use the toothed blades in the medial-lateral direction and nontoothed blades on the rostro-caudal direction. For single-level discectomies, the rostral-caudal retractors are sometimes not necessary.

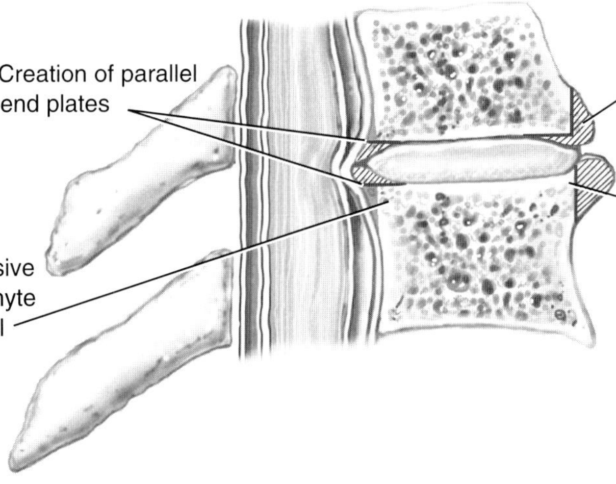

Figure 5-2. Plan for discectomy. This schematic demonstrates the essential steps for an adequate anterior cervical discectomy and fusion. Step 1 involves optimal visualization of the disc. Step 2 involves gardening of osteophytes to allow the creation of a smooth anterior vertebral surface for optimal bone plate interface to avoid stress risers. Step 3 is the creation of parallel end plates after discectomy for optimal graft bed preparation. Lastly, step 4 involves aggressive osteophyte removal to decompress the nerve roots and spinal cord.

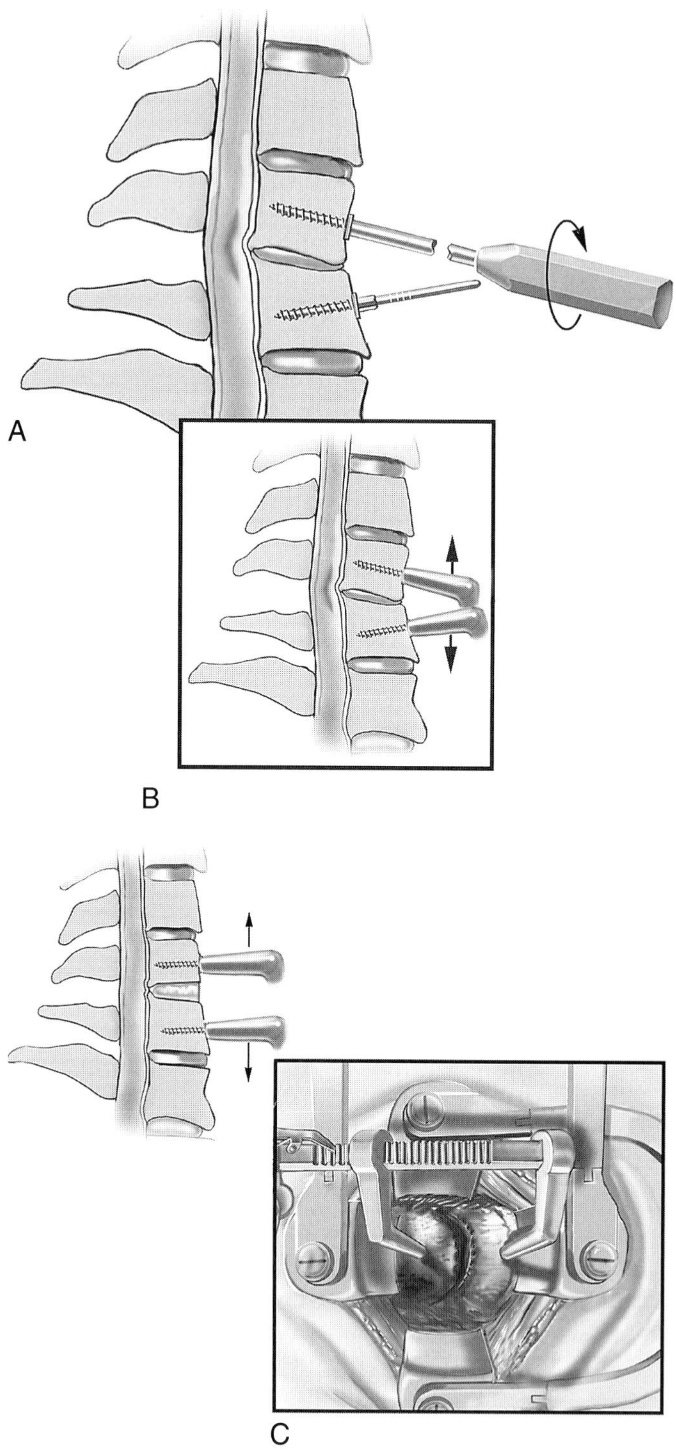

Figure 5-3, A–C. **A,** Divergent distraction screw placement. **B** and **C,** By placing distraction pins in a slightly divergent fashion, the subsequent distraction will recreate normal sagittal balance at the diseased segment and will optimize cervical lordosis.

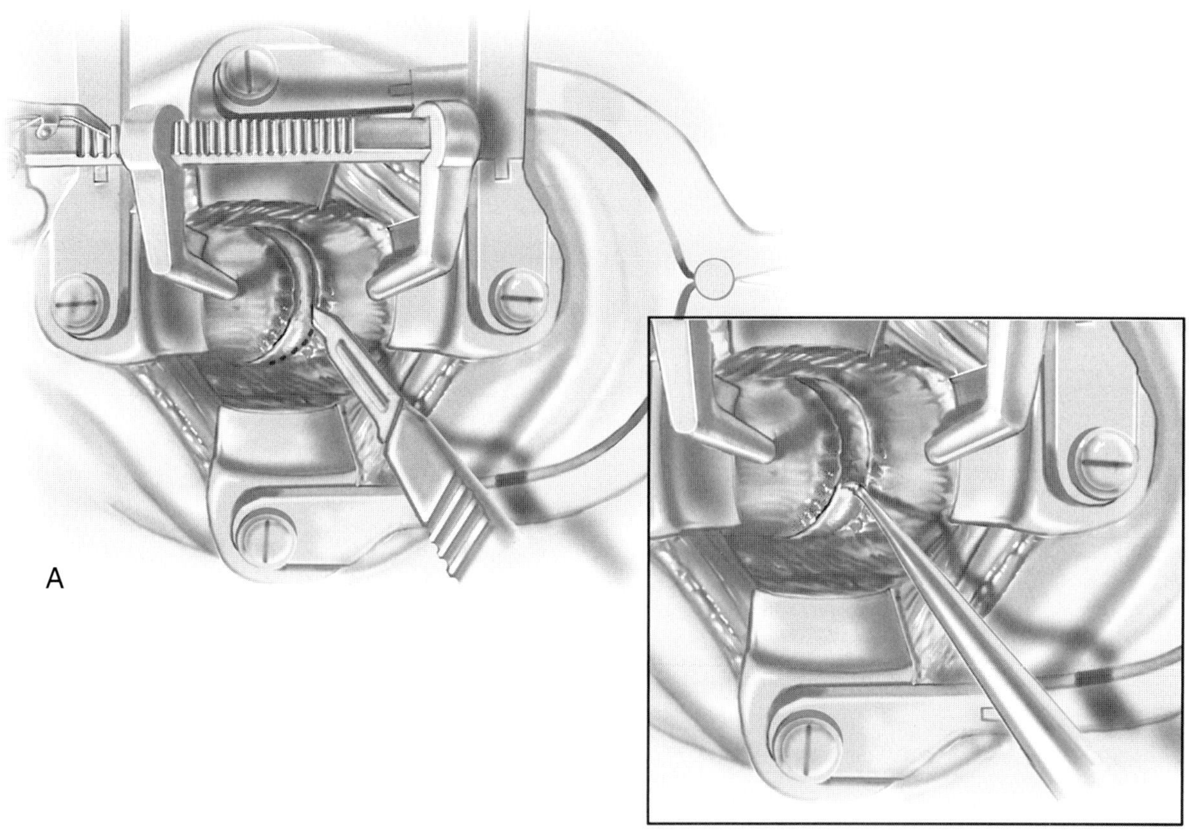

A

B

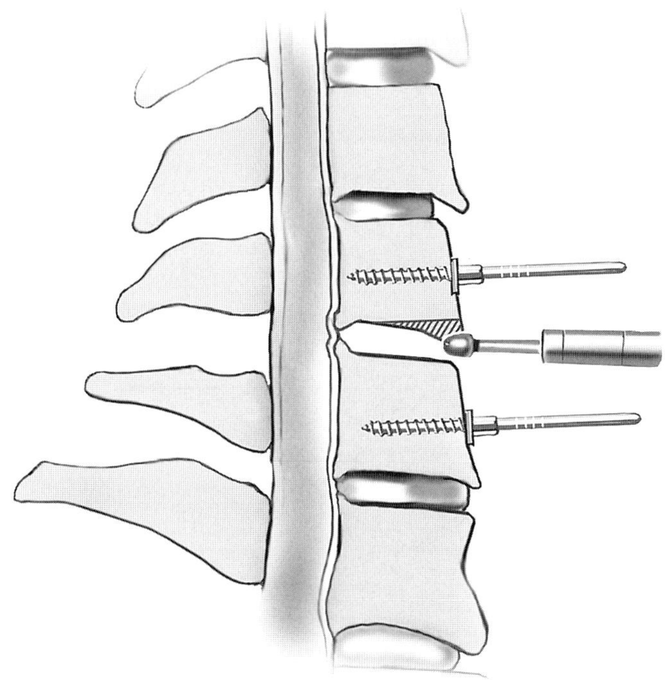

C

Figure 5-4, A–C. **A** and **B,** The annulus is then incised with a scalpel, and the anterior portion of the disc is removed with an angled curette. Then the distraction can be dialed in to the appropriate tension. **C,** For advanced spondylosis, sometimes it is necessary to remove the underlying osteophytes with a high-speed drill (Midas Rex) first for adequate visualization of the disc. This is the first step in creating parallel end plates and allows for better visualization of the remaining disc space.

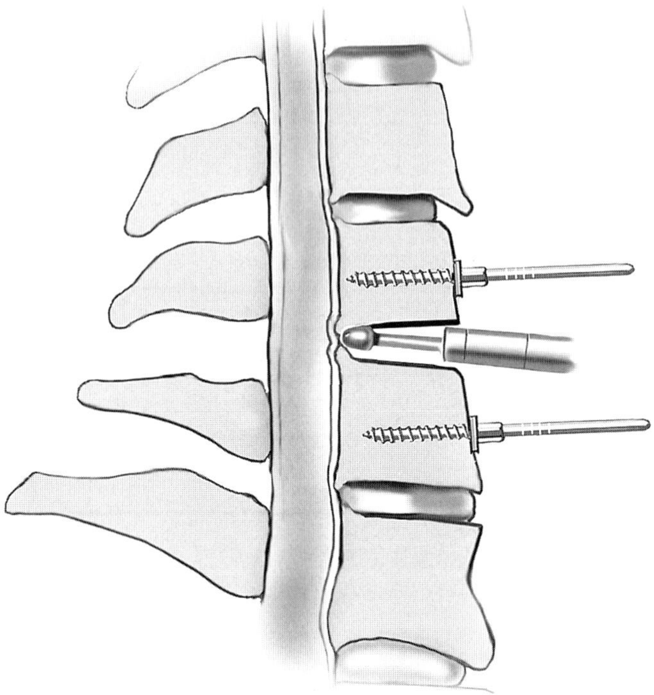

Figure 5-5. After the last portion of disc has been removed, the drill is advanced to remove the posterior osteophyte. A thin-lipped 2-mm Kerrison rongeur can also be used.

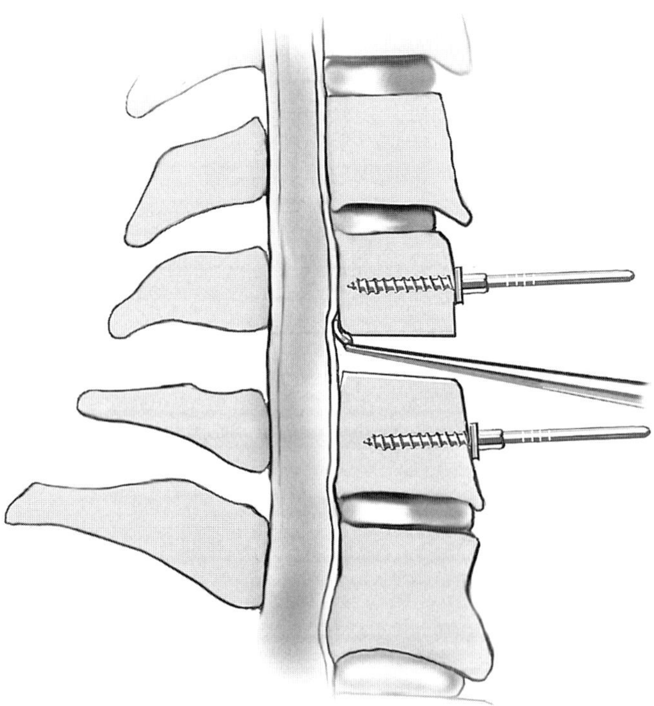

Figure 5-6. Once the posterior osteophyte has been removed with a high-speed drill, the posterior vertebral body can be palpated with a forward- or back-angled curette. This allows the surgeon to determine the depth of the vertebral body and verify that the osteophyte has been completely removed.

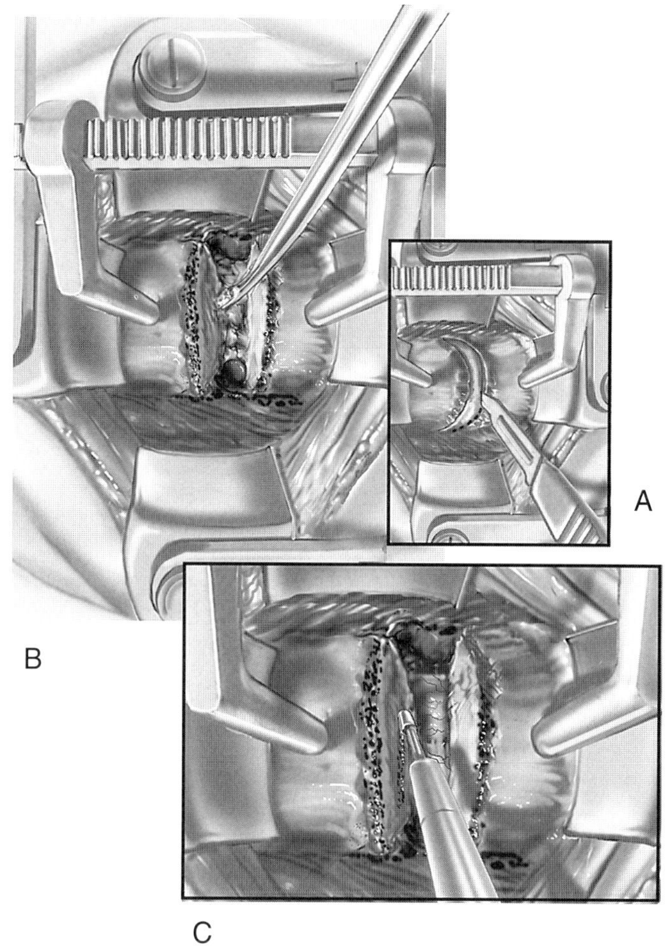

Figure 5-7, A–C. Surgical view of the removal of the posterior osteophyte wall with a high-speed drill.

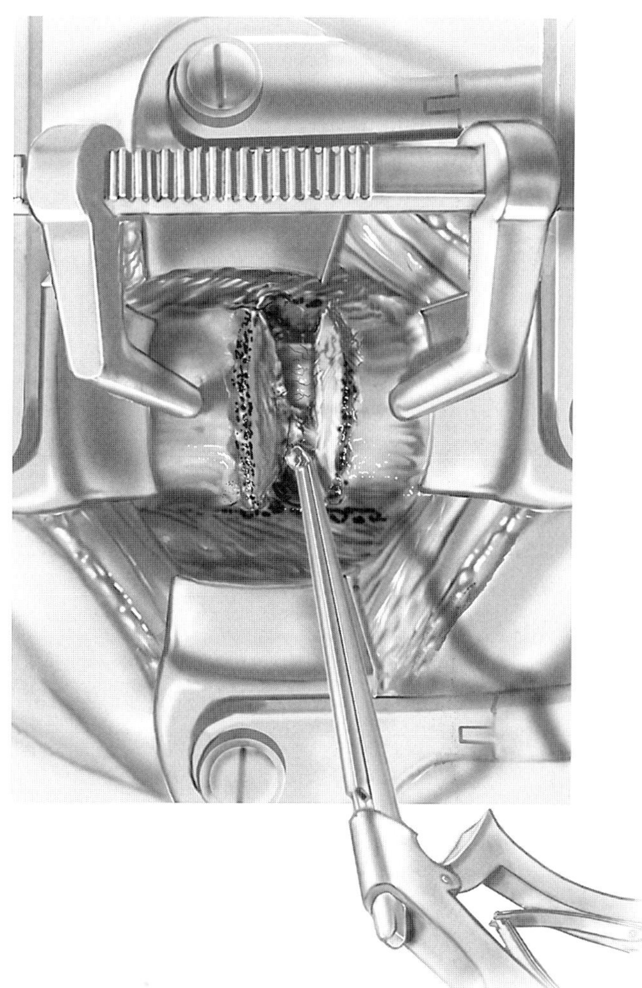

Figure 5-8. A Kerrison rongeur can be used to complete the osteophytectomy.

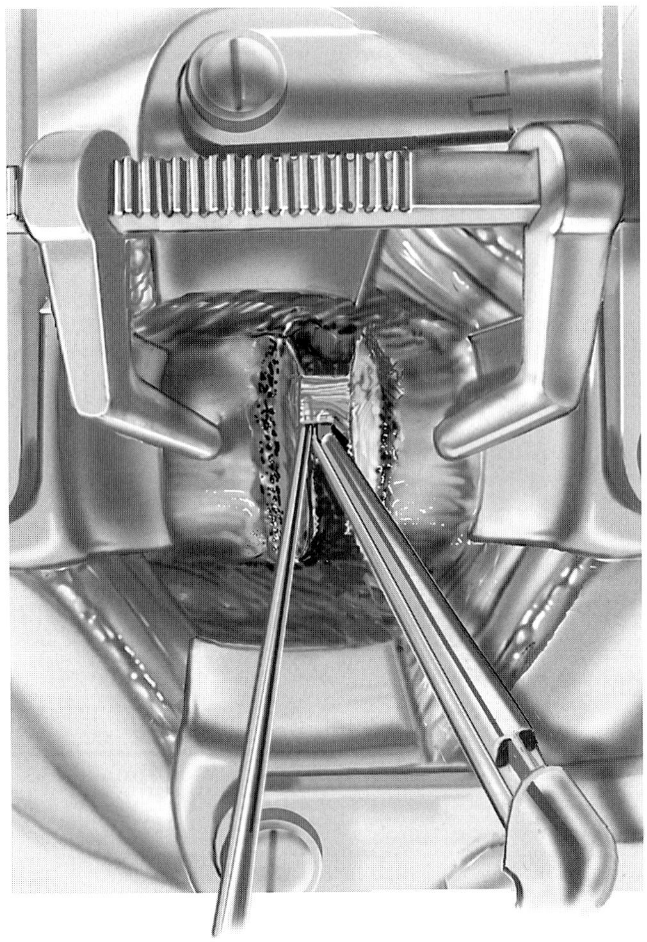

A

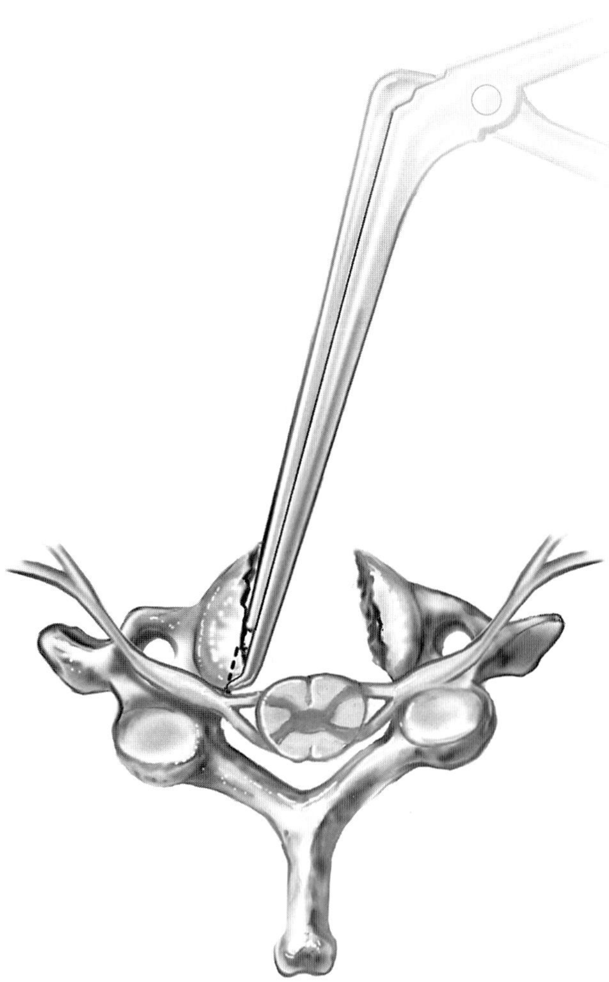

B

Figure 5-9, A and B. **A,** Once the posterior longitudinal ligament (PLL) is exposed, in most cases it should be opened with gentle elevation and sharp dissection either with a Kerrison rongeur or an angled curette. The PLL is then removed using the Kerrison rongeur. This allows for adequate visualization of a well-decompressed spinal cord and nerve roots. **B,** If foraminal stenosis is present, a foraminotomy can be performed using a 2-mm Kerrison rongeur. The shoulder of the nerve root should be well visualized coursing ventrally.

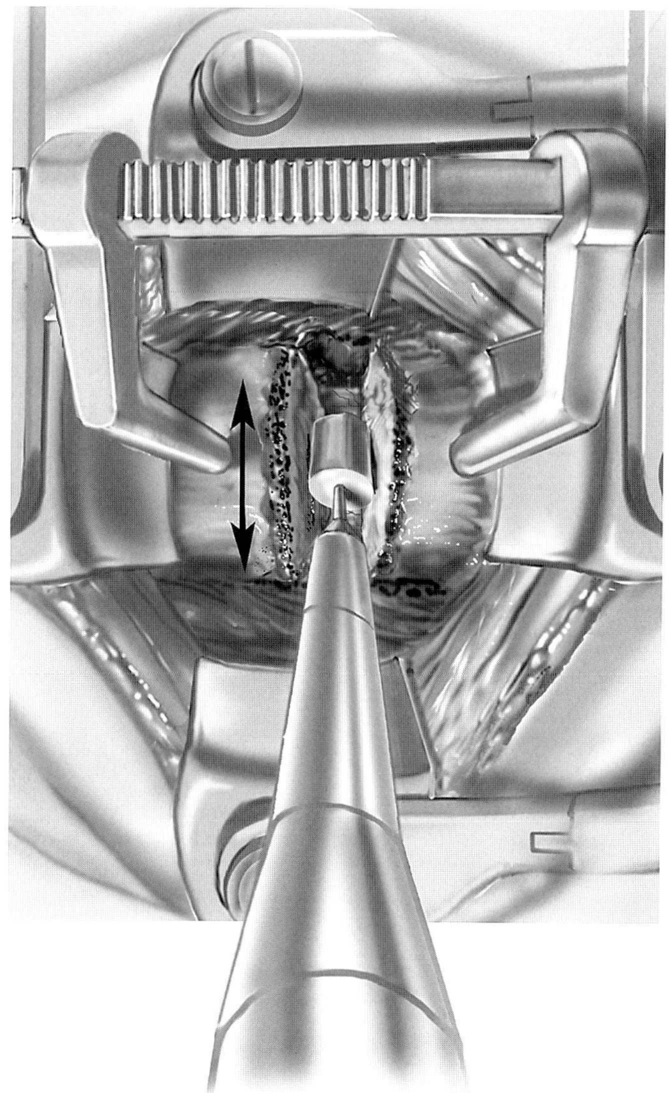

Figure 5-10. End plate preparation is performed with a Midas matchstick bit, barrel bit, or curettage to remove the cartilaginous end plate and to create the optimal biological atmosphere for the bone graft.

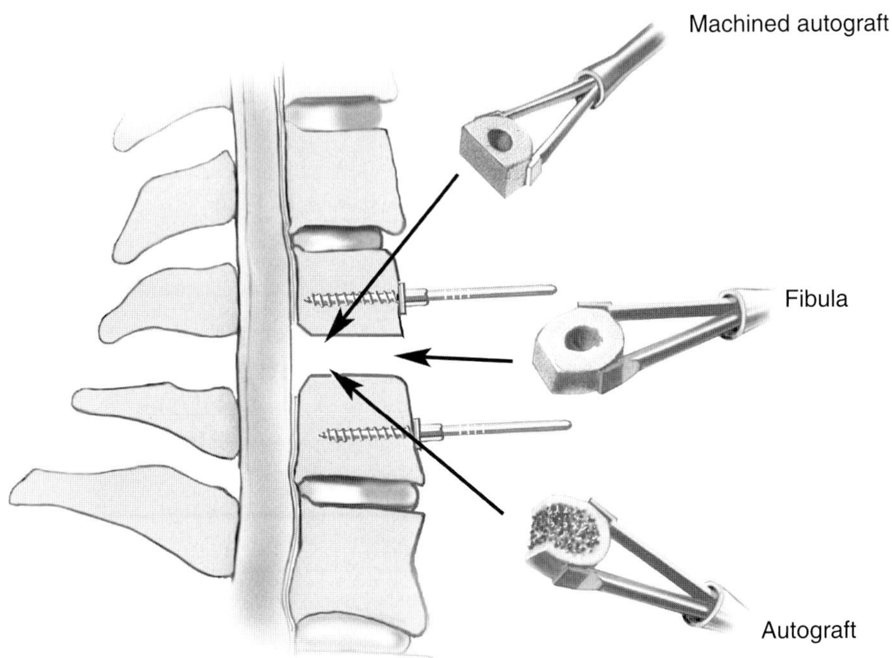

Figure 5-11. Graft materials include machined allograft, fibular allograft, autograft, iliac crest, and polyetheretherketone (PEEK) polymer with bone morphogenetic protein (BMP) options.

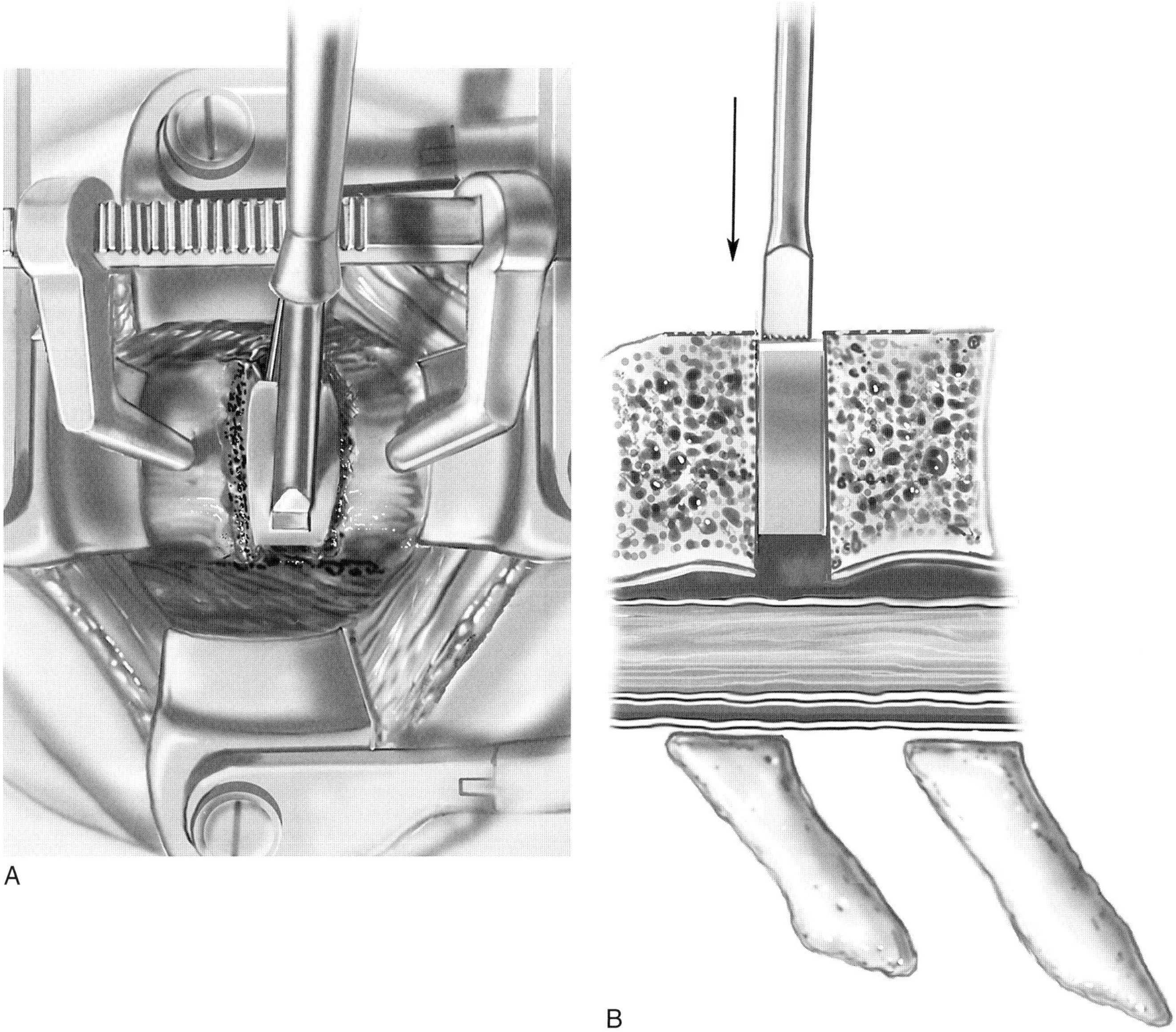

A

B

Figure 5-12, A and B. **A,** Surgical view demonstrating graft placement with tamp. Whenever we tamp bone into proper position, we support our tamp by holding a hand somewhere on a fixed point. That way, when the mallet is used to tamp the graft in, no sudden movements or changes of graft position occur. **B,** The graft is countersunk 2 mm.

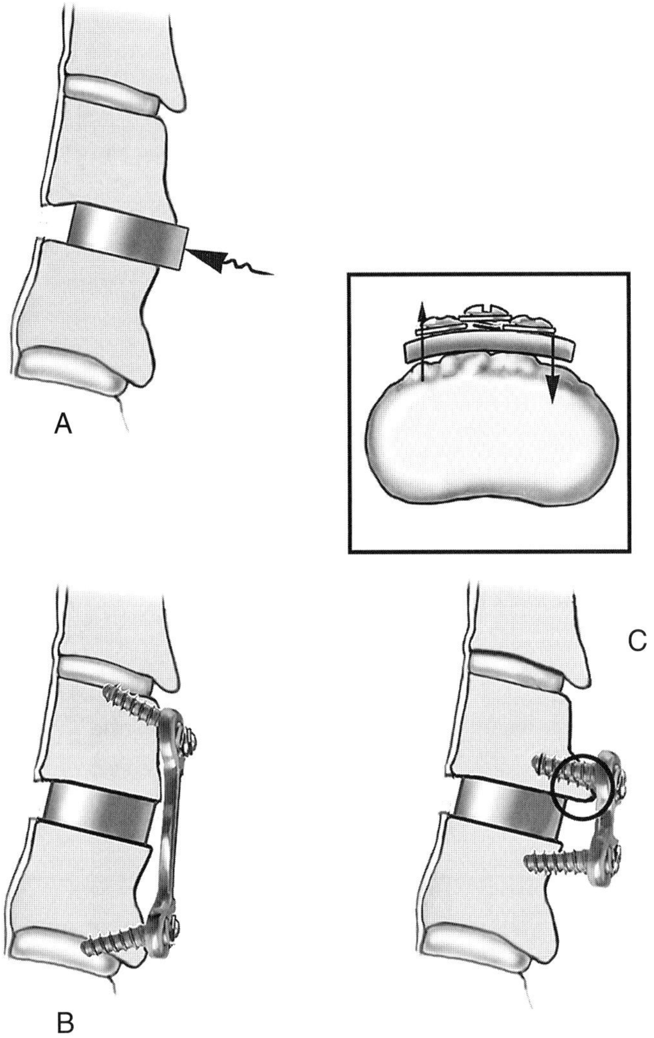

COMMON PITFALLS

Figure 5-15, A–C. **A,** The graft is not countersunk completely because the osteophyte is not completely removed. **B,** The plate is too long, causing adjacent level disc space capture. **C,** Inadequate gardening of osteophytes can cause plate rocking and stress risers either in the rostrocaudal or mediolateral directions (see *inset*).

POSTOPERATIVE RESULTS

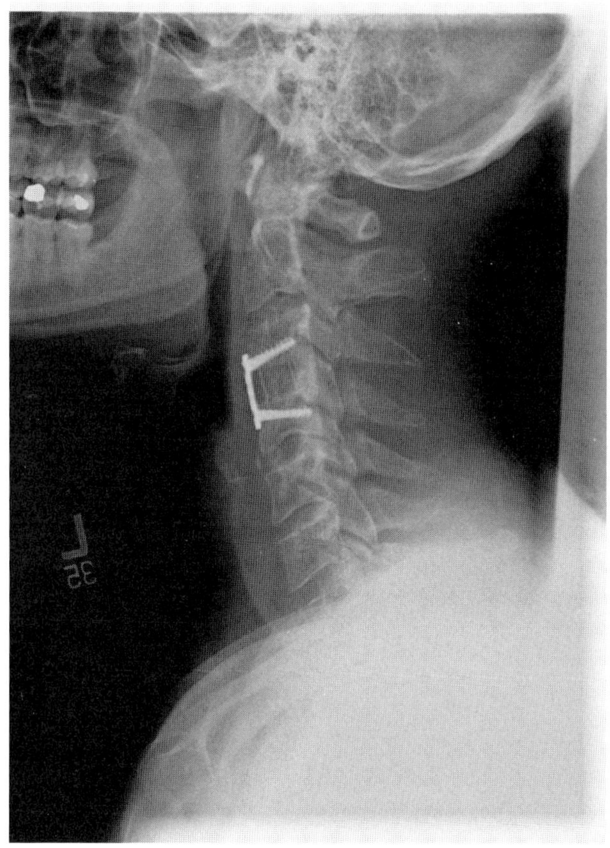

Figure 5-16. A single level ACDF with PEEK synthetic spacer, bone morphogenetic protein and small-stature plate that avoid the disc spaces above and below the fusion.

CHAPTER

VI

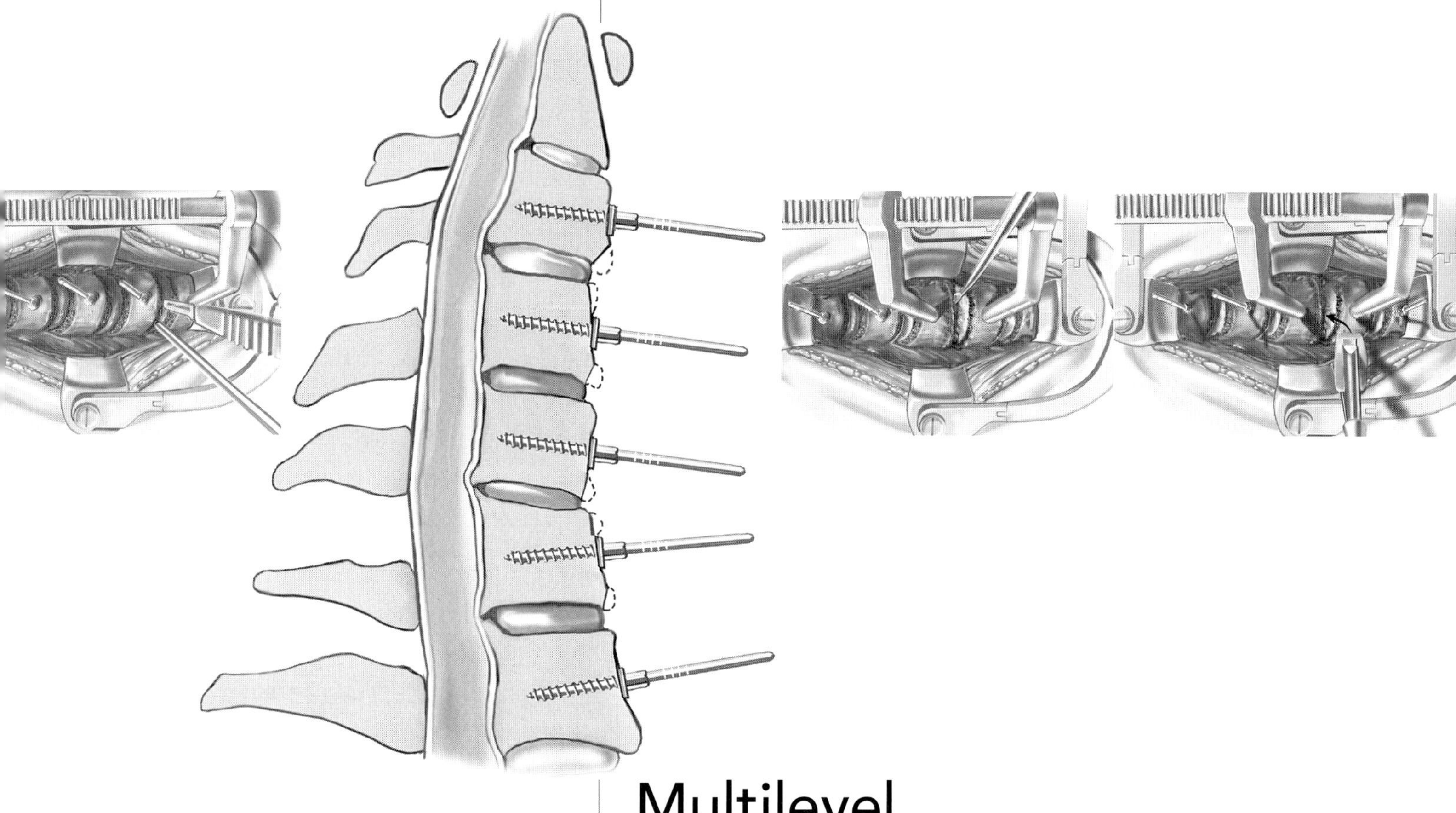

Multilevel Discectomy

The key to any multilevel anterior cervical fusion is adequate exposure. The entire anterior vertebral body face must be visualized for each segment that will be decompressed and plated. Osteophytes must be gardened to create a smooth plane on the anterior vertebral faces. Lateral exposure must define the upsweep of the uncinate process bilaterally.

In general, we have found that multilevel discectomy restores cervical lordosis better than multilevel corpectomy, and therefore we carefully use preoperative computed tomography (CT) scanning with or without myelography to assess the specific area of compression. If the compression is located at the disc level and not at the middle portion of the vertebral body, we tend to approach this with discectomies. If there is a significant amount of compression at the mid-body level, either a corpectomy or posterior approach is considered.

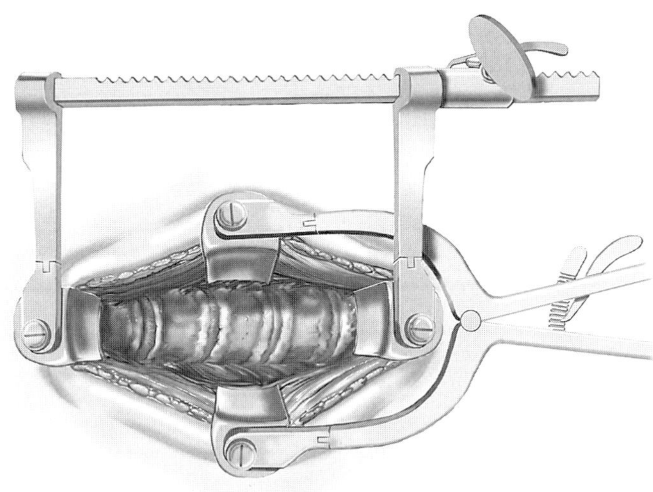

Figure 6-1. Using the releasing techniques described in Chapter 4, multilevel exposure of the cervical spine is achieved. We prefer to spend extra time releasing the soft tissues superiorly and inferiorly because this decreases the amount of retractor pressure on the esophagus and trachea, thus reducing postoperative edema. Also, for three or more level decompressions, an extra-long superior-inferior retractor is required and is not usually part of the standard Caspar set. It is a good idea to discuss this with the equipment representative before surgery. We prefer not using an esophageal temperature probe or stethescope during surgery, because this may increase the chances of dysphagia.

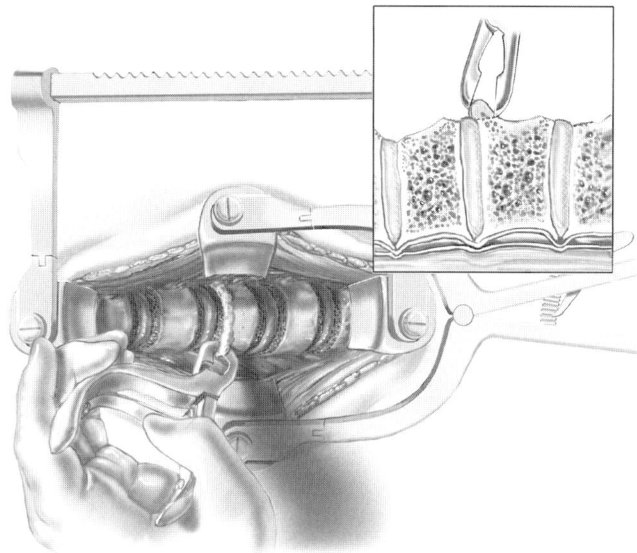

Figure 6-2. Osteophytes are gardened using a Cushing or Leksell rongeur. This must be done before placement of the distraction pins/ screws. This will allow for more accurate central placement of the screws.

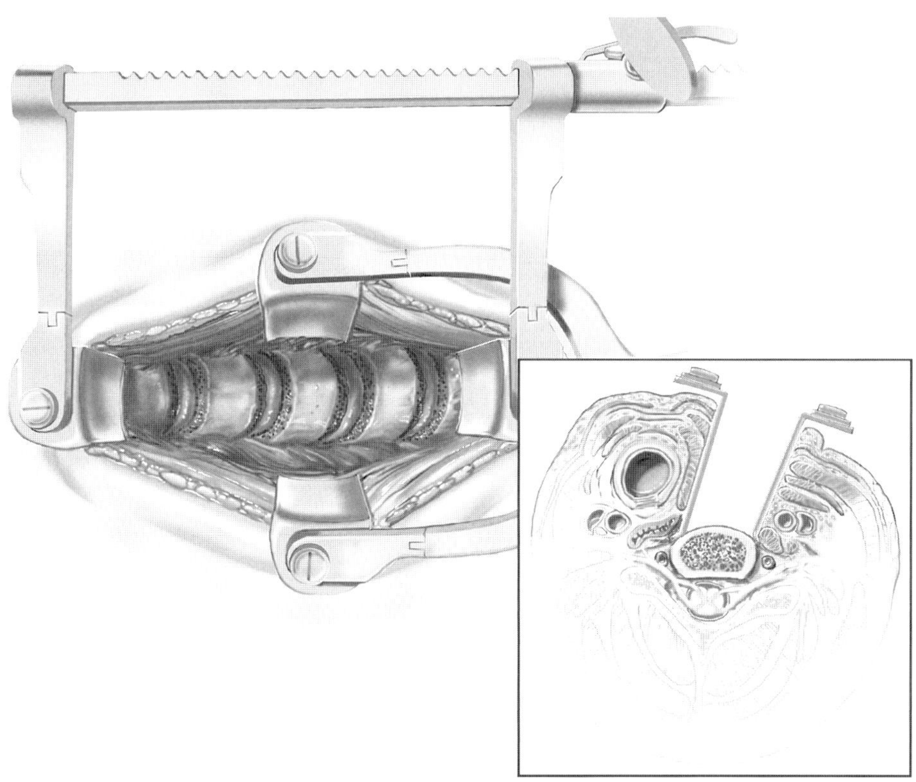

Figure 6-3. All four levels are gardened before the placement of screws. Also, the lateral disc space is cleaned of longus colli attachments to expose the upsweep of the uncinate processes bilaterally. This helps the surgeon better approximate the midline. Frequently, there are lateral osteophytes in the uncinate region that also need to be gardened.

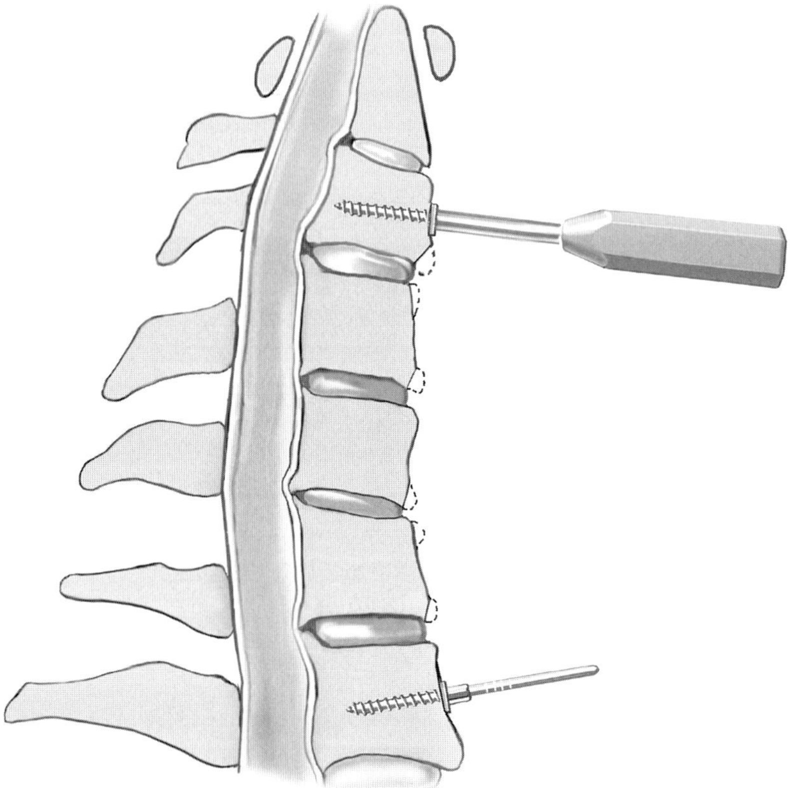

A

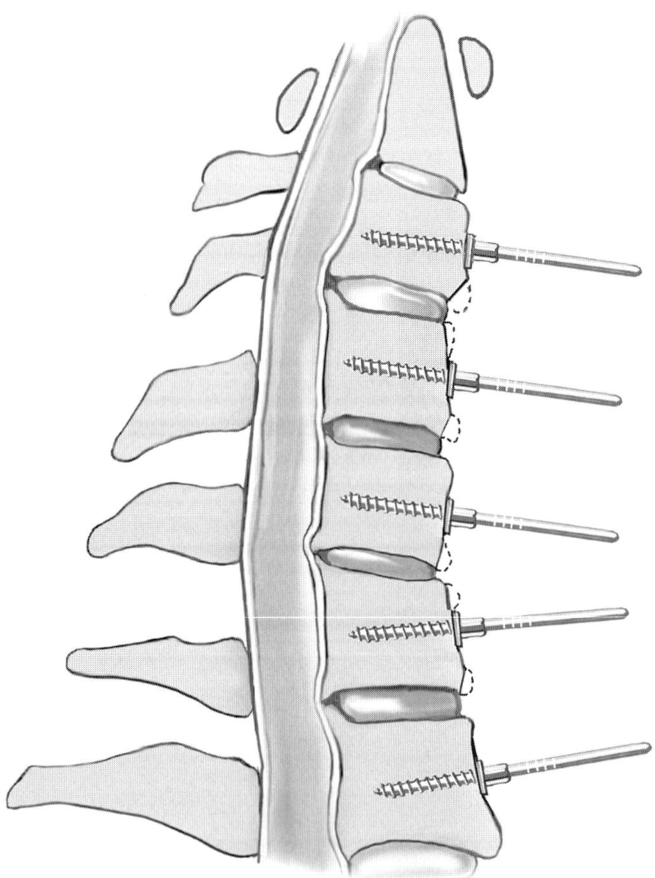

B

Figure 6-4, A and B. Caspar distraction pins are then placed sequentially into each vertebral body. A slight divergence in screw placement is obtained to "dial in" lordosis upon sequential distraction.

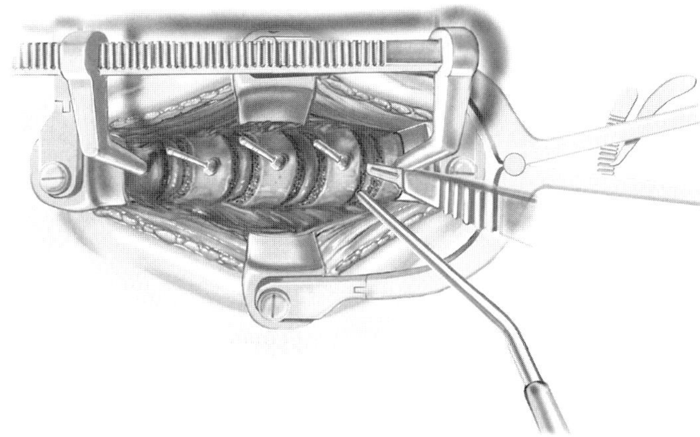

Figure 6-5. The annulus is then opened sharply, and a radical discectomy is performed with curettes and a pituitary rongeur. The discectomy can be started before distraction, but to complete the discectomy, distraction must be applied.

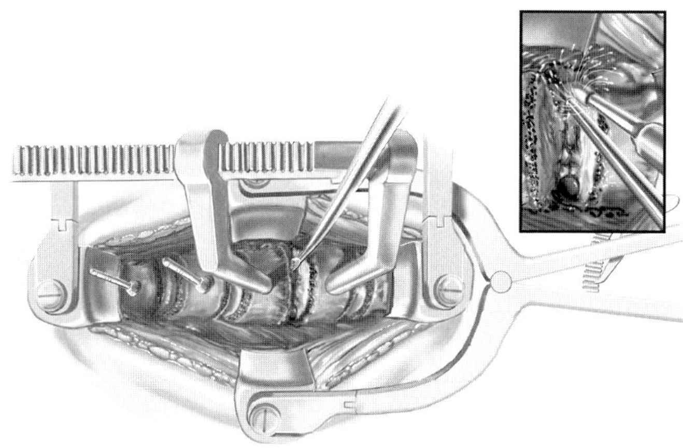

Figure 6-6. The posterior osteophytes are either curetted out or drilled out with a high-speed drill (see *inset*).

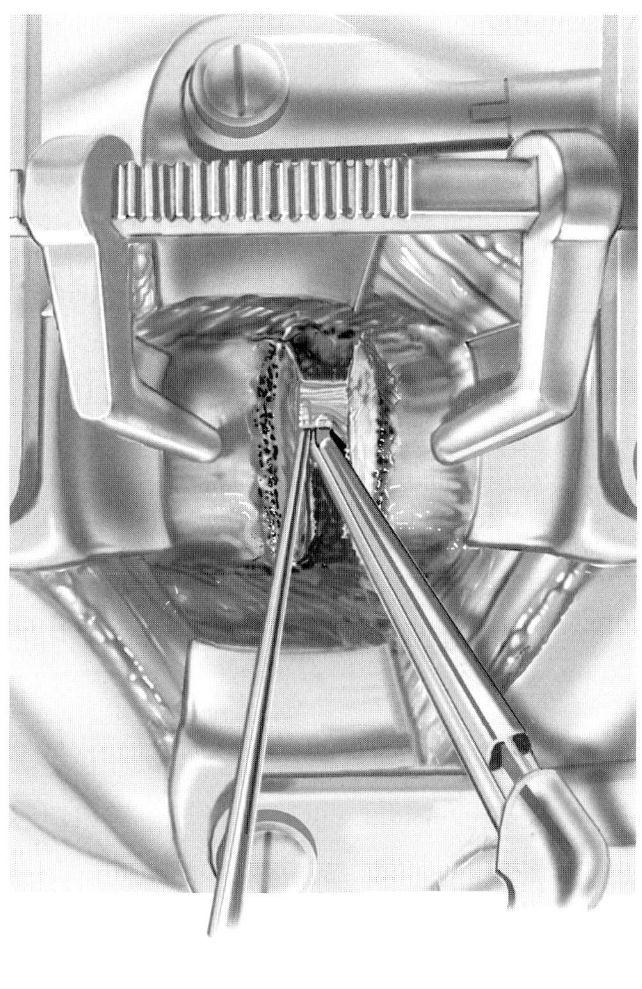

Figure 6-7. The posterior longitudinal ligament is then opened and removed to complete the decompression. Using a forward-angled curette or right-angled nerve hook, the posterior vertebral body wall can be palpated to verify an adequate decompression.

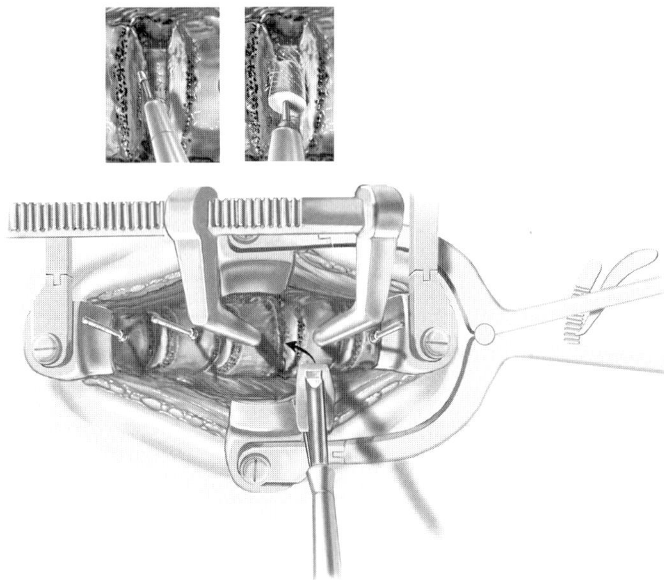

Figure 6-8. After the decompression is performed, the other levels are decompressed in a similar fashion. Once all appropriate levels are decompressed, the end plates are prepared using either a matchstick drill bit (see *left inset*) or a barrel drill bit (see *right inset*). Parallel end plates are prepared, and the premeasured and customized grafts are tamped into position.

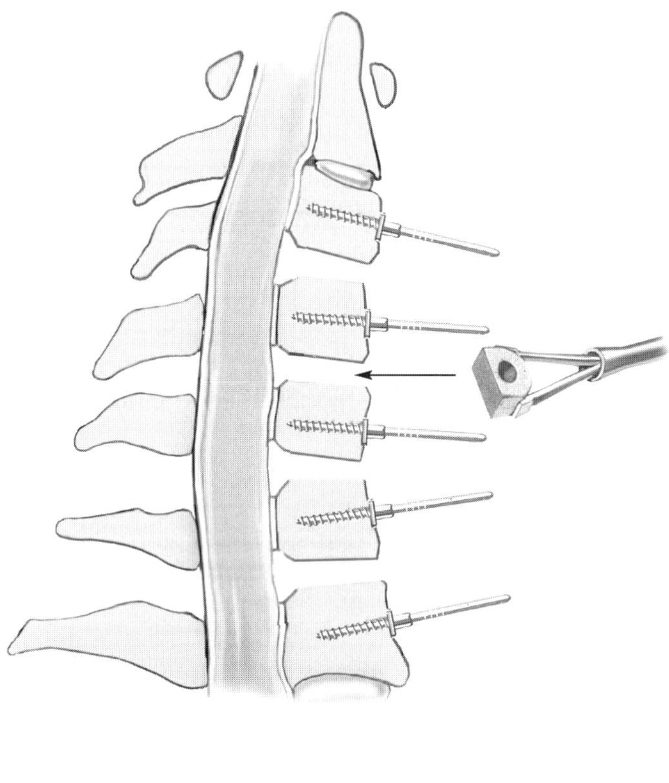

Figure 6-9. When multilevel arthrodesis is performed, the central level grafts should be tamped in first, followed by the peripheral grafts. This allows for better reproduction of sagittal balance. Keep in mind that each graft placed will slightly decrease the size of the adjacent graft sites, and care should be taken not to oversize the peripheral grafts.

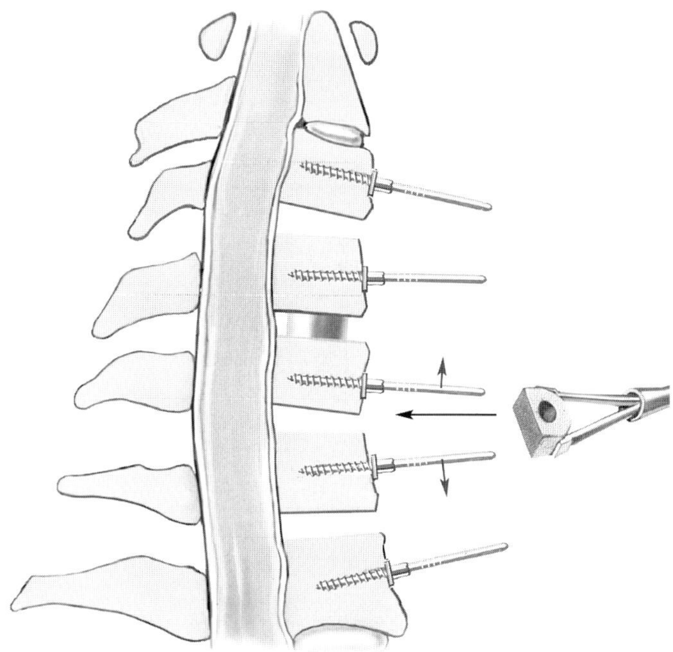

Figure 6-10. Gentle distraction is applied to the next level, and the second graft is placed.

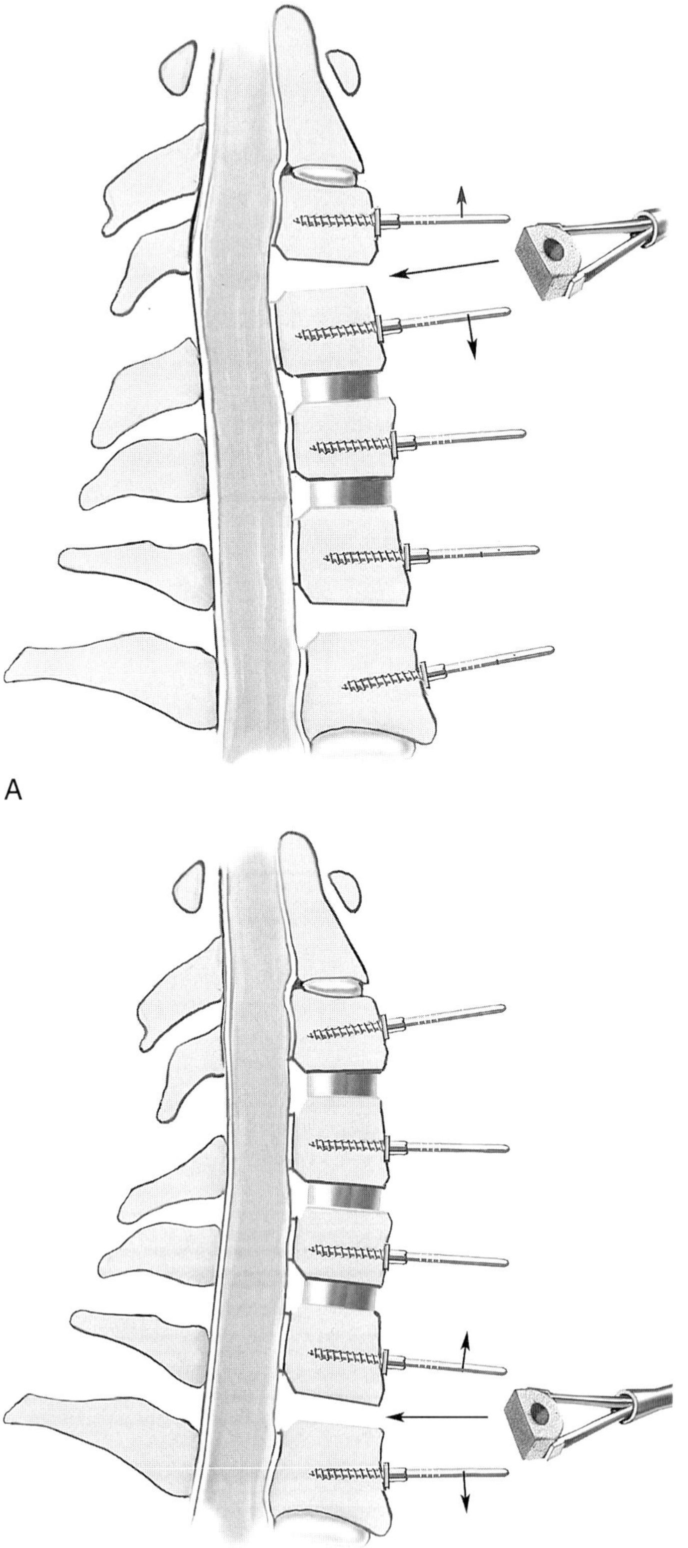

A

B

Figure 6-11, A and B. This process is continued until each level graft is in place.

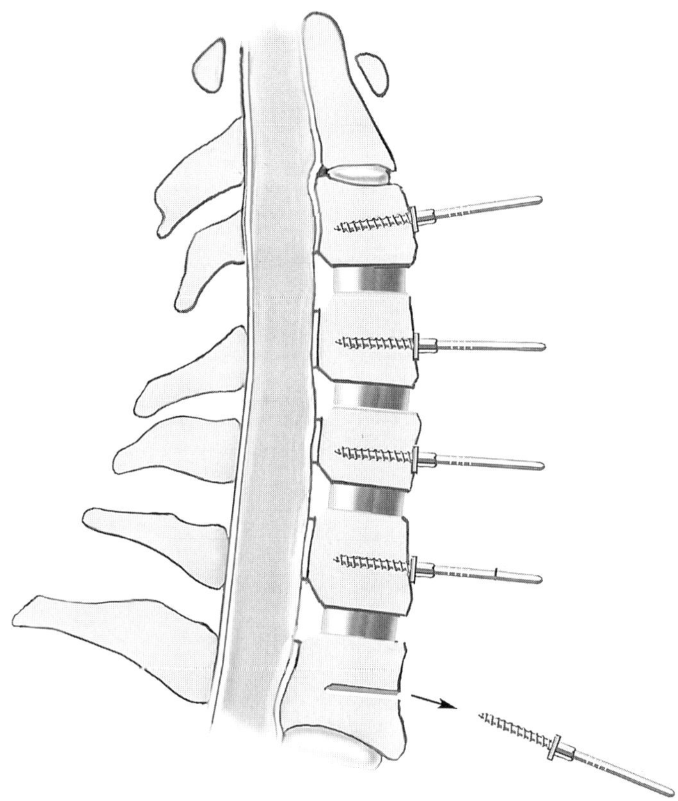

Figure 6-12. Graft position and stability are checked, and then the distraction pins are removed.

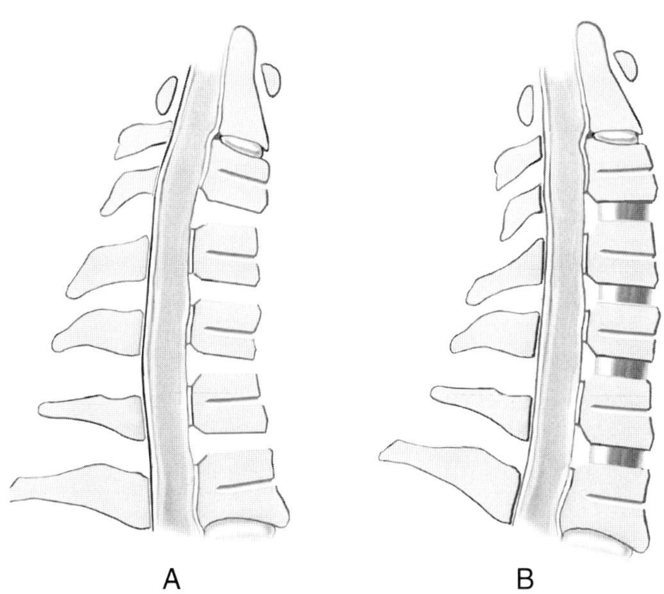

Figure 6-13, A and B. With appropriate graft sizing and distraction, preoperative cervical kyphosis and cord compression can be corrected back to better sagittal balance.

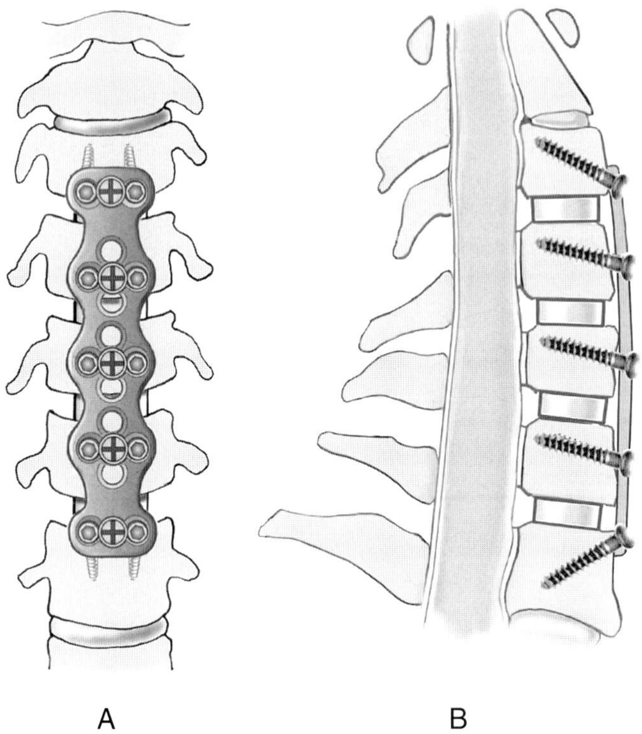

Figure 6-14, A and B. A rotational hybrid plate is then used to stabilize the spine. We prefer to use rotational (variable-angle) screws in each upper segment with locked screws on the most inferior vertebral body. This allows for a buttress plate type (construct with load sharing) at each upper level to promote osseous integration (Wolff's law).

COMMON PITFALLS

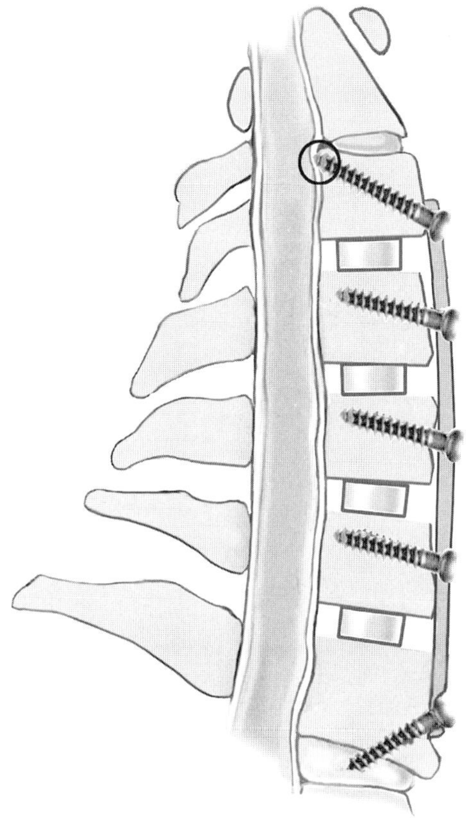

Figure 6-15. A common pitfall in multilevel plating is using a plate that is too long, causing either the superior or inferior screws to enter the adjacent disc space. This can be avoided by choosing the shortest plate possible. It is acceptable, and perhaps desirable, for the initial screw entry point to be in the subchondral bone of the vertebral body, provided the screw trajectory is appropriate and the remaining threads of the screw will capture cancellous bone. Moreover, purchase of subchondral bone is significantly stronger than cancellous bone and increases screw pullout strength.

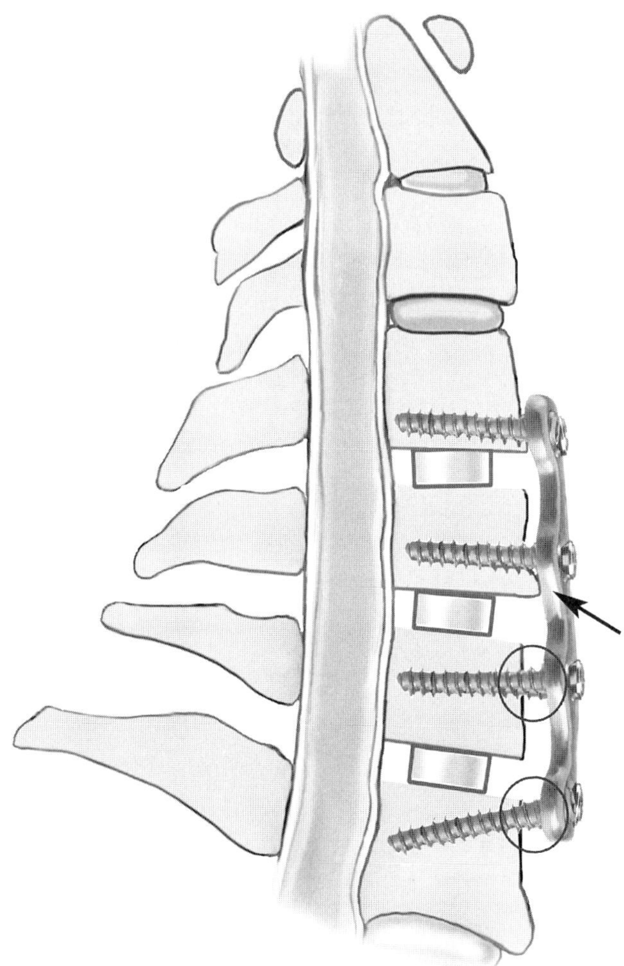

Figure 6-16. Another common pitfall is suboptimal gardening of the anterior osteophytes before performing the discectomy. If an osteophyte is still present, the plate will not sit flush on the face of the vertebral bodies; this can create stress rises and can decrease screw purchase at adjacent levels.

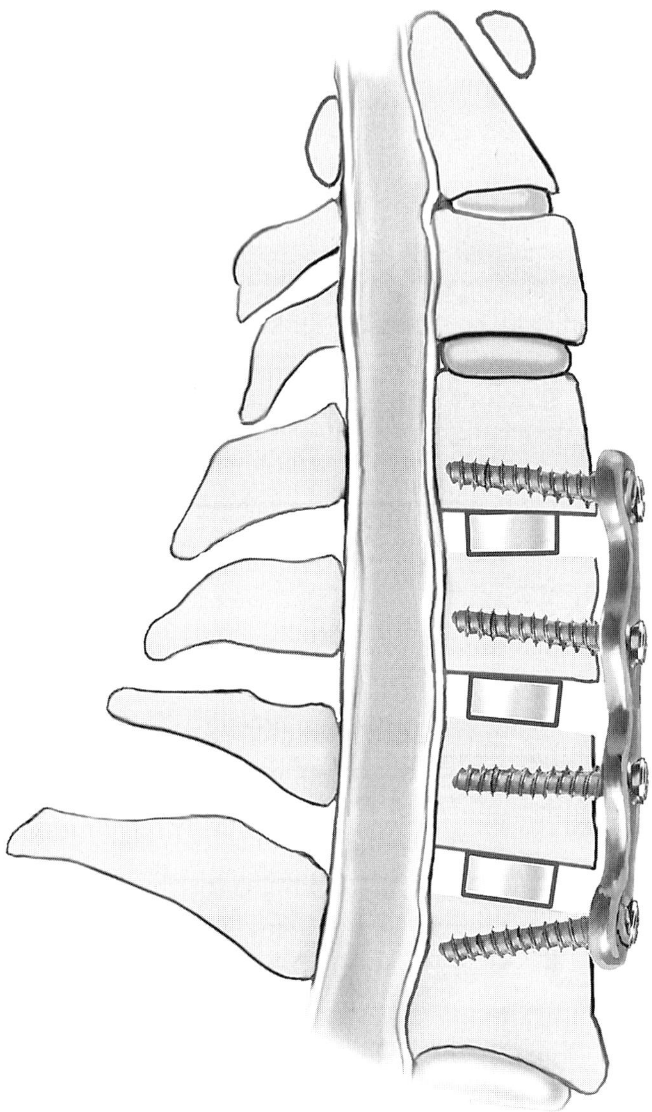

Figure 6-17. Some surgeons choose not to place screws in the intervening vertebral body segments. It has been our preference to place rotational (variable-angle) screws at each level when possible to increase the points of fixation and to decrease the chances for screw pullout. In cases of degenerative disease, rotational screws are preferred to promote load sharing. In trauma situations, it may be preferable to use fixed screws at each level to promote immediate rigid fixation, although there is no definitive study in the present literature to support this.

POSTOPERATIVE RESULTS

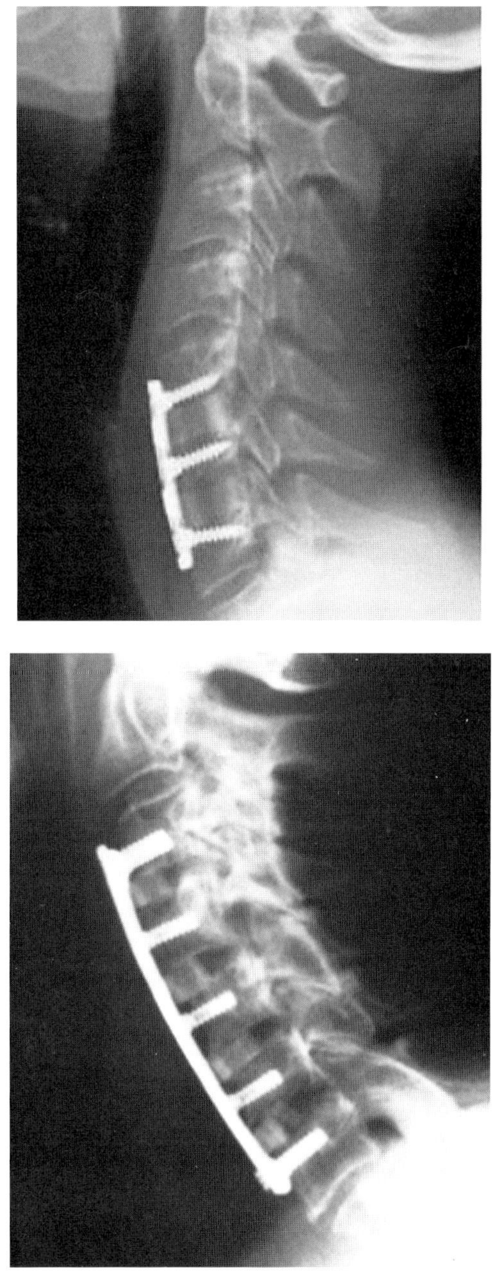

Figure 6-18. Lateral C-spine x-rays demonstrating good position of the graft, plate, and screws. Again, the desired plate length should be short enough so that it does not abut the adjacent nonfused segments.

CHAPTER

VII

Figure 7-1
can be mad
prefer a lor
level appro
and relaxin
airway eder
a smaller
used.

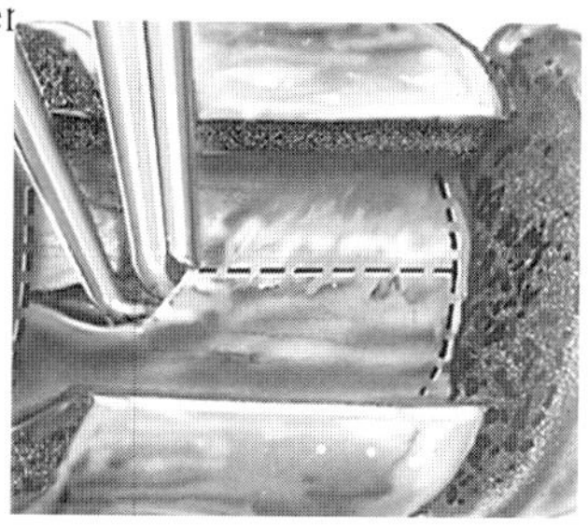

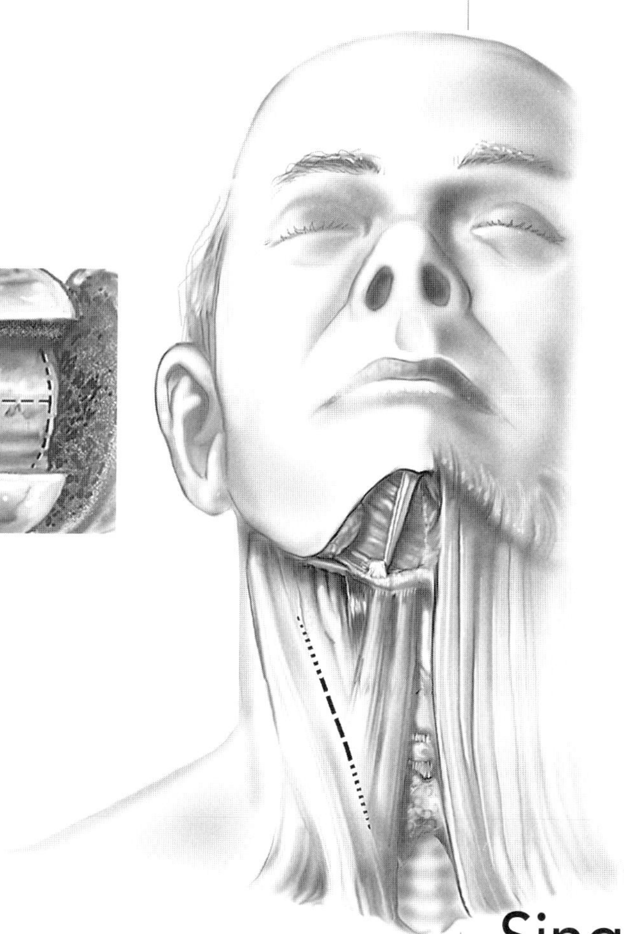

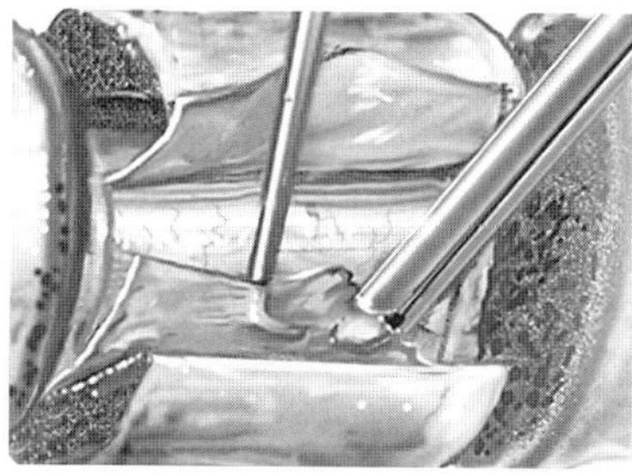

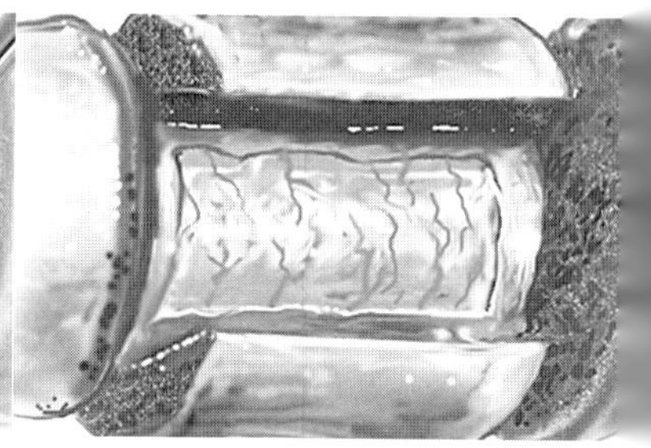

Single-Level Corpectomy

Figure 7-
anterior ve
for adequa
body for
important
so that the
the anter
prominenc

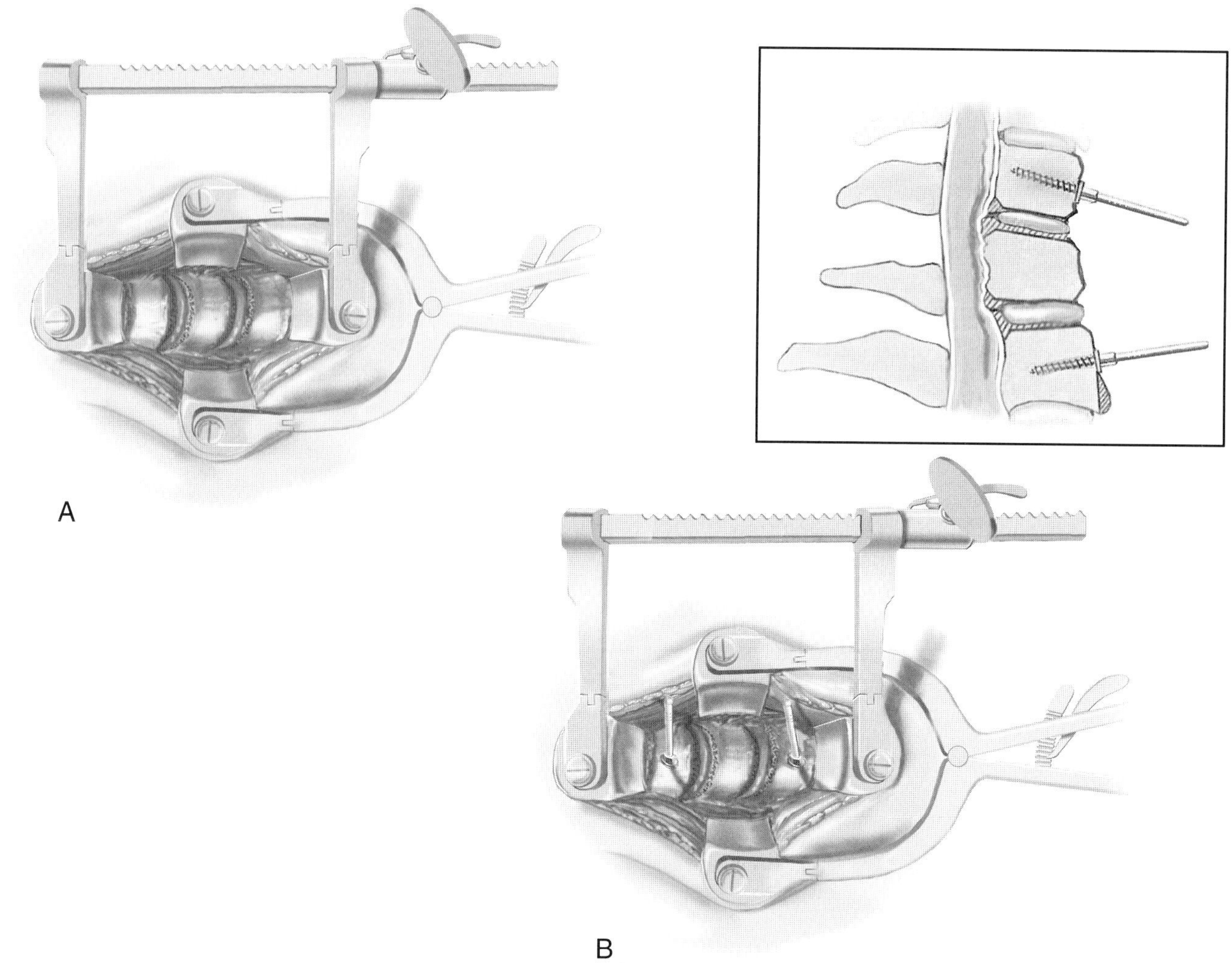

A

B

Figure 7-3, A and B. Once the vertebral bodies have been gardened **(A),** the distraction pins can be placed in a divergent direction **(B)** to reapproximate sagittal balance when distraction is dialed in.

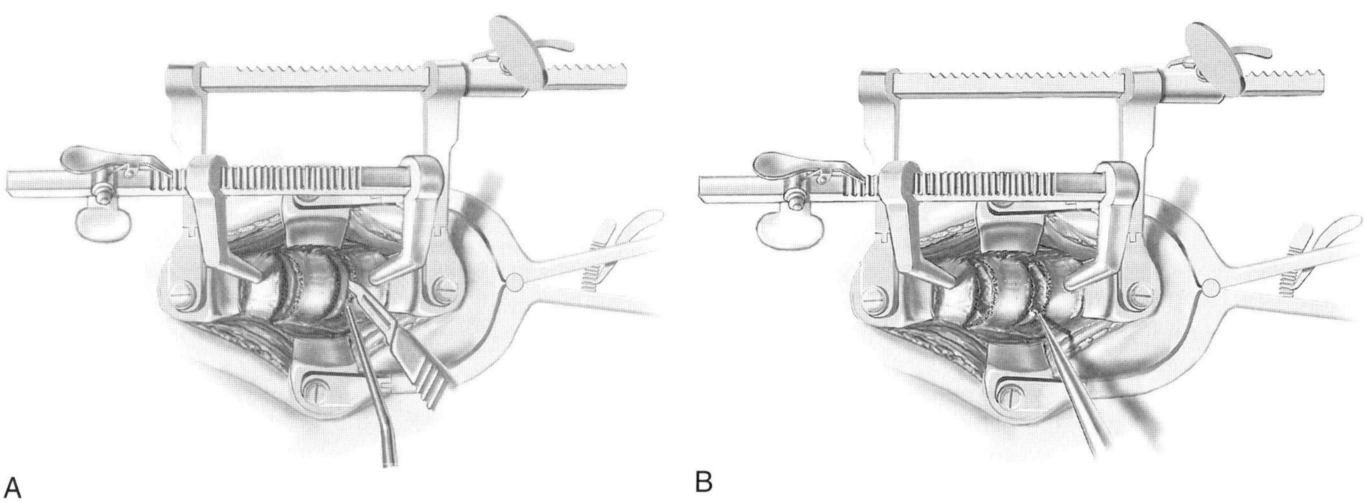

A

B

Figure 7-4, A and B. After distraction, radical anterior cervical discectomies are performed at the disc spaces adjacent to the vertebral body that will be removed. Before vertebrectomy, we try to perform a complete discectomy with the exception of the removal of the posterior longitudinal ligament (PLL). This makes bony removal easier when drilling is performed.

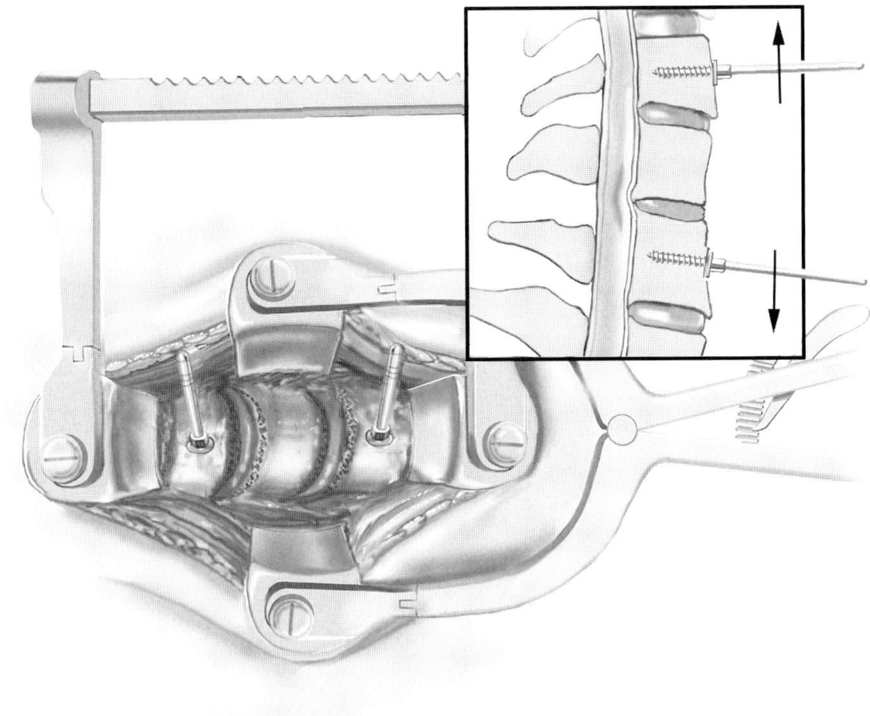

Figure 7-5. Distraction can be increased slightly after discectomy. This can improve sagittal balance because the anterior longitudinal ligament (ALL) has been removed and the spine is released from these ligamentous constraints. Care must be taken not to overdistract the segment, which can cause an inordinate amount of posterior cervical/interscapular pain and can also cause spinal cord injury.

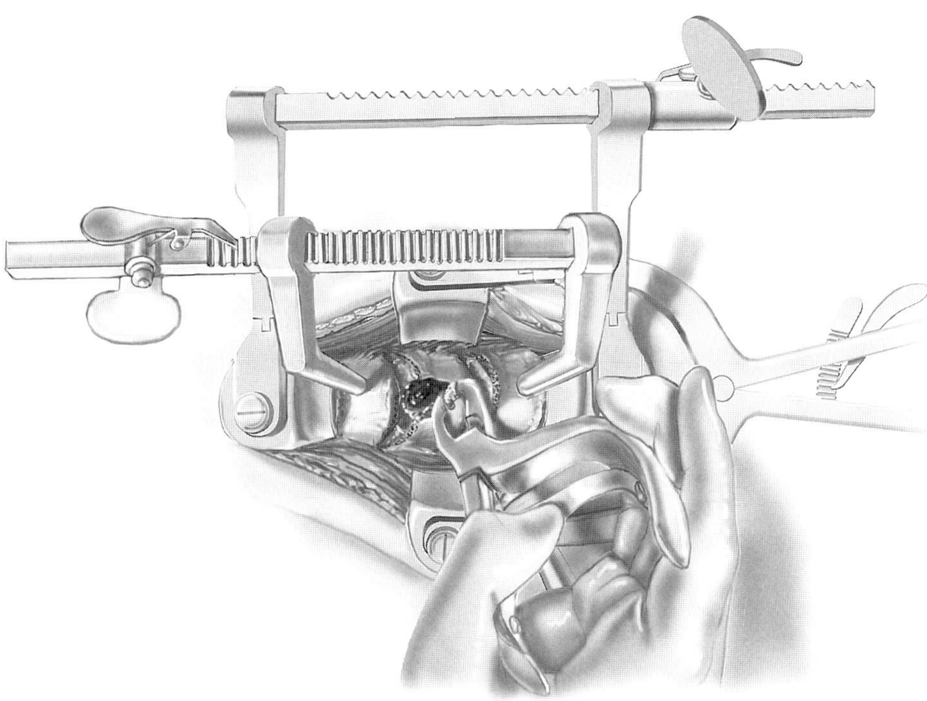

Figure 7-6. Once complete discectomies are performed, the vertebrectomy can commence. Before using a Midas Rex barrel bit, a Cushing or Leksell rongeur is used to bite the vertebral body down for the initial part of the anterior vertebrectomy. Bone from the rongeur is saved and used to pack into the strut graft or cage to be placed. This technique also begins the trough for the drill bit to sit in and therefore decreases the chances for drill skiving the soft tissues.

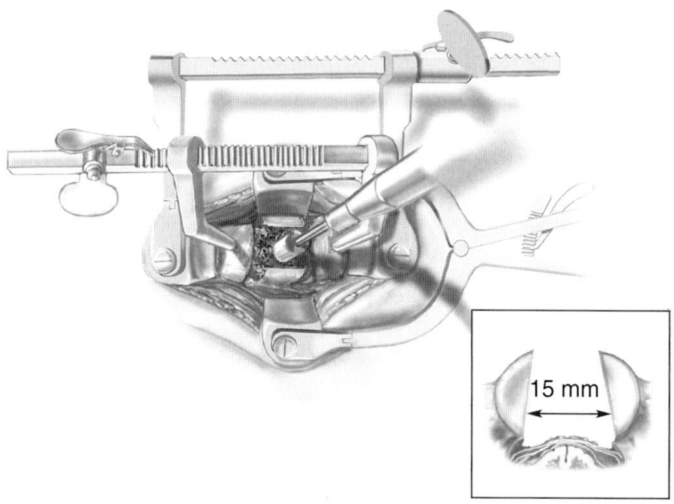

Figure 7-7. The vertebrectomy channel is deepened with a Midas Rex barrel bit, which creates an even trough down to the posterior cortex. The initial trough is created by the rongeur. Gentle sweeping motions with the drill bit will remove bone with a symmetric pattern to get down to the PLL. **Inset,** A 15- to 19-mm-wide trough is created to allow for adequate cord decompression.

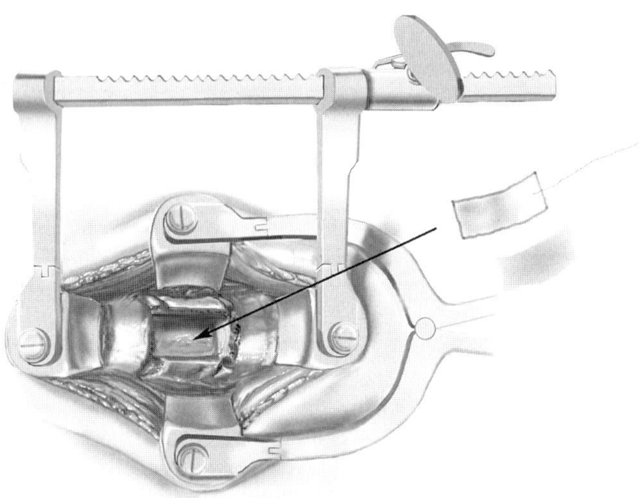

Figure 7-8. A $^1/_2$-inch × $1^1/_2$-inch cottonoid paddy is used to measure the trough. The paddy is 13.5 mm wide, and the trough should be slightly wider than this to approximate a 15-mm width. The particular width is dependent on the patient's anatomy and pathology (i.e., central versus foraminal stenosis).

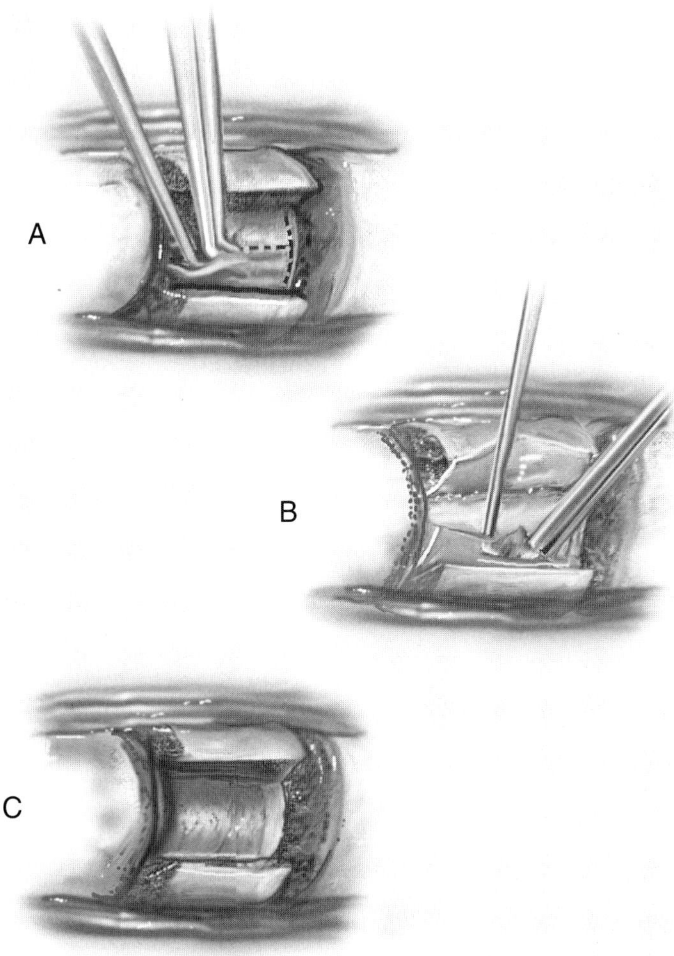

Figure 7-9, A–C. Once the posterior cortex is drilled off and the PLL is identified, the fibers of the PLL are split with a right-angled nerve hook and removed with a Kerrison rongeur. The PLL is best removed using a "cereal box" opening technique in which the flaps of the PLL are cut with the rongeur in the shape of the capital letter "I." The cord is decompressed, and the PLL can be removed safely without any further spinal cord pressure or manipulation.

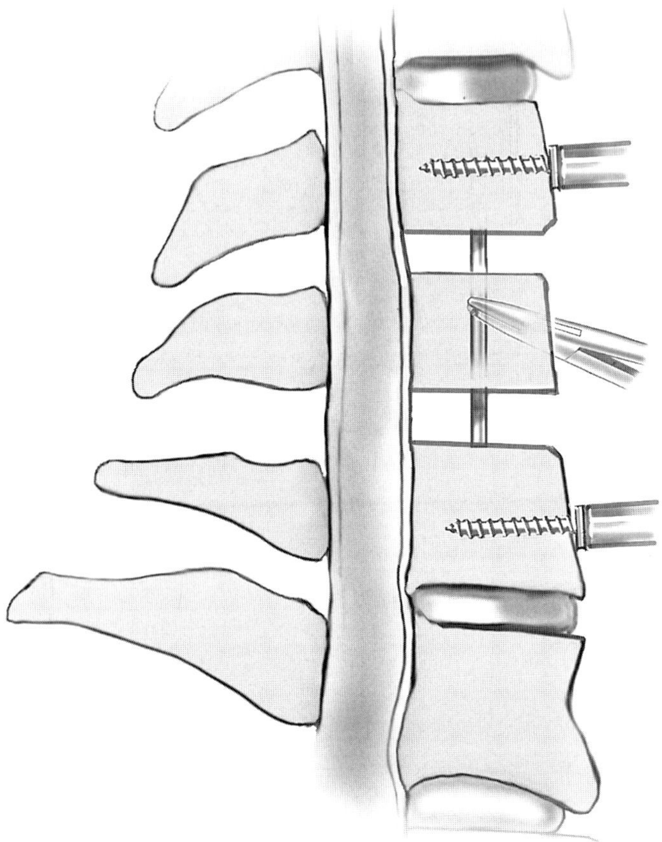

Figure 7-10. After the spinal cord is decompressed and the end plates have been prepared, a "West Virginia" measuring stick (tailored wooden cotton swab) is fitted into the corpectomy site to approximate the bone graft length. This approximates the length of the bone graft to be used.

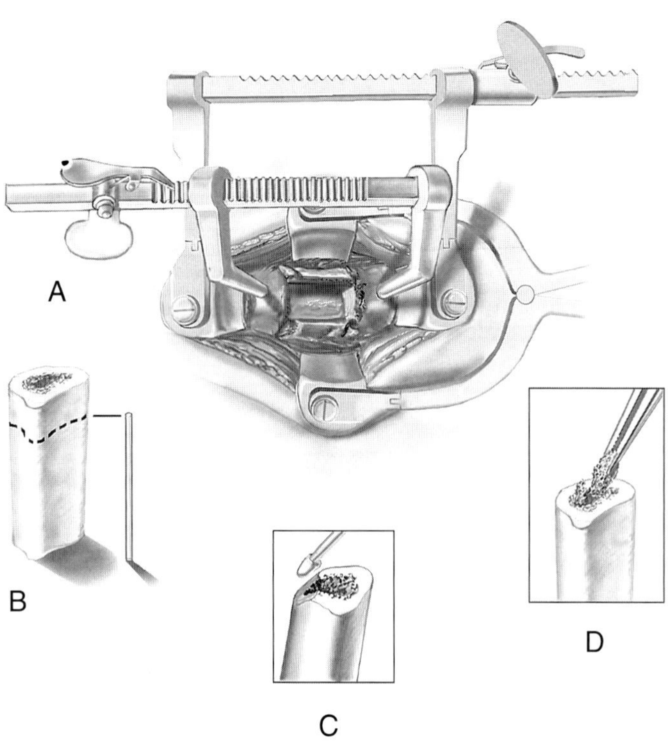

Figure 7-11, A–D. A, The spinal cord is decompressed, and end plates are prepared for placement of graft. **B,** The fibular allograft shaft is tailored to the appropriate length of the "West Virginia" measuring stick. Conversely, autograft can be used as well. **C,** A ramp is created on the inferior portion of the graft to facilitate tamping. **D,** An autologous graft harvested from the vertebral body is packed into the medullary portion of the shaft. If the central portion of the strut graft is too small to pack bone, the area can be enlarged by drilling a small channel in from the top and bottom of the graft.

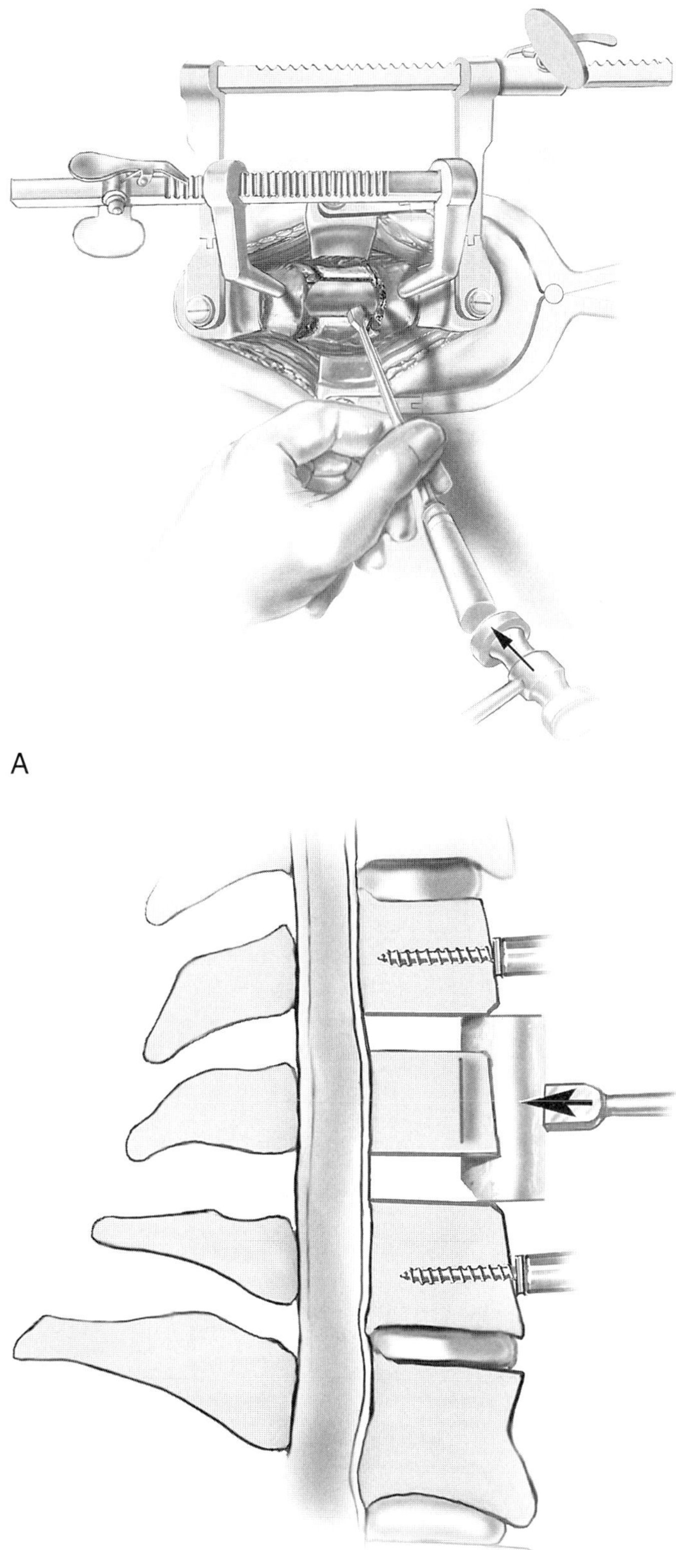

A

B

Figure 7-12, A and B. The fibular allograft is tamped into position and countersunk 2 mm into the prepared site. Note the location of the insertion ramp.

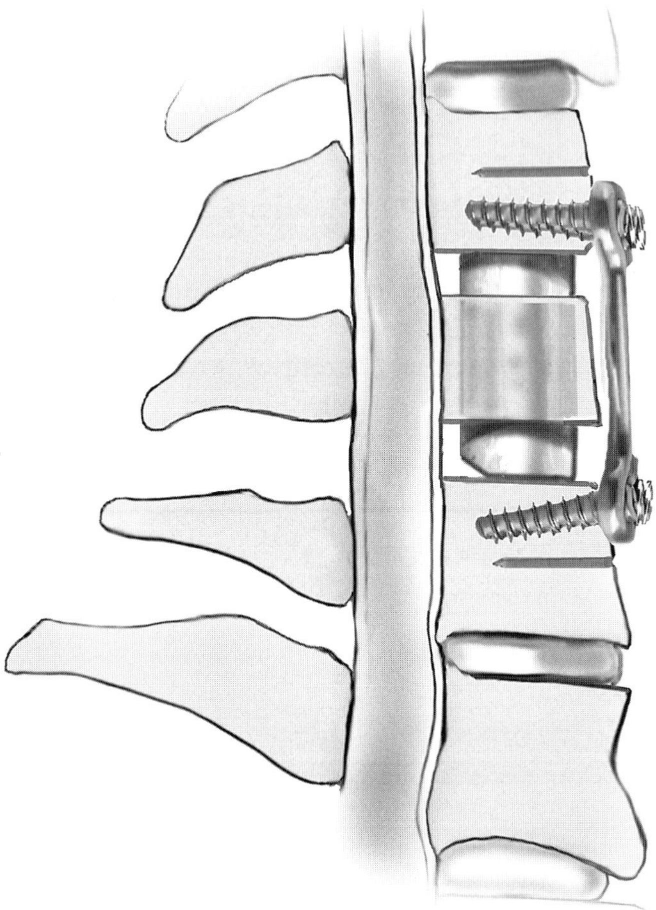

Figure 7-13. The plate is then affixed to the spine and secured with screws of appropriate length.

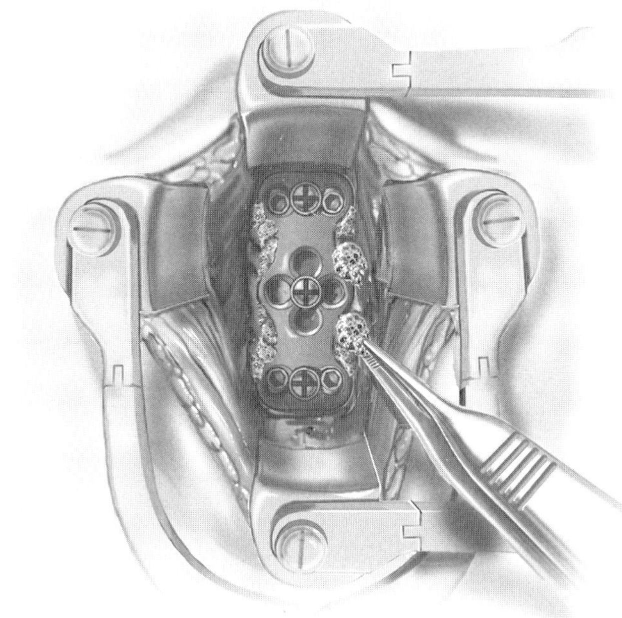

Figure 7-14. Additional autograft is packed into the sides of the corpectomy site.

COMMON PITFALLS

- Proper strut graft length is critical for optimal arthrodesis. One common pitfall is to customize the graft slightly larger than is measured. If a graft that is too long is tamped into position, there can be overdistraction and possible canting of the graft off to one side.
- Proper width of the graft is also important because the graft width should be small enough to allow a nerve hook to be passed behind the graft. This allows for additional bone to be placed laterally and allows for any epidural or bone bleeding to extravasate out of the arthrodesis bed, rather than being contained within thc fusion bed, which could cause epidural compression.

POSTOPERATIVE RESULTS

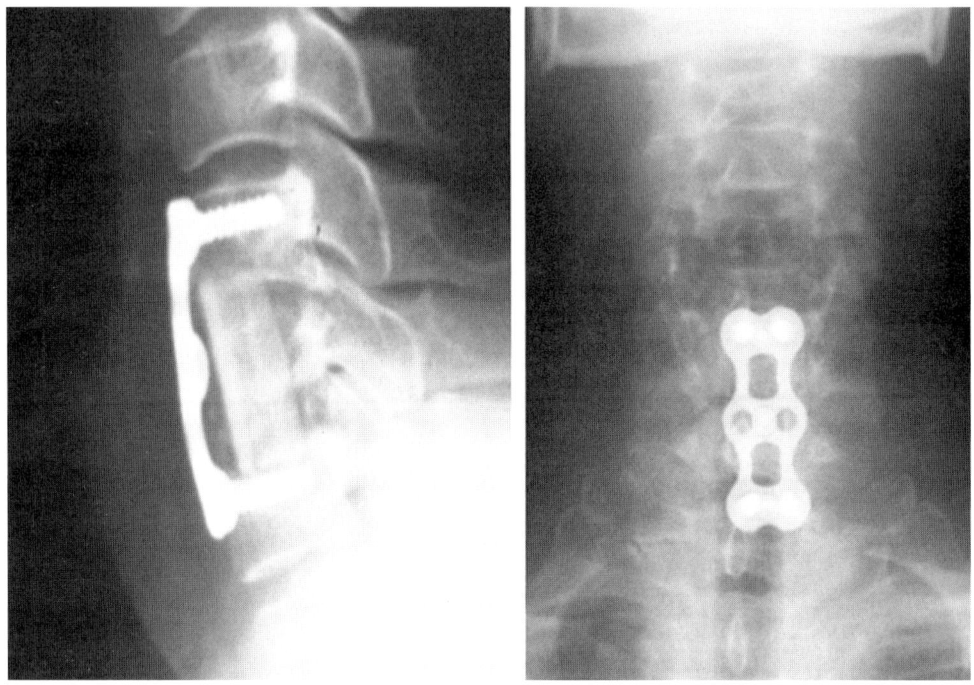

A B

Figure 7-15, A and B. Lateral and anteroposterior C-spine x-rays demonstrating a single-level anterior cervical corpectomy and fusion with plate fixation. Because fixed screws were chosen superiorly and inferiorly, forming a more rigid construct, note good incorporation of the strut graft at the superior and inferior levels with minimal telescoping of the graft.

CHAPTER VIII

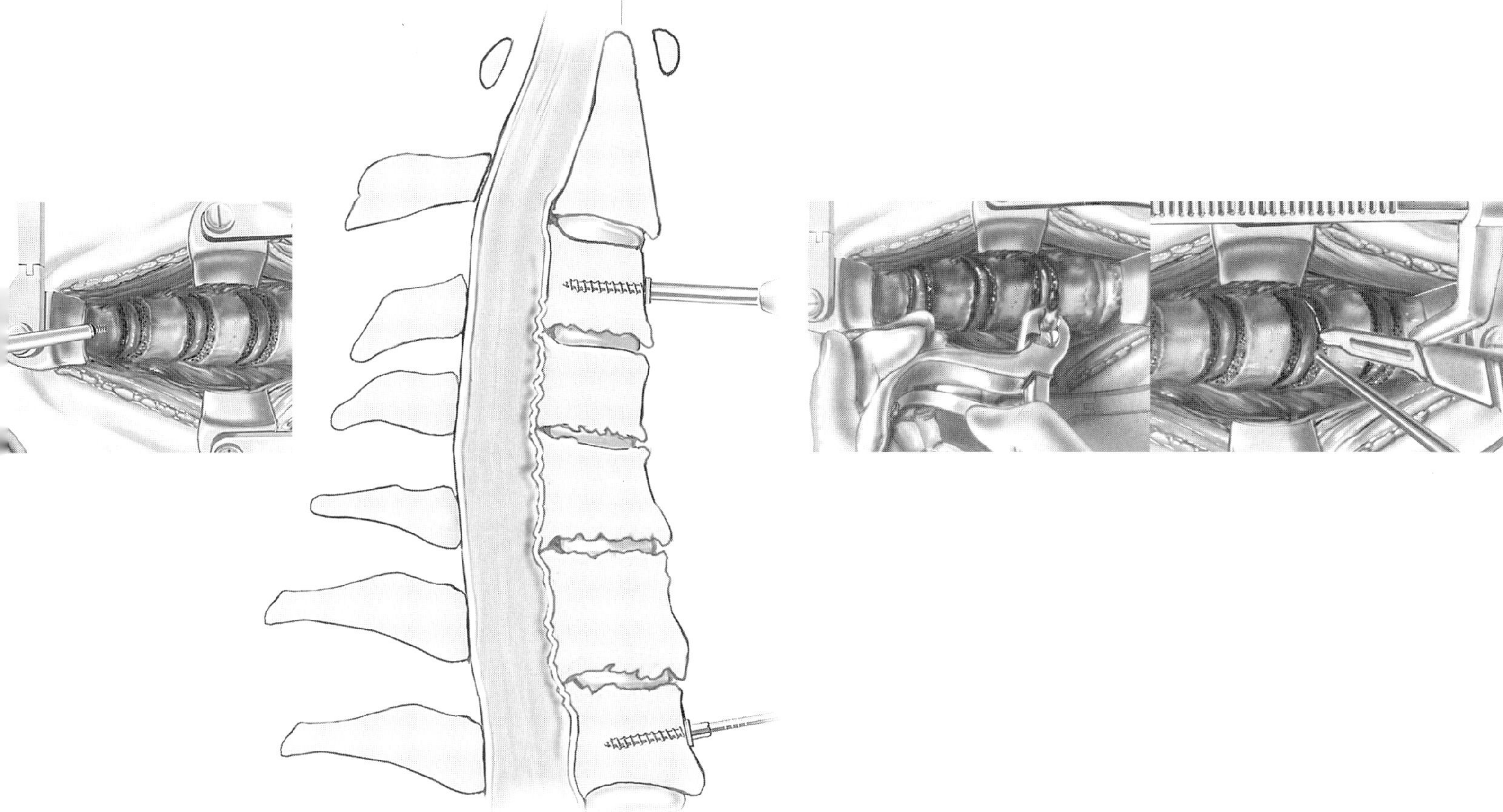

Multilevel Corpectomy

Probably the most important consideration when planning a multilevel corpectomy is whether or not a posterior supplementation is needed. The literature regarding this question is scant and not definitive. For patients with multilevel disease due to ossification of the posterior longitudinal ligament, a purely posterior approach could even be considered.

We generally use posterior supplementation in patients undergoing greater than two-level anterior corpectomies. It has been our experience that the graft- and hardware-related complications from "stand-alone" multilevel anterior corpectomies increase because of a strain on the graft and hardware to "do too much of the work." With posterior supplementation for multilevel corpectomies, the anterior graft-related and hardware-related complications decrease and the fusion rate increases. Posterior supplementation can also be considered for two-level corpectomies. In special situations, in can be considered for single-level corpectomies.

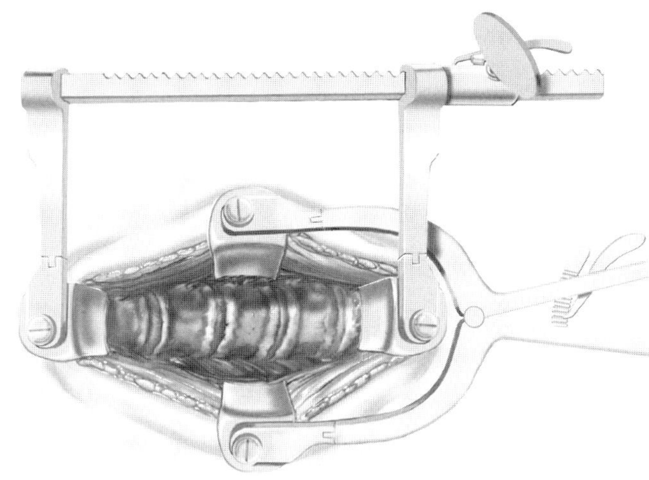

Figure 8-1. Before scheduling this type of a case, the retractor equipment should be checked to make sure the extra-long retractors and distractors are part of the existing set. Additional retraction systems, such as the Thompson-Farley spinal retraction system, may be necessary to gain adequate exposure. Retractors are placed after extensive releasing techniques to expose the appropriate level.

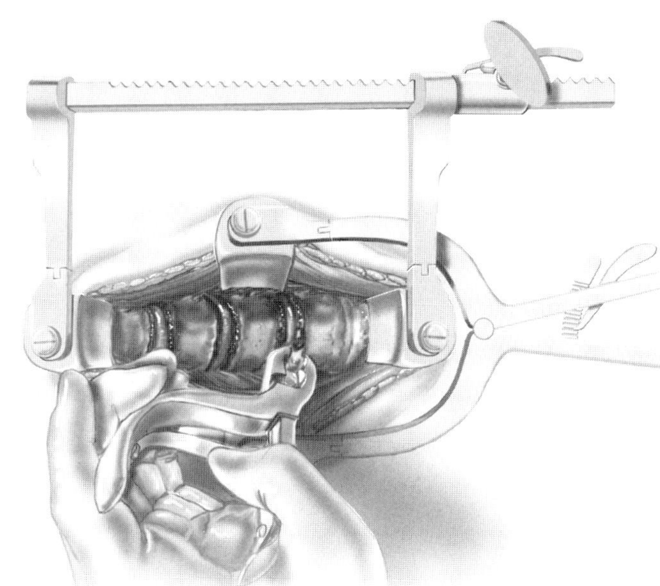

Figure 8-2. Anterior osteophytes are gardened to prepare the vertebral bodies for placement of distraction pins.

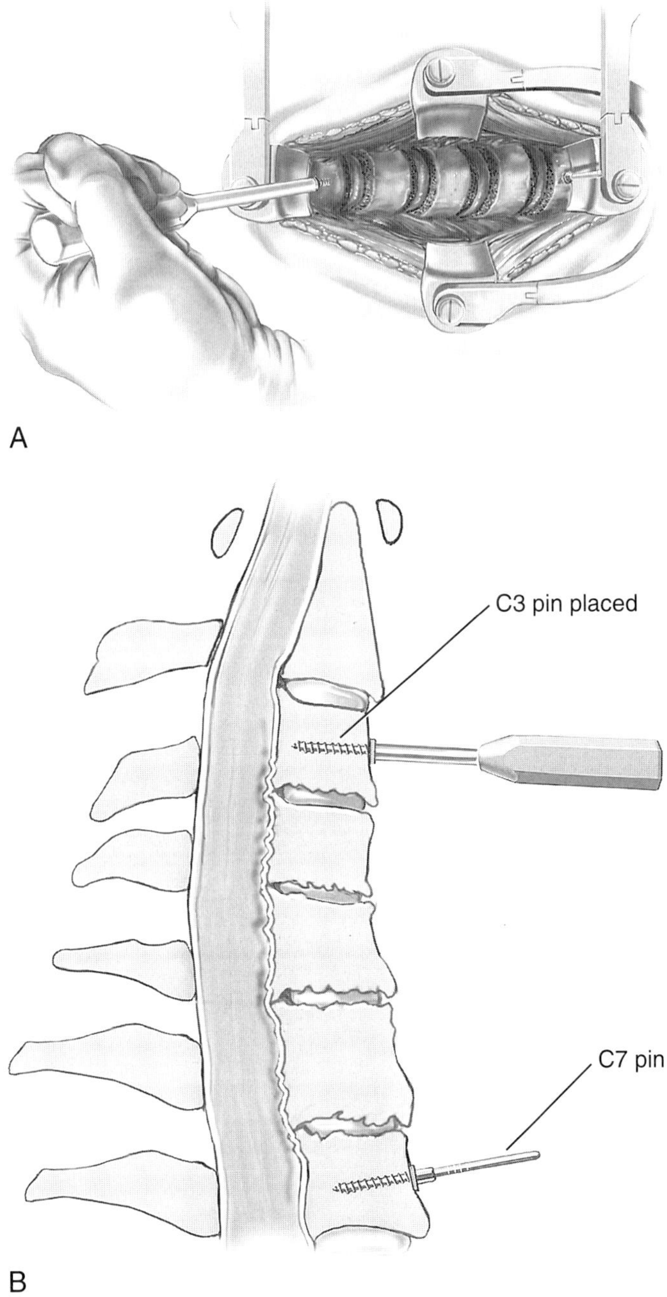

Figure 8-3, A and B. Distraction pins are placed in the cephalad and caudal vertebral bodies that will be incorporated in the plate.

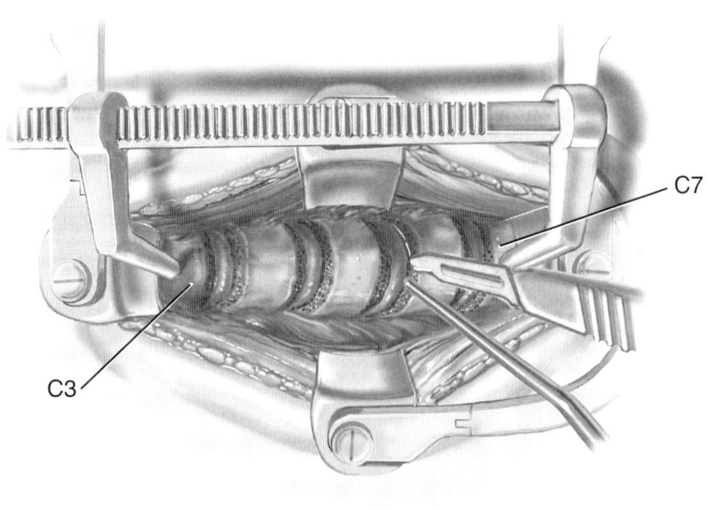

Figure 8-4. After distraction is dialed in slightly and the gardening is complete, radical discectomies are performed at each intervening segment. It is easier to clean the cartilaginous end plates before corpectomy, which provide a better fusion surface area.

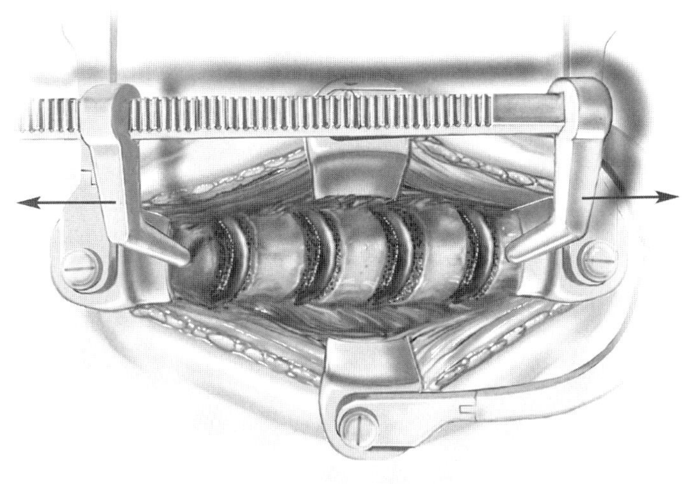

A

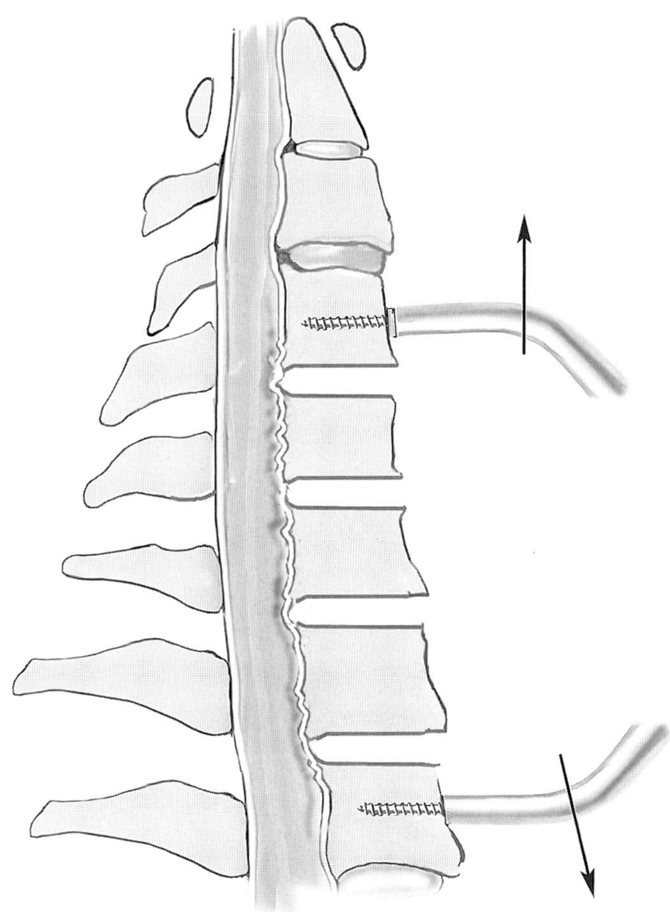

B

Figure 8-5, A and B. After the anterior longitudinal ligament (ALL) and posterior longitudinal ligament (PLL) have been opened and disc material has been removed, distraction can be increased slightly to restore sagittal balance.

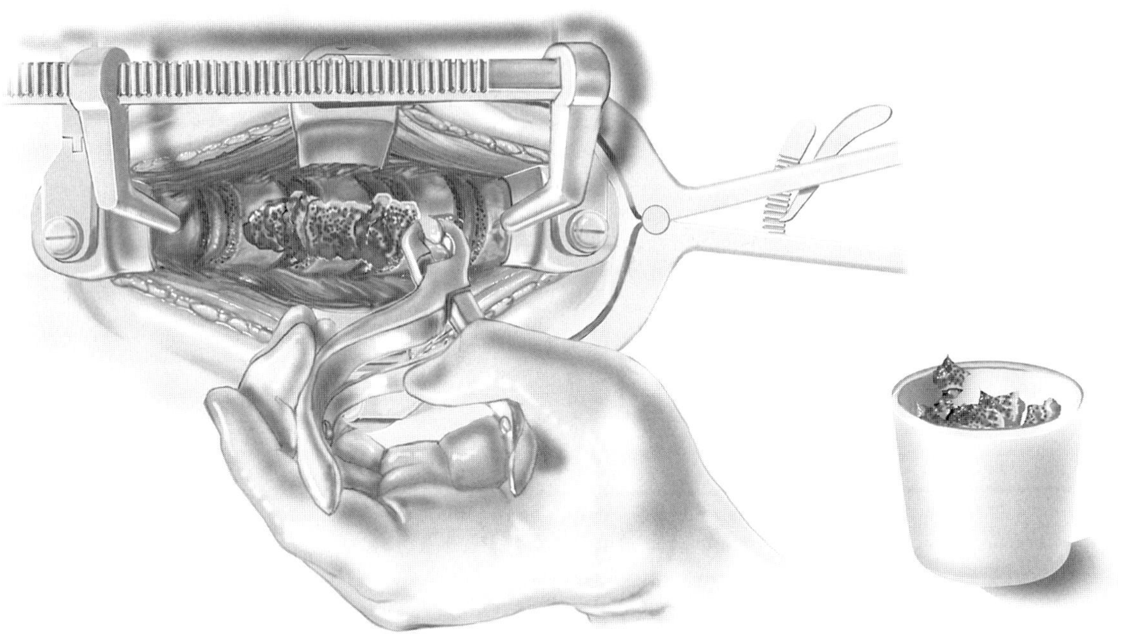

Figure 8-6. The corpectomy trough is then created with a Cushing or Leksell rongeur, and the products of decompression (autograft) are saved for packing of the strut graft or cage.

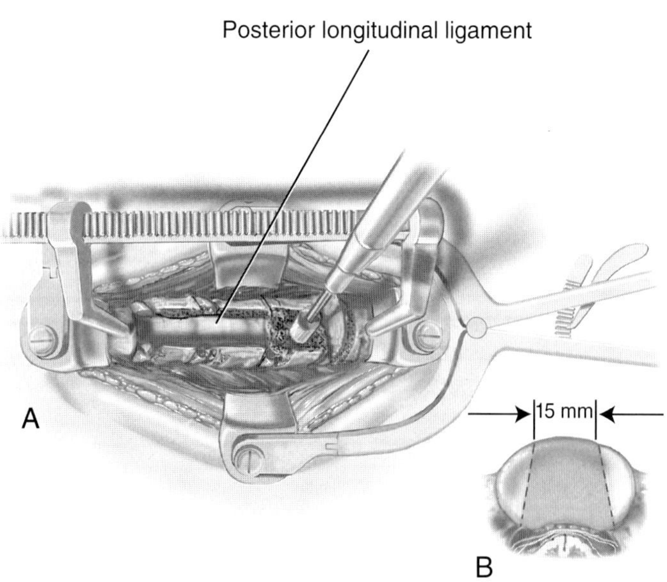

Figure 8-7, A and B. **A,** Using a Midas Rex barrel bit, the corpectomy trough is enlarged and deepened down to the PLL. **B,** A 15- to 19-mm wide trough must be created to adequately decompress the spinal cord. The trough is smaller anteriorly and widened posteriorly like an Erlenmeyer flask.

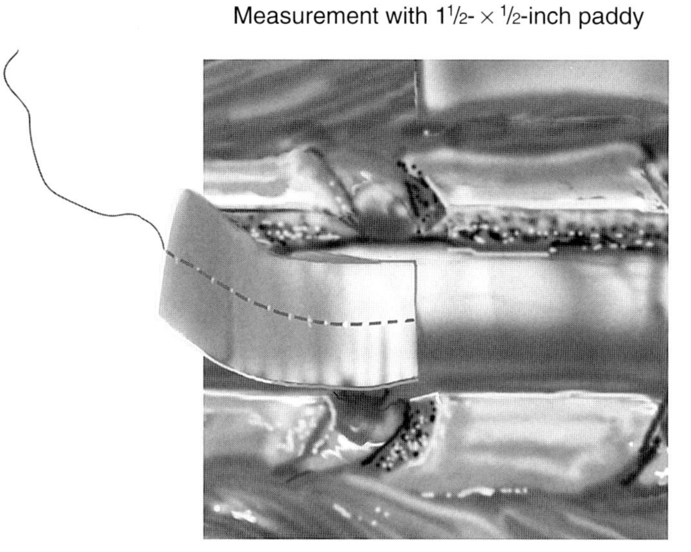

Figure 8-8. A 1½- × ½-inch paddy is used to approximate the appropriate width of corpectomy.

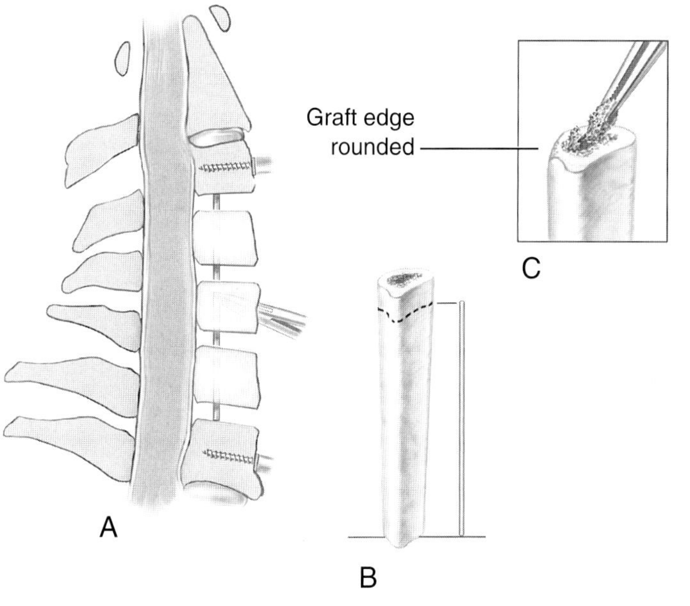

Figure 8-9, A–C. Using a "West Virginia" measuring stick (tailored wooden cotton swab) or caliper, a graft of appropriate length is measured, contoured, and cut for the graft site. The strut graft is packed with morselized autograft.

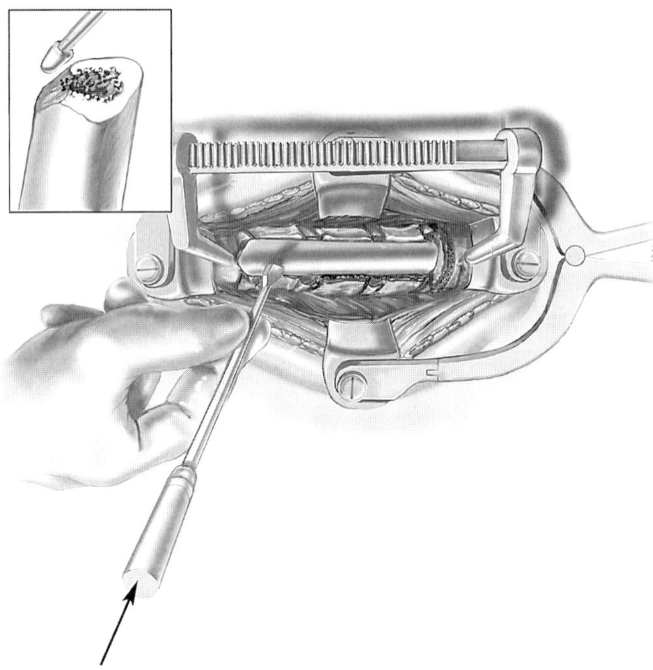

Figure 8-10. A ramp is cut on the leading edge of the graft to facilitate mortising. The graft is then tamped into position into the distracted segment.

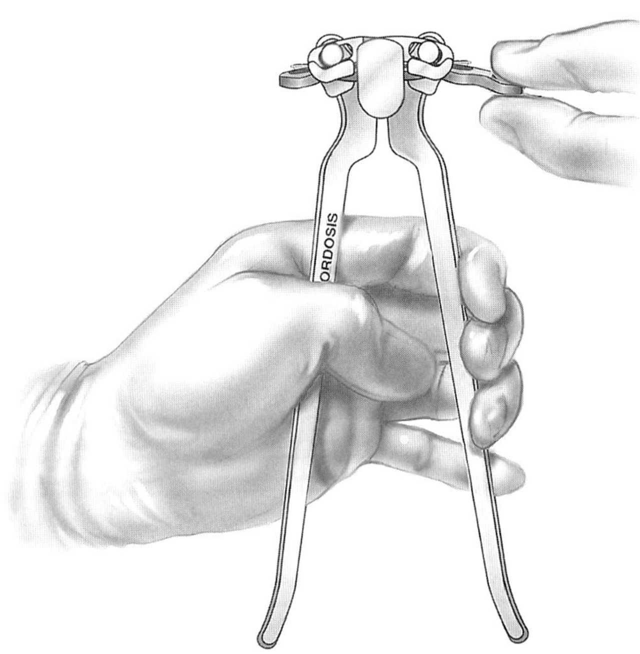

Figure 8-11. For multisegment fixation, the plate often needs to be contoured with bending to increase the lordosis of the plate. Sometimes the plate lordosis actually needs to be decreased.

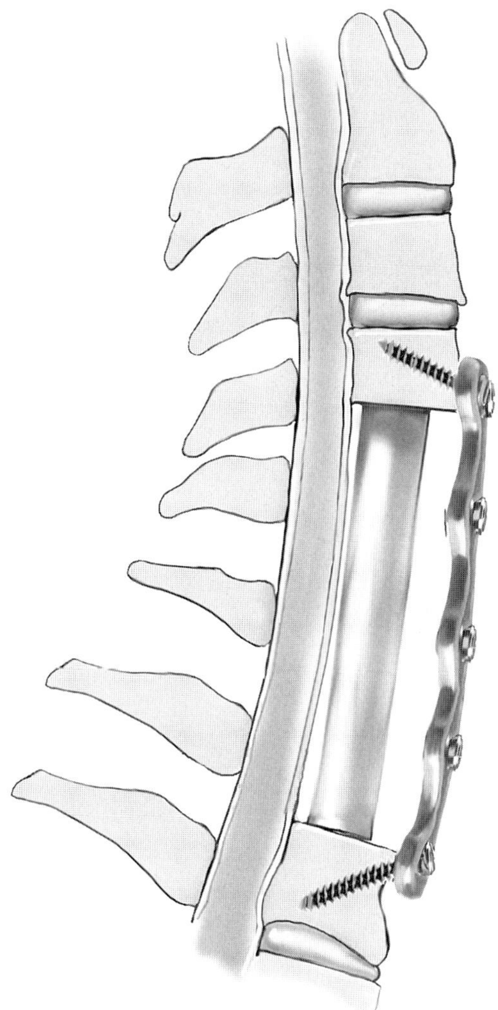

Figure 8-12. Lateral view of the anterior plate with correct positioning graft and screws.

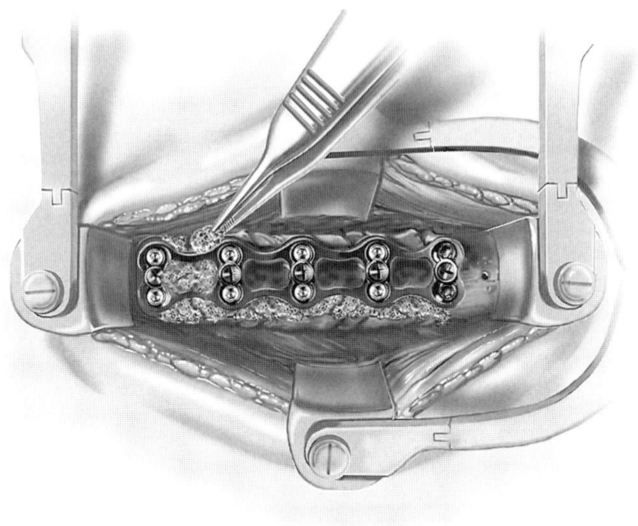

Figure 8-13. Autologous morselized graft is packed into the sides of the bone graft in the lateral gutter.

COMMON PITFALLS

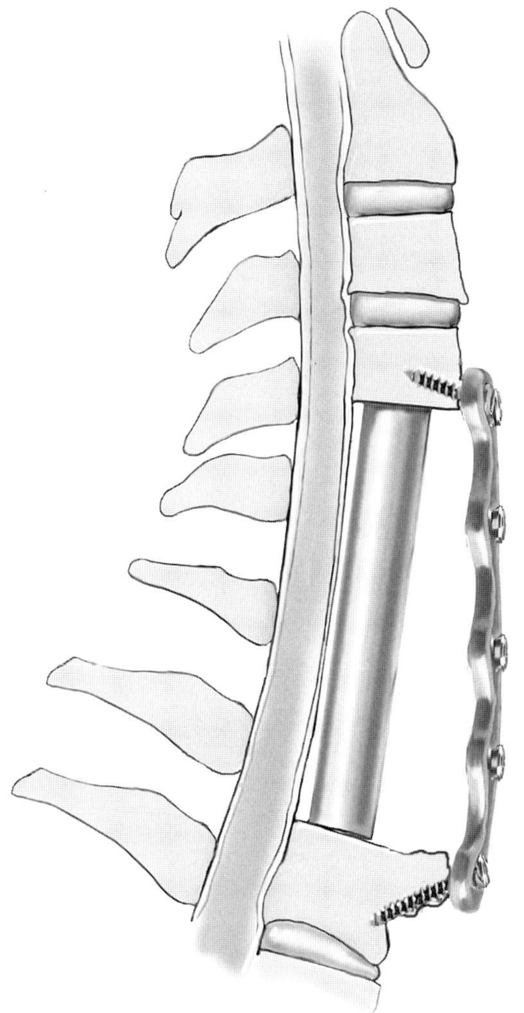

Figure 8-14. A common pitfall is incomplete gardening, which results in poor vertebral body purchase of screws or plate rocking and stress risers. This can increase the chances of plate or graft kickout.

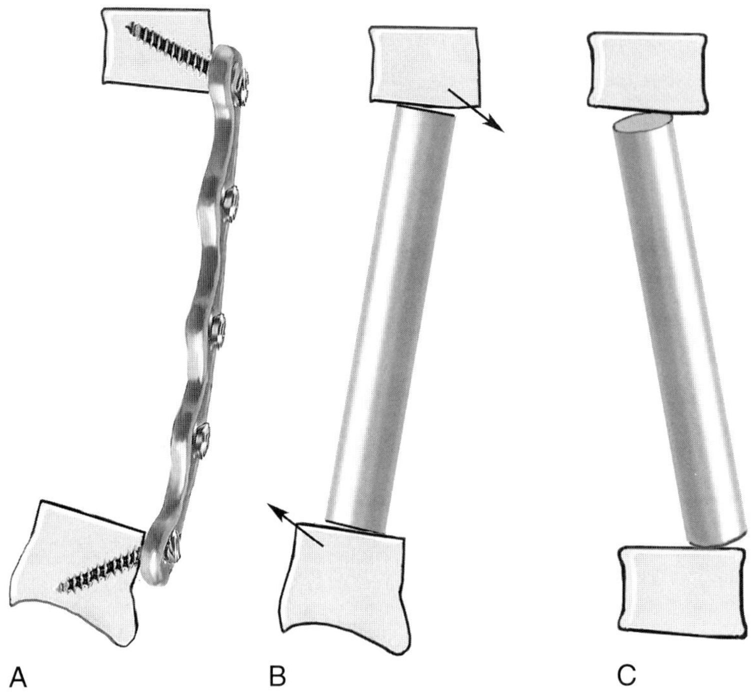

Figure 8-15, A–C. Another common pitfall is improper graft sizing. **A,** If the graft is too short, when distraction is removed the graft may not be tightly opposed to the bony surfaces, thus decreasing the chances for good graft incorporation and subsequent fusion. **B** and **C,** If the graft is too long, it will create a shifting torque either in the anteroposterior plane or in the coronal plane, predisposing graft or plate kickout. Good plating cannot make up for poor carpentry. An appropriately sized graft must be fitted.

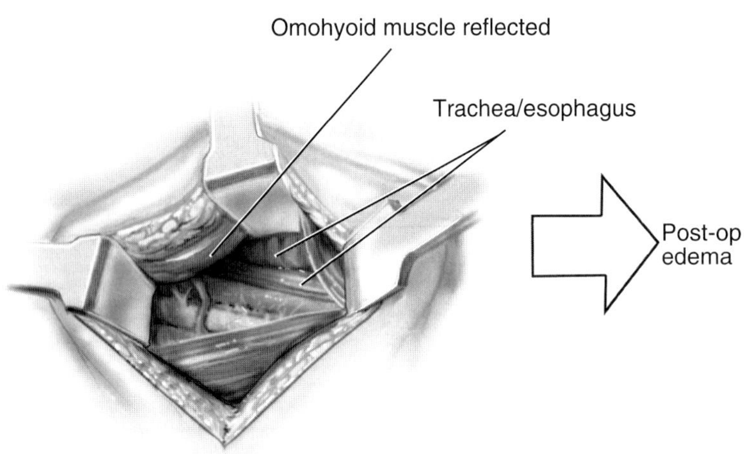

Figure 8-16. If the omohyoid muscle is not divided, or if the soft tissue planes have not been adequately dissected and released, increased pressure is placed on the trachea and esophagus. This increased retractor pressure can result in more significant postoperative edema, which may preclude early extubation after surgery or cause stridor.

POSTOPERATIVE RESULTS

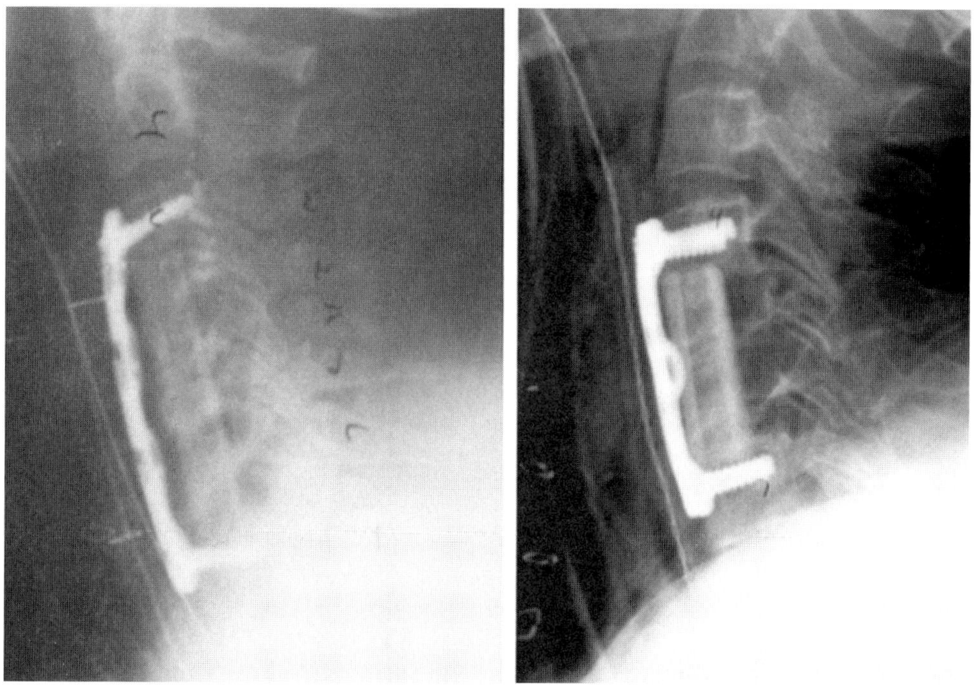

Figure 8-17. Lateral views of multilevel anterior cervical corpectomy and fusion with plate fixation.

CHAPTER

IX

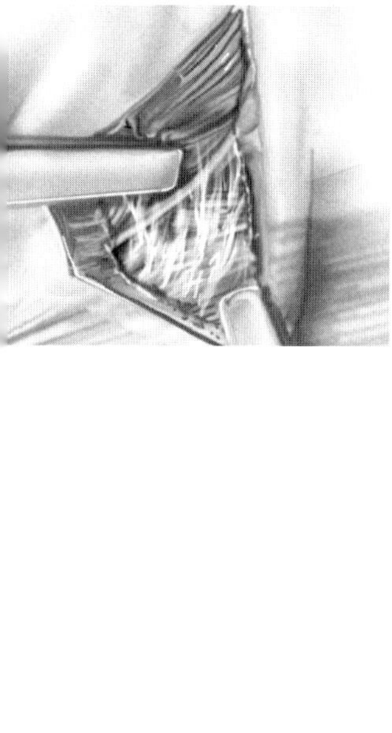

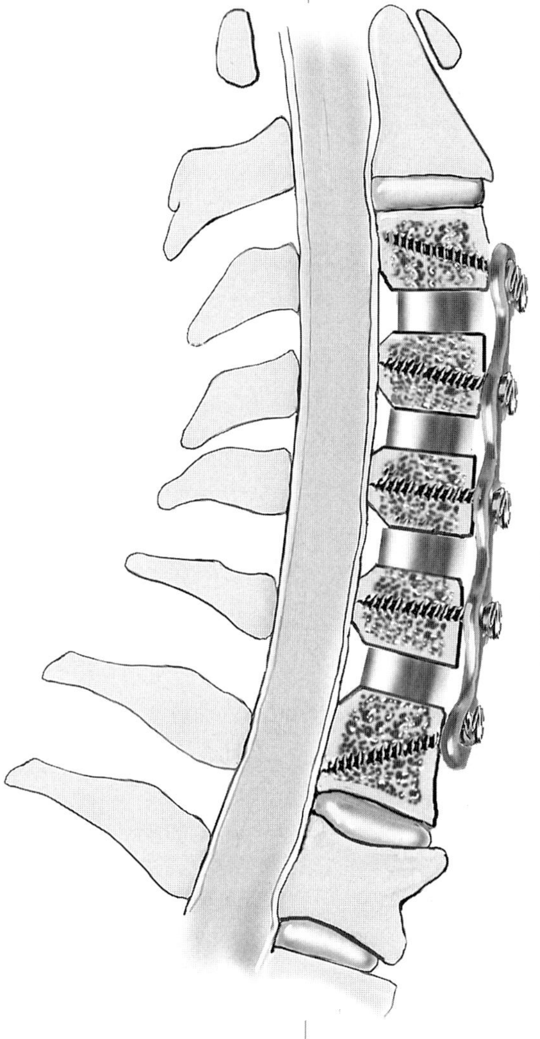

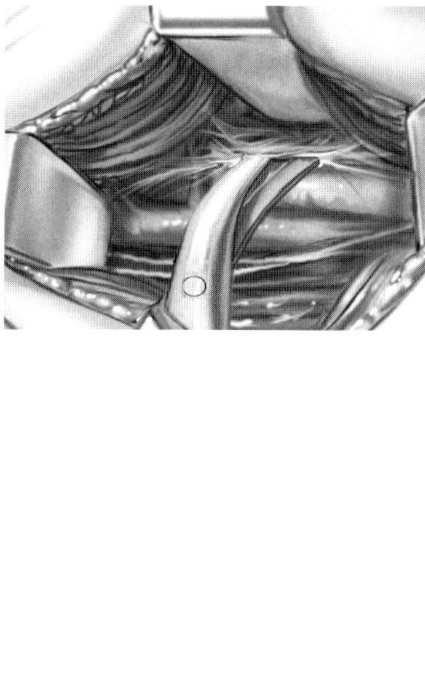

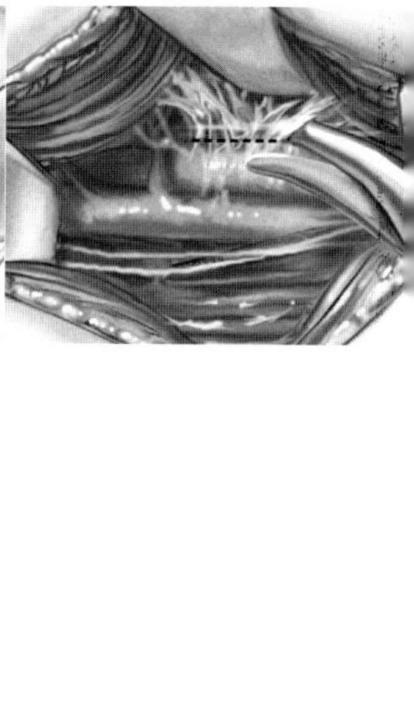

Special Situations: Anterior

This chapter discusses a few "tricks of the trade" for certain techniques that the spine surgeon encounters less frequently. These techniques have been picked up over the years and are an amalgam of the authors' experiences. Upper cervical disc herniations in the C2-C3 area are rare and require a slightly modified approach and exposure.

Bicortical purchase was a technique commonly used when anterior plates were first introduced because there were no locking screw mechanisms to prevent screw back-out. Dr. Caspar introduced this technique to avoid this complication. With more advanced plating and screw technology, bicortical screw purchase is no longer necessary to prevent screw back-out, but it still offers a superior screw purchase and may still be desired in patients with long anterior screw constructs.

Reexploration of the anterior cervical region also warrants further discussion. Side of approach and dissection are important considerations when evaluating these patients.

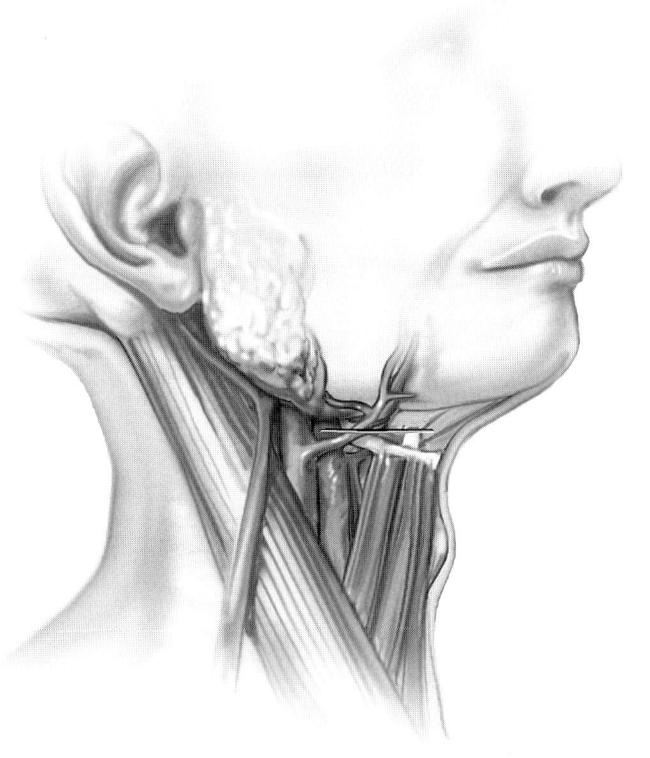

Figure 9-1. For C2-C3 discectomy, a similar anterior cervical incision is planned about one to three fingerbreadths below the angle of the mandible. The lateral aspect of the incision should touch the medial border of the sternocleidomastoid muscle. This will give the surgeon a good landmark for deeper dissection. Care should be taken to identify and preserve the mandibular branch of the facial nerve.

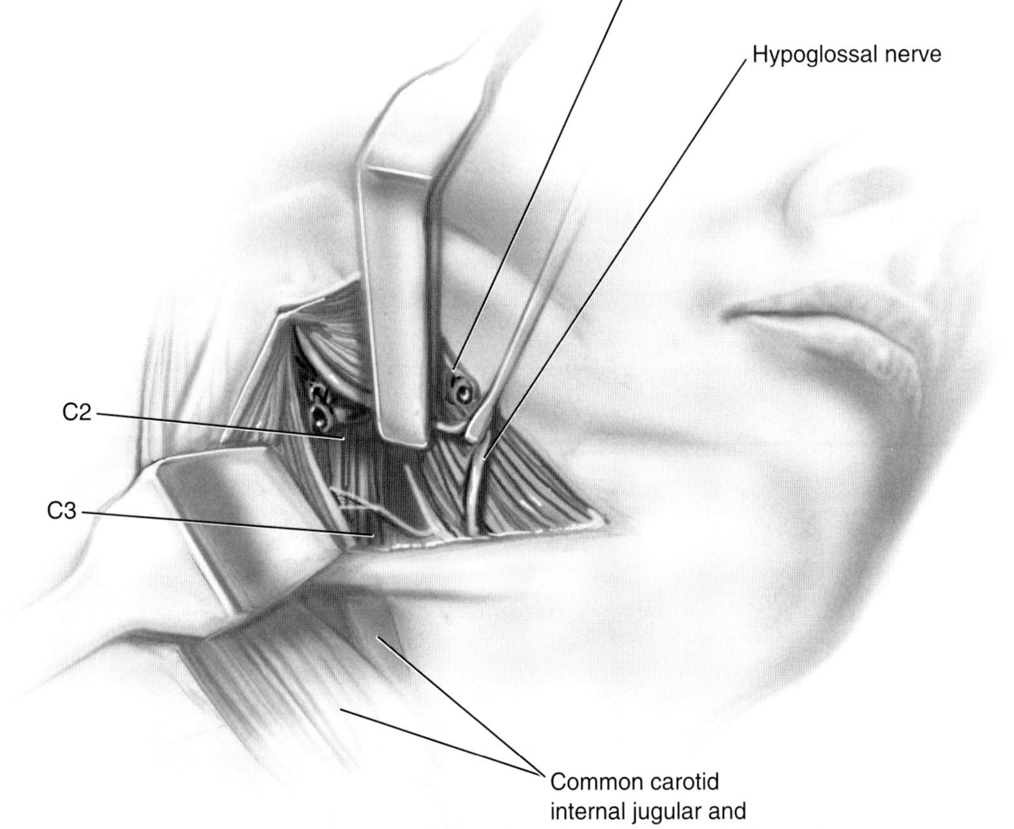

Figure 9-2. The investing sheath of the sternocleidomastoid is opened, and the avascular plane between the sternocleidomastoid and carotid sheath is dissected laterally and the trachea and esophagus medially. The common facial vein is encountered and divided. Careful attention is paid to identifying and preserving the hypoglossal nerve, which lies just beneath the posterior belly of the digastric muscle. The posterior belly of the digastric muscle and the hypoglossal nerve are retracted superiorly. Frequently, lymph nodes can be encountered in this area, and the submandibular gland lies superiorly and medially. The superior laryngeal nerve may be occasionally visualized inferiorly because it commonly arises from the vagus nerve at the C3-C4 level. Most of these structures can be dissected and retracted medially or laterally. Occasionally, a large lymph node must be removed for better visualization.

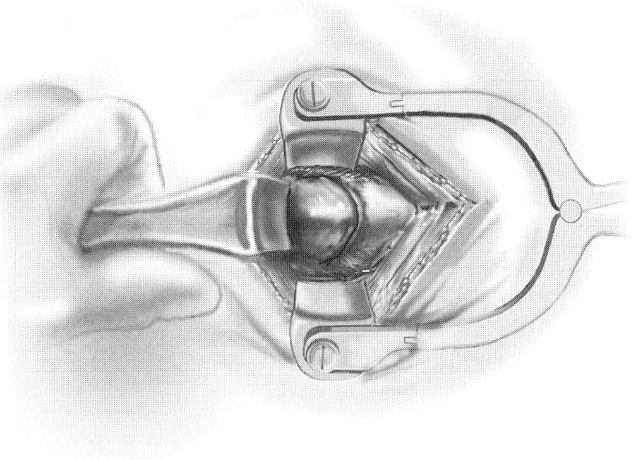

Figure 9-3. Intraoperative exposure of C2-C3 disc space with retractors in place. An assistant with a handheld retractor in the superior direction is usually necessary to obtain the adequate dissection. Sometimes the superior-inferior retractor will not sit well for exposure, and an assistant must continually hold the retractor for placement of the C2-C3 plate.

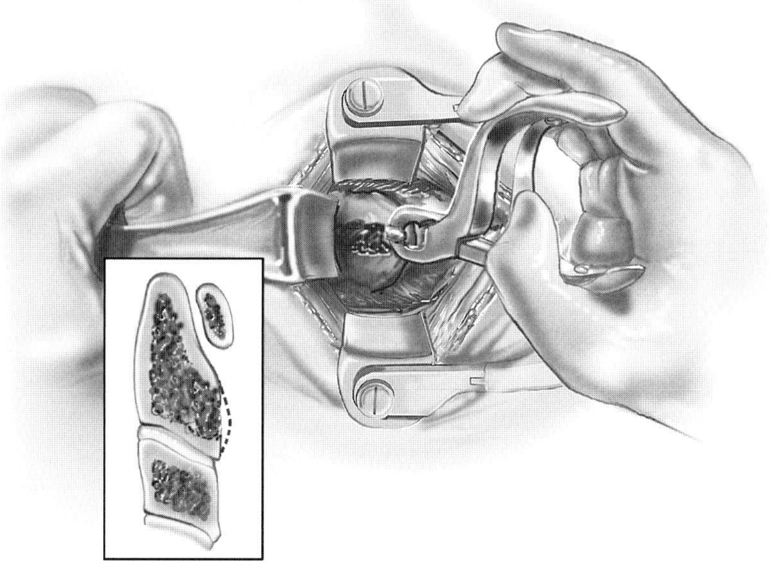

Figure 9-4. The anterior face of C2 has a keel on it that must be gardened to create a flat surface for plating. Therefore, it is important to premeasure the screws for the C2 body. This can be done best on a preoperative computed tomography (CT) scan. It can also be measured with a depth gauge. There is usually a significant insertion of the longus colli musculature at these levels that must be reflected adequately to gain optimal bony exposure. The vertebral arteries turn slightly more medial in this region, and careful dissection in the medial-to-lateral direction is critical.

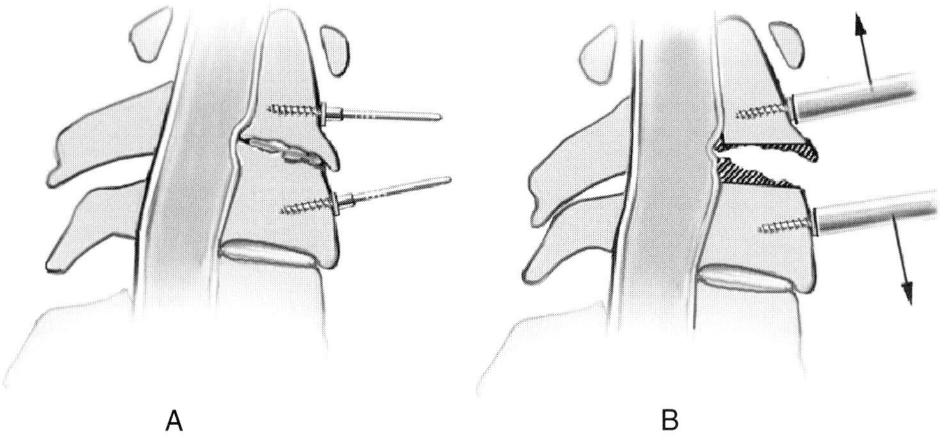

Figure 9-5, A and B. A, Caspar distraction screws are placed in C2 and C3 in divergent directions. **B,** Distraction is then applied to recreate sagittal balance and open the disc space for visualization and discectomy.

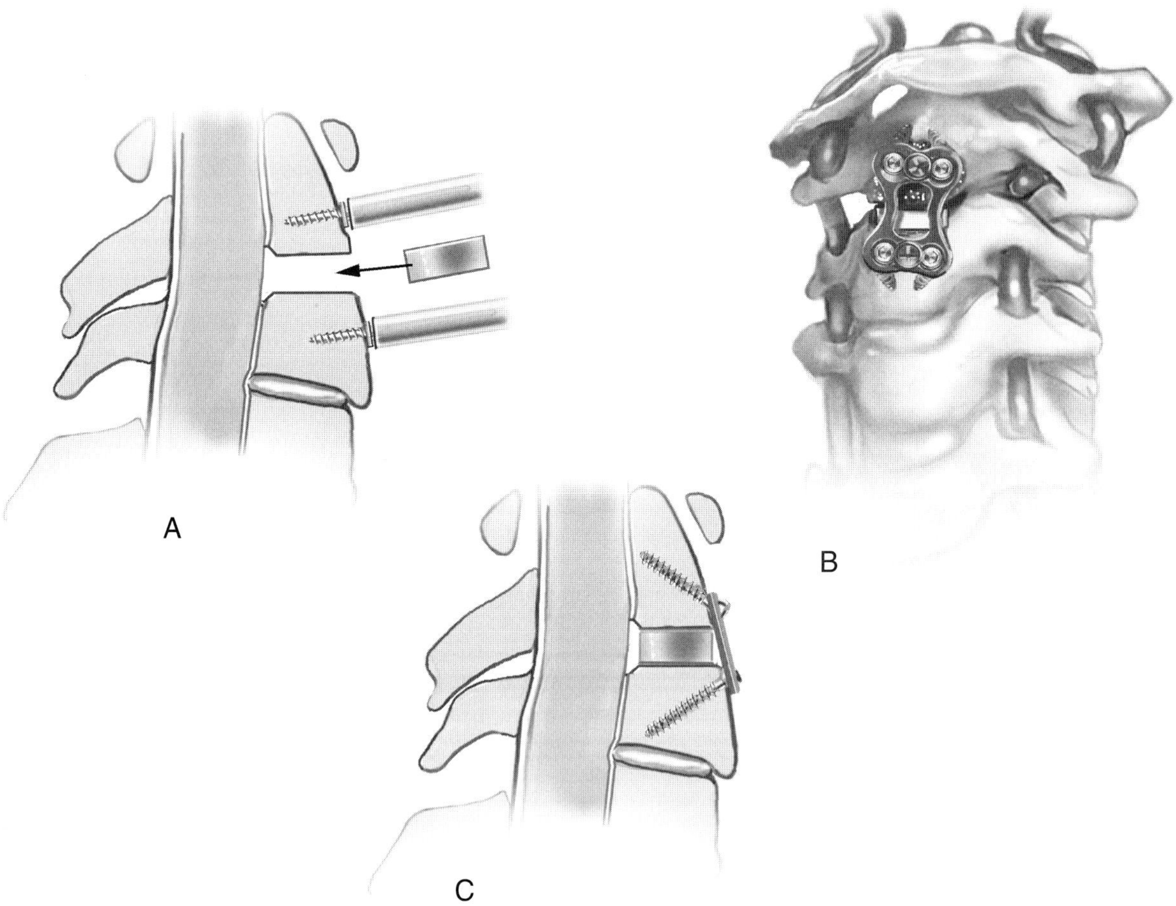

C2-C3 DISCECTOMY

Figure 9-6, A–C. After a completed discectomy, decompression, and end plate preparation, the appropriately sized graft is tamped and countersunk into position. Cervical plate fixation is optional. Premeasuring screw length on preoperative CT scan for optimal length is recommended.

BICORTICAL PURCHASE FOR LONG-SEGMENT FIXATION

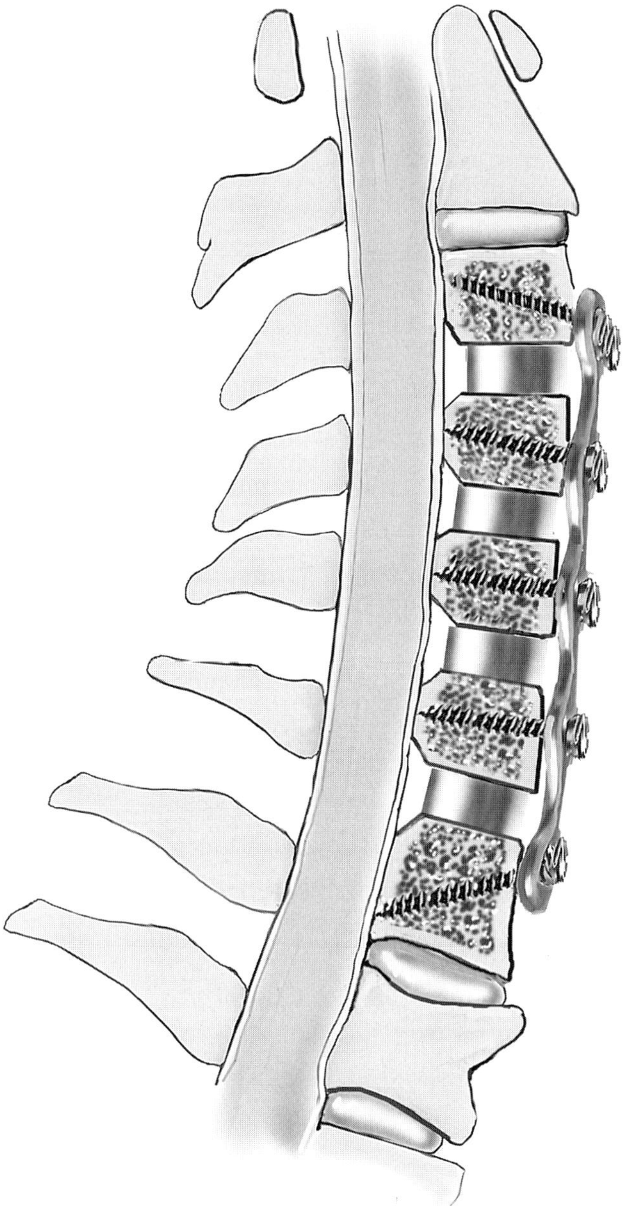

Figure 9-7. To increase stability, bicortical screw purchase is an option for long-segment plate fixation for multilevel discectomy or corpectomy. This technique affords significantly better screw purchase and decreased chances for plate migration. We recommend obtaining preoperative CT scans to premeasure screw length, and consider intraoperative C-arm or frameless spinal stereotaxis for screw placement.

REEXPLORATION CONSIDERATIONS

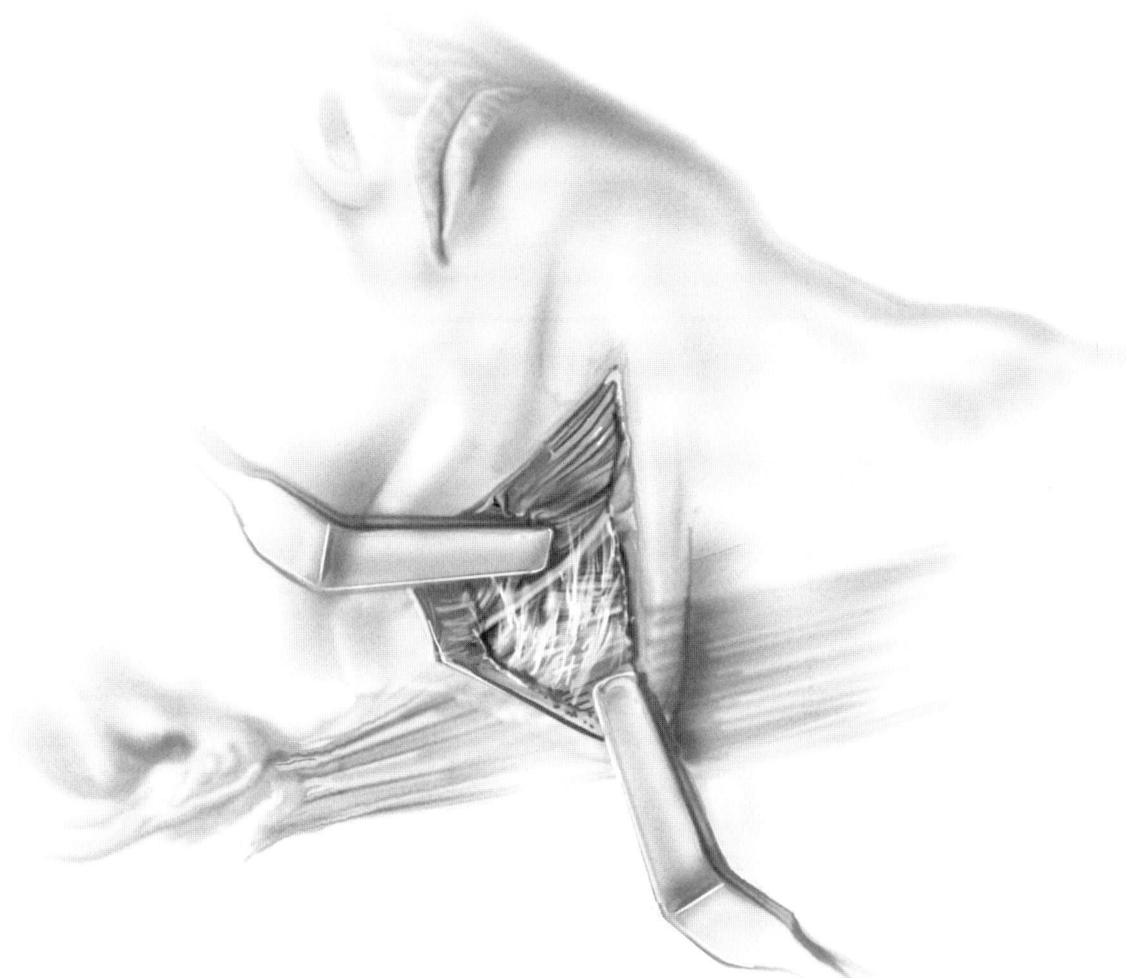

A

Figure 9-8, A. In patients who have had prior anterior cervical surgery that requires reexploration, we recommend an approach from the same side as the previous surgery. Although the dissection is slightly harder, in general the difficulties are minimal. If an approach is contemplated from the other side, we recommend an ear, nose, and throat evaluation with direct laryngoscopy before surgery. This will verify normal vocal cord function bilaterally. If this is not done, an occult recurrent laryngeal nerve palsy from the previous operation may not be detected. **A,** Depending on the level to be approached, the prior incision can be opened, or a new incision above or below can be chosen, depending on the level. Usually there is focal scarring on the area of the investing sheath of the sternocleidomastoid that can be freed by dissecting unscarred tissue above and below the adhesion. Then the two normal areas can be connected with sharp dissection.

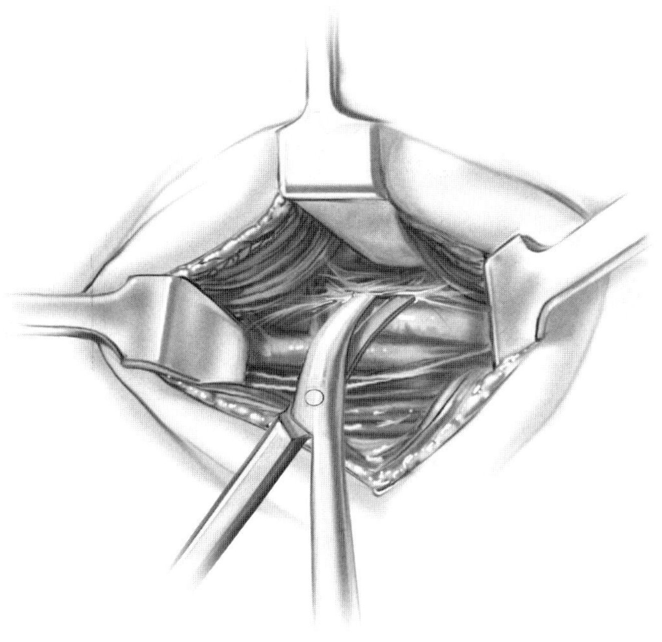

B

Figure 9-8, B. Using a combination of sharp dissection and gentle blunt dissection over the scarred area, the tissues can be released. Tension bands are dissected deeper and freed with sharp dissection, first from above and below the scar in the normal planes and then extrapolated to the prior surgical area.

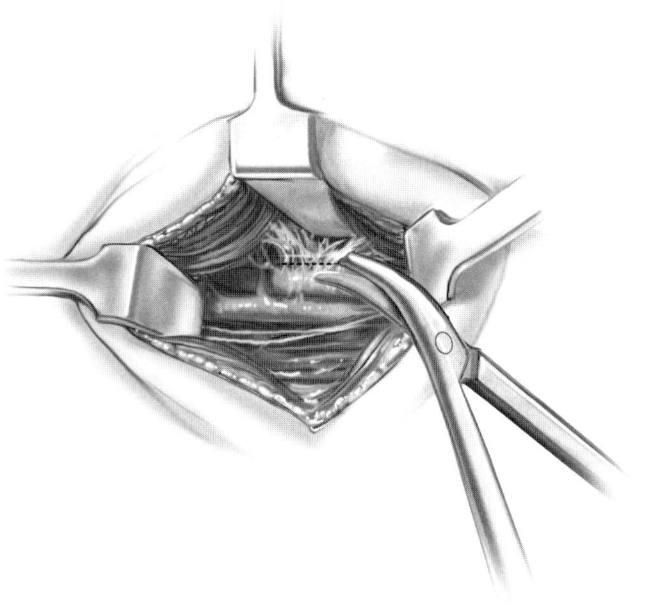

C

Figure 9-8, C. Once the carotid sheath is identified, a sharp dissection plane is created just medial to the sheath. This plane can be carried down to the longus colli musculature. The prevertebral fascia is usually thicker and more vascular on reoperation but can be cauterized and cut sharply. If an anterior plate has been placed at the prior operation, the plate can be identified by palpation and dissected free for exposure.

COMMON PITFALLS

- Sometimes it is difficult to identify the hypoglossal nerve during the upper cervical dissection, and the nerve can be injured. Usually the nerve lies just under the posterior belly of the digastric muscle and can be identified there. Also, it is important to garden the keel of C2 so that there is a smooth surface for plate fixation.
- If bicortical purchase is desired for added stability, it should be performed with image guidance or C-arm fluoroscopy. Also, a preoperative CT should be obtained to premeasure screw length.
- The most common pitfall of reexplorations in the anterior cervical region is poor exposure due to inadequate releasing techniques of the scar tissue and surrounding structures. It is critical to obtain wide exposure for reexplorations because scar tissue can obscure the surgeon's view, and a wider exposure can allow for more normal anatomical landmarks for orientation.

POSTOPERATIVE RESULTS

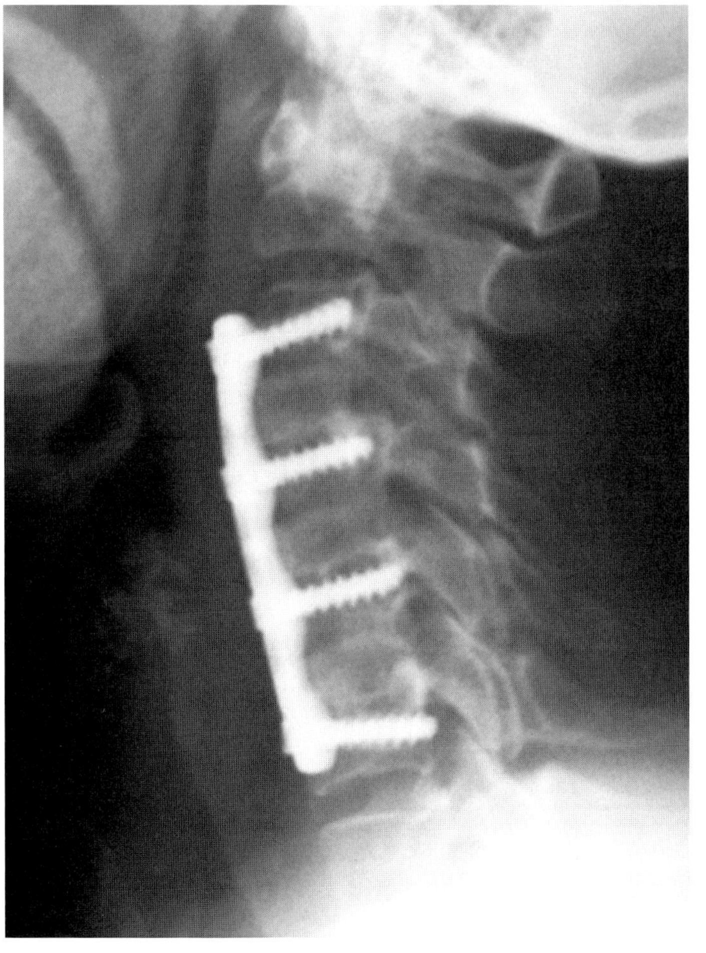

Figure 9-9. At C5 and C6, bicortical screws have been placed in this long-segment construct. Bicortical purchase increases pullout strength and significantly strengthens this long-segment construct.

CHAPTER

X

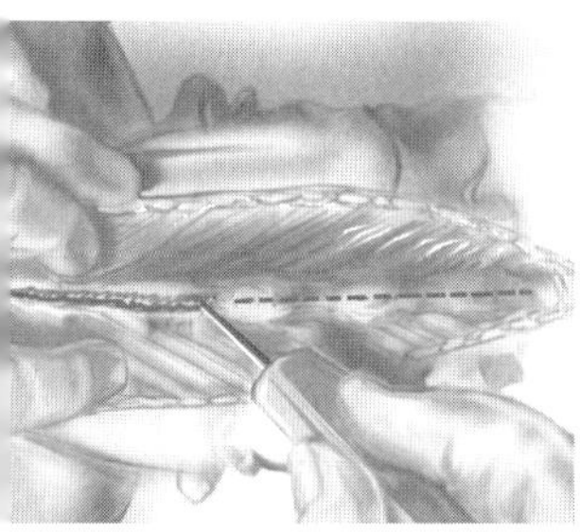

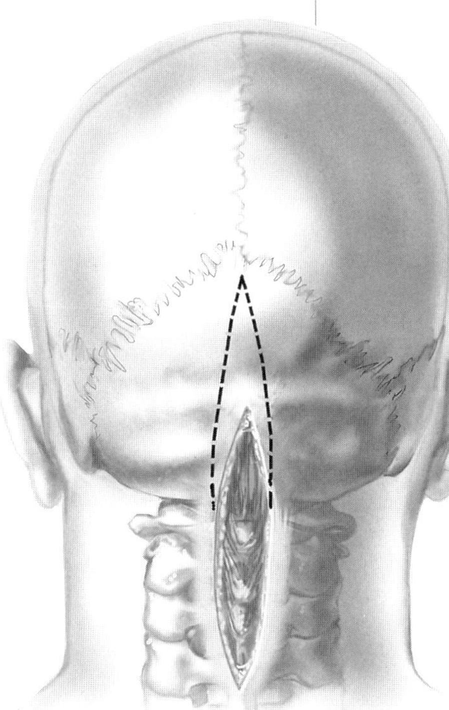

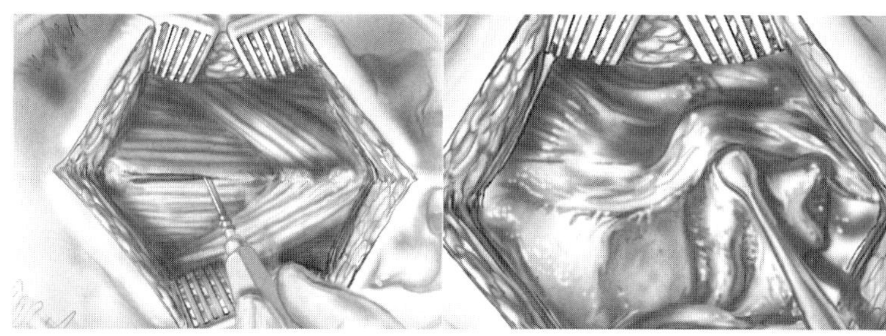

Positioning and Exposure for Posterior Cervical Approaches

For virtually all posterior procedures, we use the Mayfield three-point head fixation system. This allows for reliable stability and the ability to place the patient's neck in the appropriate position for the procedure to be performed. For instance, a military tuck position is desired for C1-C2 fixation, as opposed to gentle lordosis for a posterior cervical fusion.

The arms are tucked inferiorly and trapped with a long sheet. The sheet is secured by two perforating towel clamps and tucked so that the iliac crest is available for draping into the surgical field. Great care should be maintained to verify that all intravenous (IV) lines are working and all appropriate pressure points are padded before draping. Occasionally, an IV line will be kinked during tucking of the arms and will require repositioning before starting the case. The bed is placed in a reverse Trendelenburg position to bring the neck up into the surgical field, making exposure easier for the surgeon.

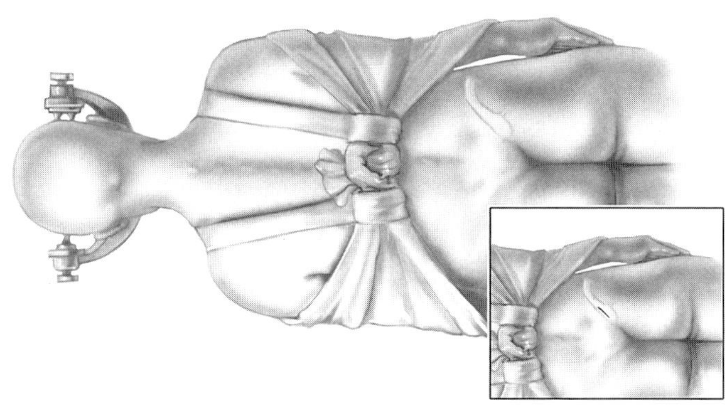

Figure 10-1. This overhead view of a patient positioned for a posterior cervical approach demonstrates several important positioning principles. The three-point head fixation device is used with the patient's arms tucked. Critical features for three-point head fixation include pin purchase around (but not cephalad to) the superior temporal line and avoidance of the squamous portion of the temporal bone. Before positioning, the head should be carefully but firmly checked to make sure there is no pin slippage. As the head is positioned, it is best to use the auditory meatus to judge the appropriate balance and vertical tilt to avoid any rotation. An extra long sheet is placed over the chest rolls, crisscrossed, and tied with perforating towel clamps. Adequate padding is placed in the region of the ulnar nerve. The shoulders are then pulled inferiorly with tape that is secured to the sides or bottom of the bed or to sheets tied together to sling the arms. This will expose the posterior/superior iliac spine if autologous graft is required for fusion.

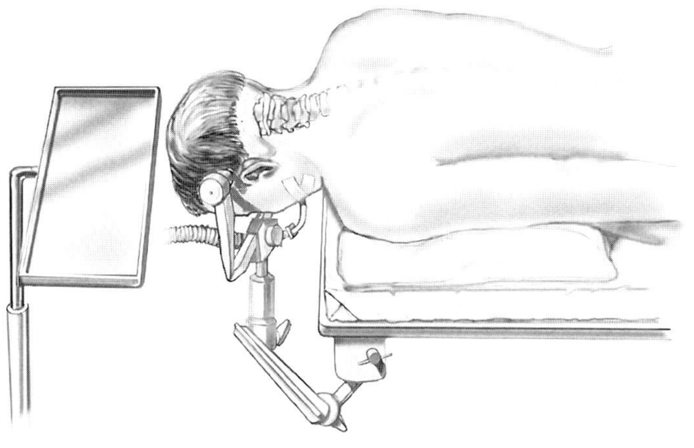

Figure 10-2. Lateral view demonstrating the position of the patient to maintain proper sagittal alignment. Lateral fluoroscopy or plain x-rays can be obtained to verify proper alignment when appropriate (i.e., fracture dislocations). Flexing the knees and dialing in a reverse Trendelenburg position optimizes the bed position for surgeon comfort during the procedure. A Mayo stand is positioned between anesthesia and the patient and is draped into the field. This allows anesthesia access to the patient's head and prevents the surgeon from placing undue stress on the patient's head.

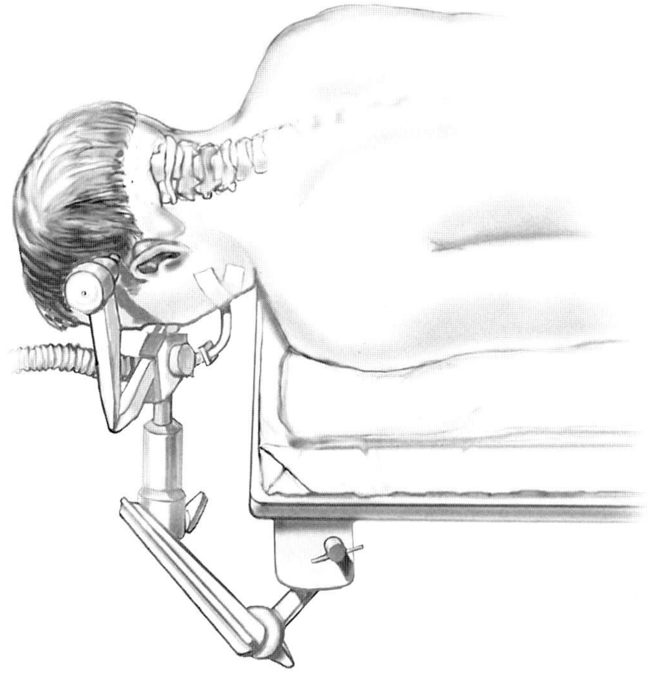

Figure 10-3. This military tuck position is particularly important for C1-C2 transarticular screw fixation. This allows the proper trajectory into the C2 pars.

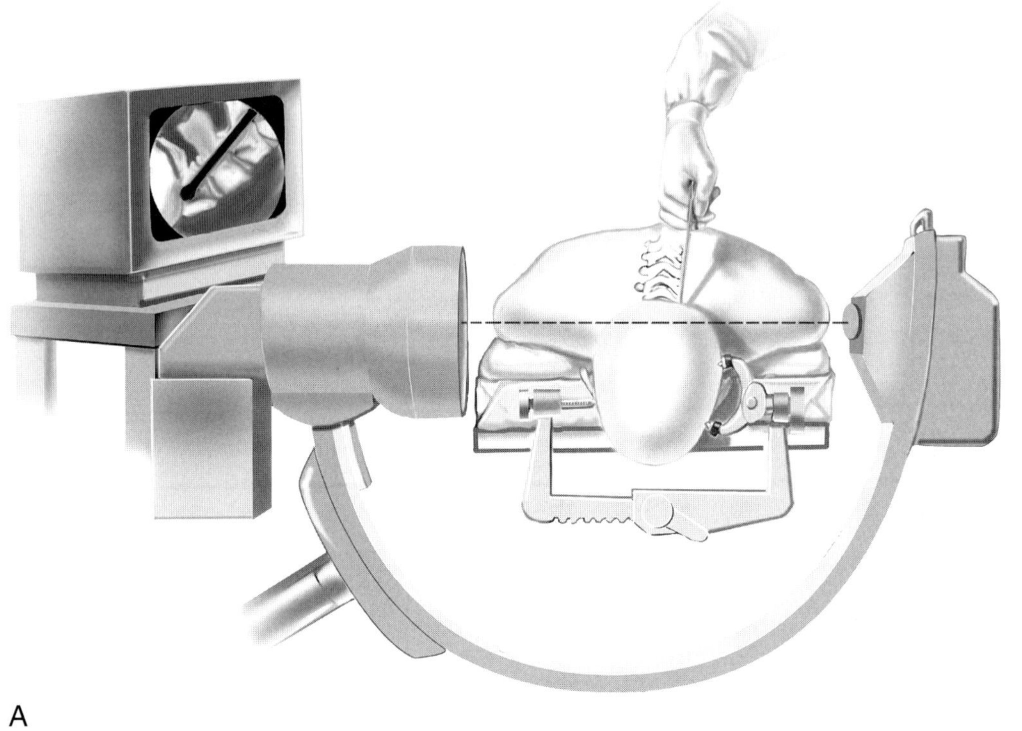

A

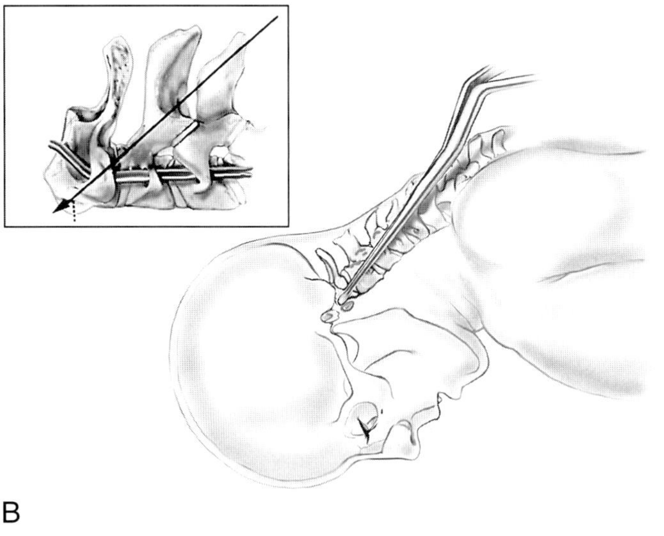

B

Figure 10-4, A and B. **A,** Using an external instrument, a fluoroscopic image can be checked to predict the feasibility of achieving the appropriate drill trajectory for C1-C2 transarticular screw fixation. **B,** Another demonstration of the military tuck position, which allows proper alignment of the C2 pars (*inset*). This position is critical for this procedure. Before any skin preparation or draping, the appropriate trajectory can be measured with a surgical instrument on the lateral aspect of the patient's neck, and any appropriate adjustments can be made.

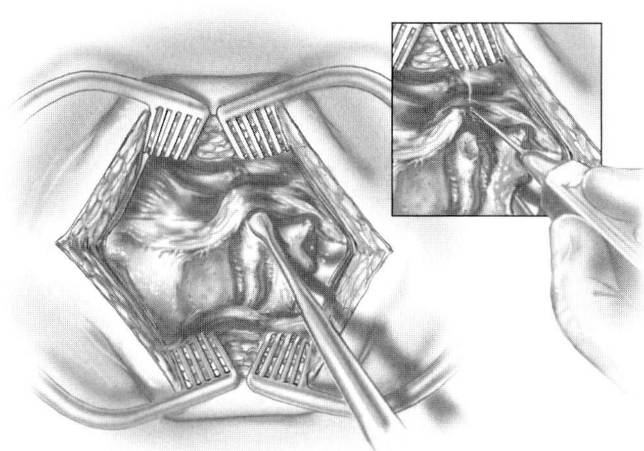

Figure 10-8. Gentle subperiosteal dissection can be used to expose the lamina of C1 and C2 in the occipital region. We prefer to use monopolar cautery on the occipital bone and C2 and the medial portions of C1 (see *inset*). When exposing the lateral portion of the C1 ring, blunt dissection with a sponge wrapped around the surgeon's index finger can afford excellent exposure. This can also be accomplished with a Penfield No. 2 dissector.

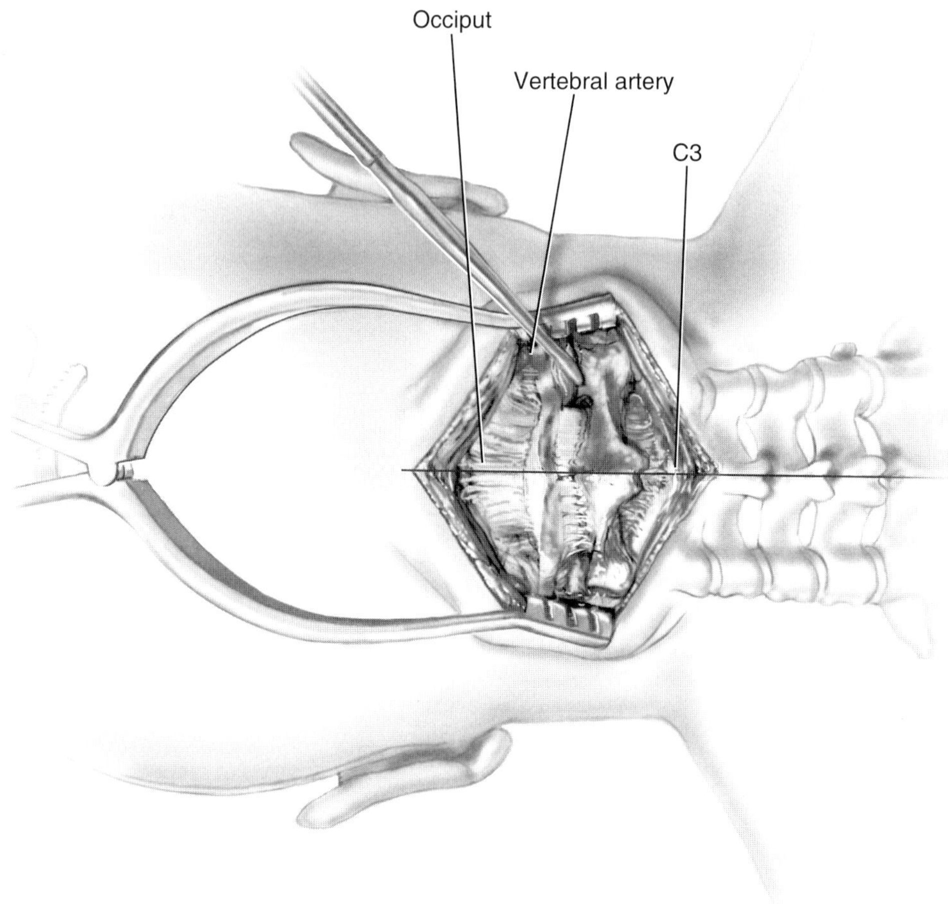

Figure 10-9. The appropriate exposure for C1-C2 transarticular screw fixation. Notice the entire superior and medial aspect of the lateral mass of C2 is exposed, with careful preservation of the C2-C3 joint. The C2 pars should be carefully dissected with bipolar cautery and a Penfield dissector to clearly visualize the pars up to the C1-C2 joint. Significant venous bleeding can be encountered at times, and this is usually controlled with absorbable gelatin sponge (Gel Foam). With careful dissection, and by staying close to the cortical bone of the C2 pars, bleeding can often be minimized. Avoid dissection of the lateral border of the C2 pars because this puts the vertebral artery at risk and increases the amount of venous bleeding.

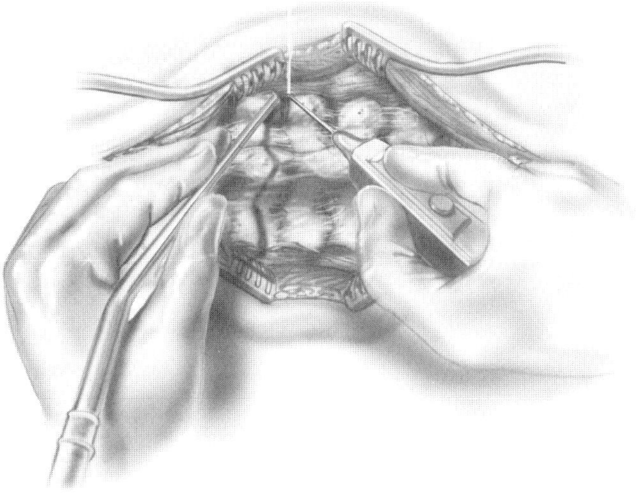

Figure 10-10. If subaxial cervical spine exposure is required for arthrodesis, a subperiosteal dissection is carried out to the lateral masses bilaterally. The entire lateral mass must be exposed if a planned fusion procedure is to be performed. This will expose the entire facet joint and will allow the surgeon to obtain a better anatomical landmark for screw placement. Exposure may be more limited for a simple decompressive technique.

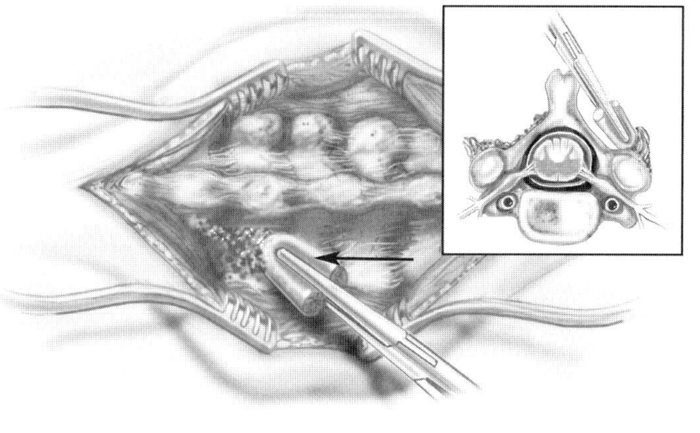

Figure 10-11. Occasionally, a Kittner dissector can be used to remove any remaining soft tissue on the exposed lamina (see *inset*). This "polishing" allows for a cleaner surface area when the decortication is performed and increases the surface area for fusion.

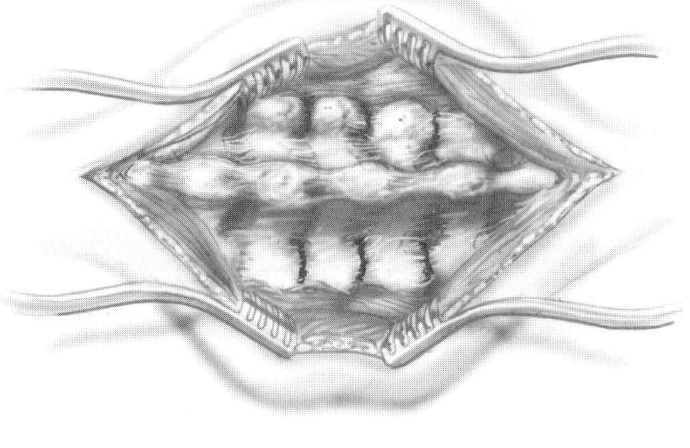

Figure 10-12. For facet fusion, after completed subaxial cervical spine exposure, the appropriate facet joints are denuded of soft tissue and synovium using monopolar cautery, curettes, and possibly a drill. We prefer a high-speed drill with a mini-matchstick bit. For arthrodesis, aggressive decortication should be used, allowing substantial room for placement of morselized autologous bone.

COMMON PITFALLS

- Before locking the Mayfield into position, the surgeon must make sure there is generous space between the fixation device and the patient's nose and forehead. This extra space is important because if there is any looseness in the Mayfield frame, there could be contact with the patient's face in the prone position, causing a pressure ulcer. The anesthesiologist should check the patient's face frequently during the surgery to verify clearance between the face and the frame.

CHAPTER

XI

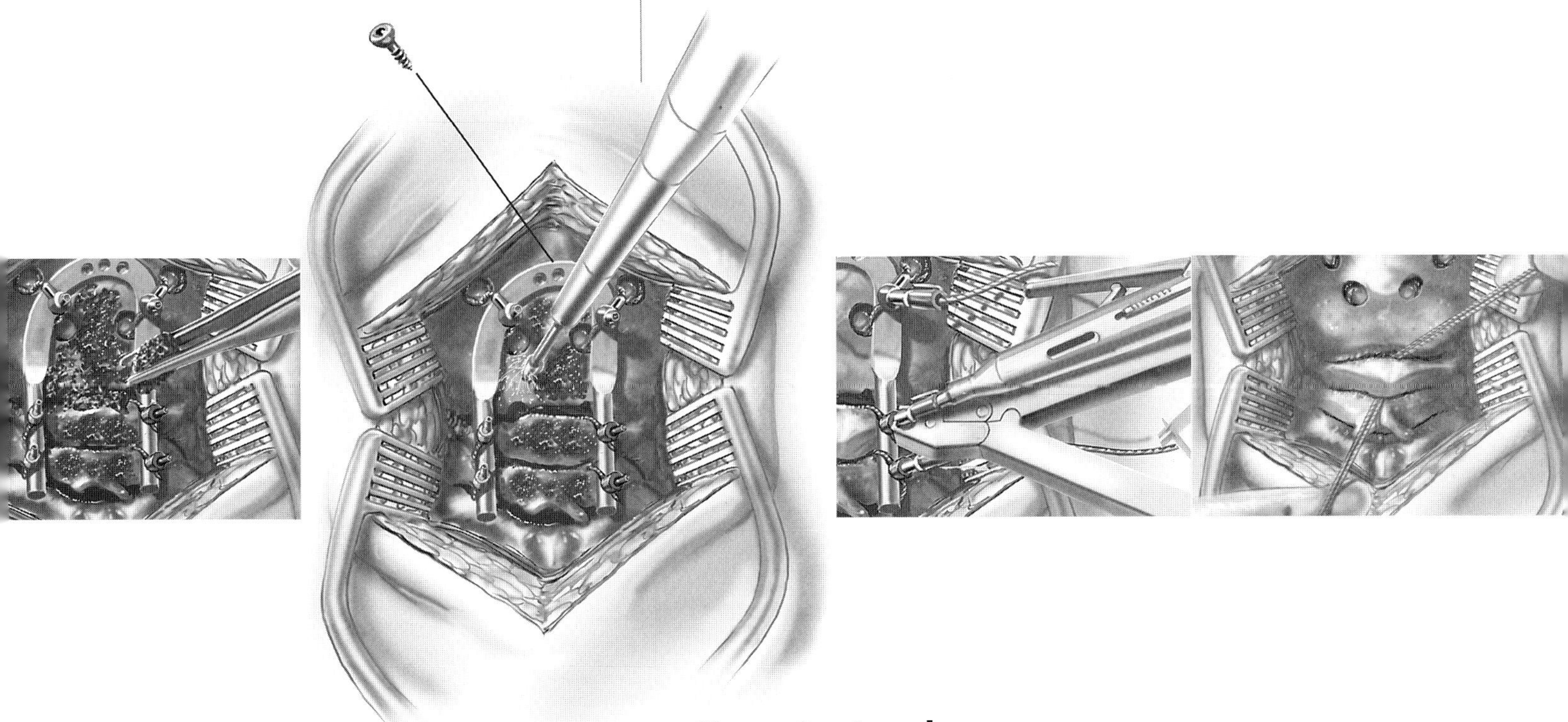

Occipital-Cervical Fusion: Loop and Cable Technique

Occipital-cervical fusion exposure was illustrated in Chapter 10 (see Figures 10-1, 10-5, and 10-7). This chapter and Chapter 12 focus more on the fusion technique. This chapter discusses the loop and cable technique; Chapter 12 discusses the rod and screw construct. Either technique can be used. We typically carry the construct from the occiput to C2 or C3. However, when the pathology dictates, arthrodesis can be extended to the thoracic spine. We usually prefer the rod and screw constructs.

Assuming a planned O-C2 fusion, the proposed incision plan for an occipital-cervical fusion should encompass the inion superiorly and the spinous process of C3 inferiorly. An incision of this length will allow the surgeon to adequately expose the occipital region and C1 through C3 levels. If an occipital-to-lower-cervical fusion is considered, the incision will need to be carried more inferiorly. For the purposes of illustration, this chapter will focus on occipital-to-C2 fusion, and Chapter 12 will focus on occipital-to-C5 fusion.

Using either monopolar cautery or sharp dissection in a subperiosteal technique, the occipital bone, C1 ring, and C2 lamina are exposed. Occipital bone exposure should encompass the inion to the foramen magnum in the superior/inferior direction and the origin of the occipital condyle laterally. Exposure of the C1 ring should include approximately 1.5 to 2 cm lateral to the midline. This will adequately expose the region for sublaminar wire passing without compromising the vertebral artery. The C2 lamina should be exposed with routine subperiosteal dissection. In cases of significant instability, great care must be used to prevent manipulation of the spine with gentle dissection. Occasionally, these patients may have significant spinal movement even with gentle retraction.

LOOP AND CABLE TECHNIQUE—OCCIPITAL-CERVICAL FUSION: OCCIPUT TO C2

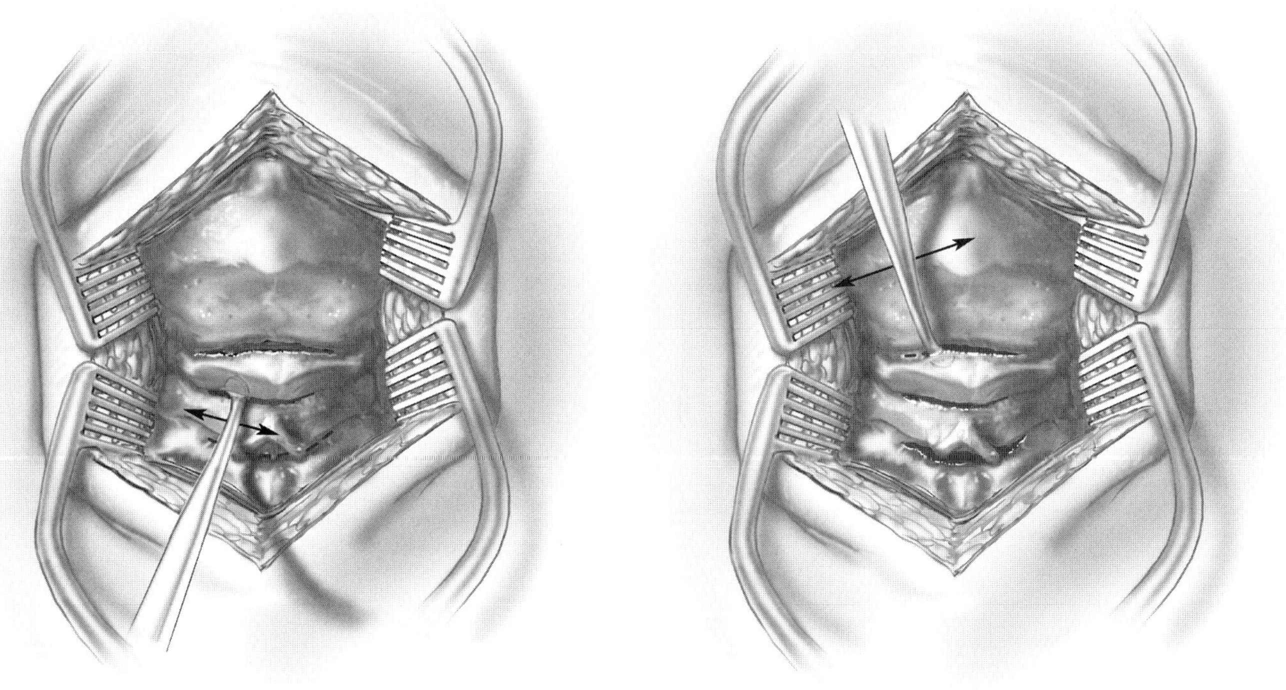

A B

Figure 11-1, A and B. Once adequate subperiosteal dissection is obtained, a forward-angled curette is used to undermine the C1 ring both superiorly and inferiorly. The C2-C3 interspinous region is cleared of all soft tissue with a rongeur, and the foramen magnum is also cleared of all soft tissue with a forward-angled curette. Using a gentle sweeping motion (two-handed technique), soft tissues must be completely dissected for safe passage of sublaminar wires. This must be completely performed at both C1 and C2.

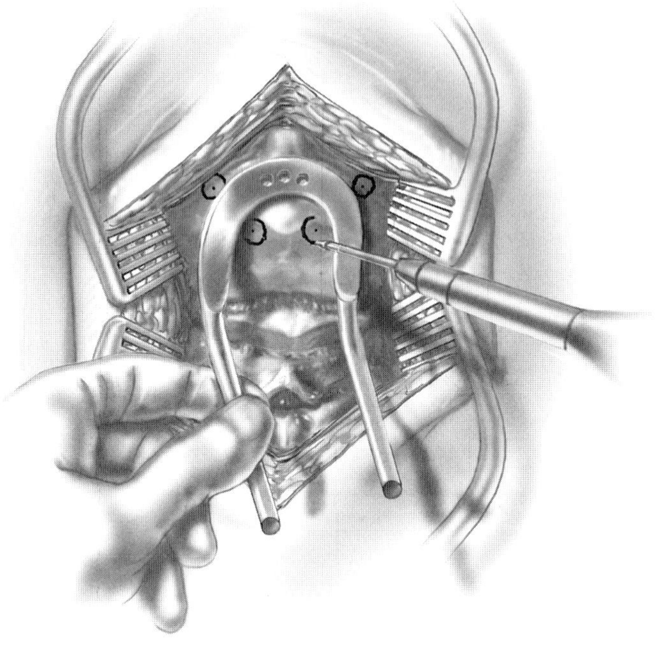

Figure 11-2. A titanium loop (OMI Medical, Cincinnati, OH) is then brought into the field and placed on the occipital bone so the surgeon can estimate the position of the burr holes. The appropriate position is marked, the loop is removed, and burr holes are created that straddle the position of the loop. Before creating the burr holes, optimal contouring and lengthening of the implant should be performed. A template (endotracheal tube stylet) can be used.

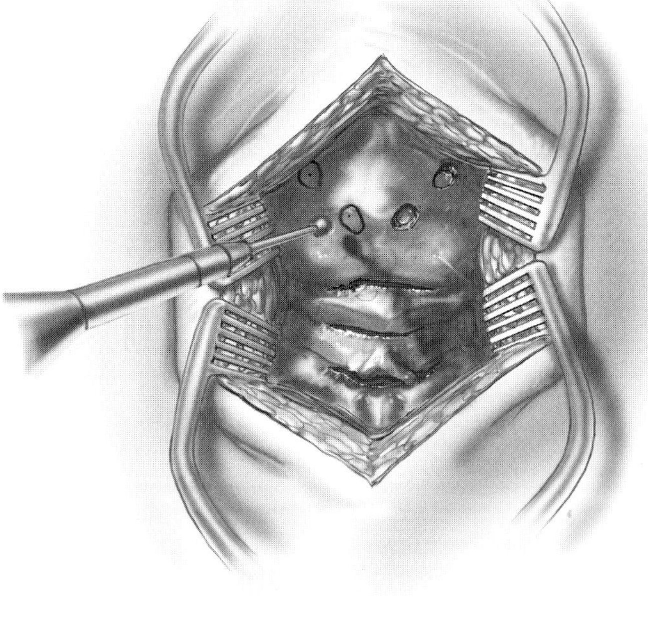

Figure 11-3. Burr holes are drilled using a high-speed drill with careful attention to preserving the dura. If cerebrospinal fluid (CSF) is encountered, the burr hole is simply waxed and can still be used. The surgeon must make a mental note to do this at the completion of the procedure. This will occasionally be necessary in older patients. The burr holes should be fairly large and spaced approximately 1 cm from one another. As long as the burr holes are spaced 1 cm apart, a generous hole can be made that will facilitate easy passage of the wire. Small burr holes can make passing the subcortical wires very difficult. The burr hole is then enlarged and beveled using a 2- to 3-mm Kerrison rongeur to facilitate passage of the cable with a curved leader.

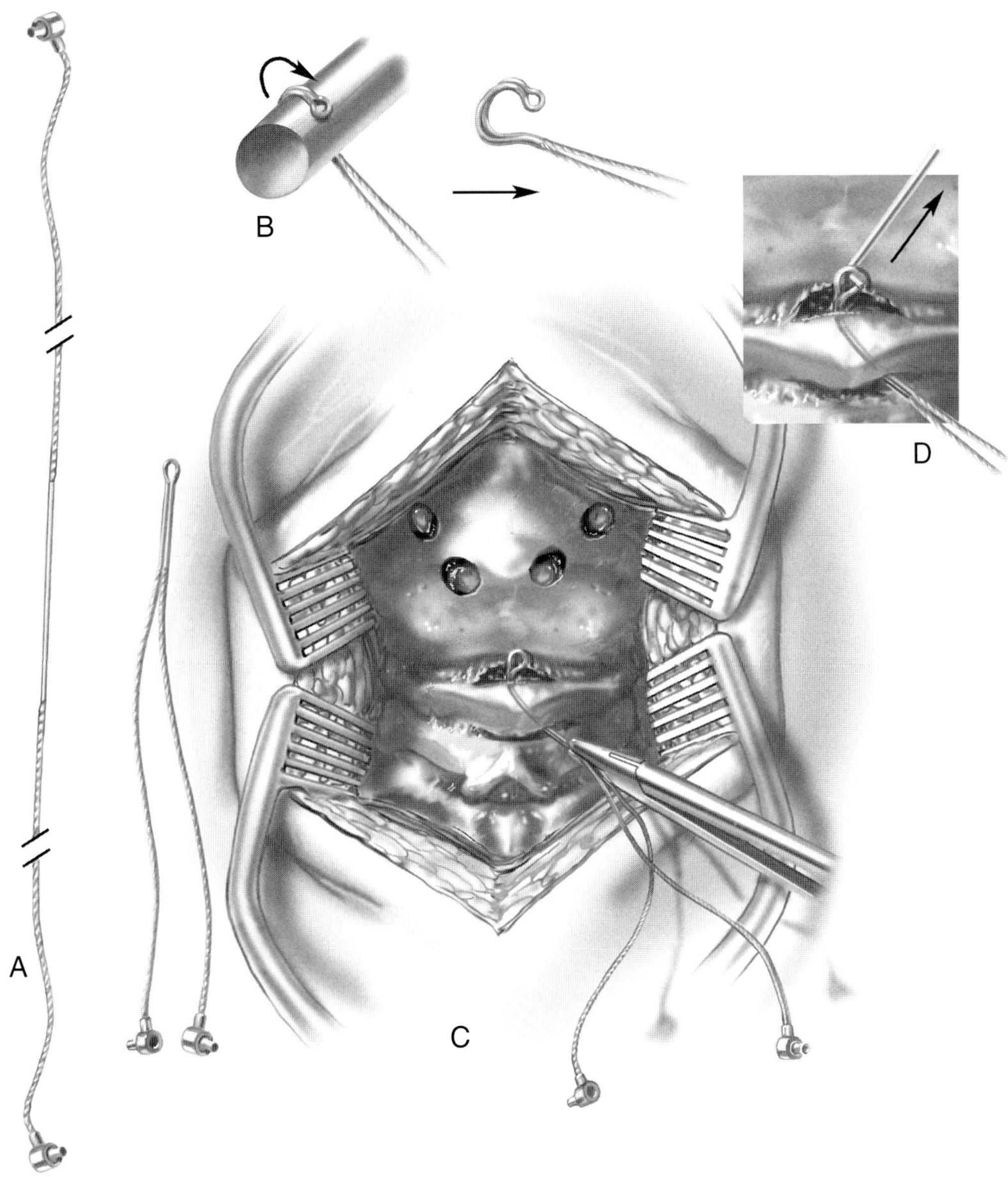

Figure 11-4, A–D. Next, a double-ended cable (Atlas, Medtronic Sofamor Danek, Memphis, TN) is customized for passage. **A,** The wire leader is folded in half on itself, creating a small loop using a needle driver. **B,** Then, using the back-ended handle of a Cobb dissector, this loop is bent to approximate the curvature of C1. **C,** Using a needle driver, the loop is then passed under C1 and hooked with a 90-degree-angled nerve hook. **D,** The wire is then passed using a "push me, pull me" technique to allow the flexible portion of the cable to pass through the sublaminar space. Although a firm pull is required to allow the cable to pass, the surgeon should take care to avoid undercutting the C1 lamina. This occurrence is particularly common in children and in patients with osteoporosis. Although the cables are soft and flexible, they can still cut bone if significant tension is applied.

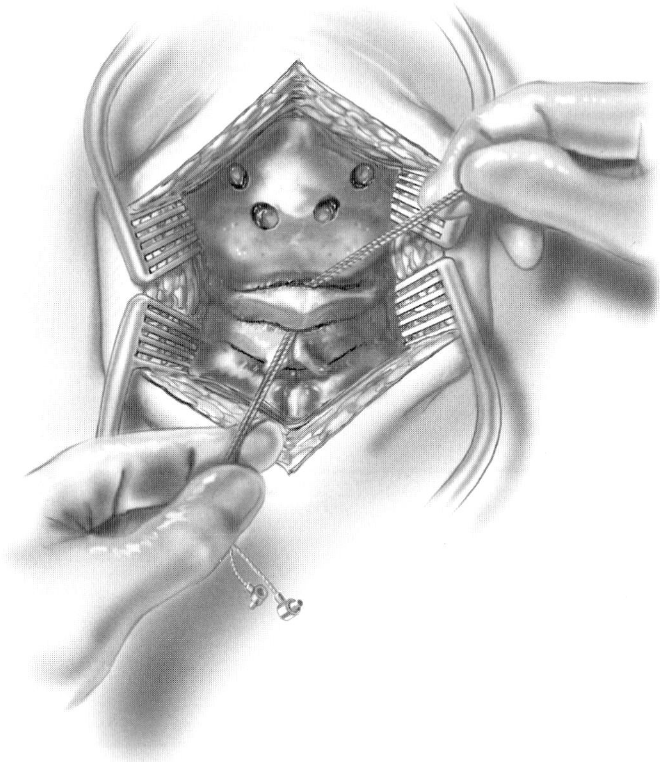

Figure 11-5. Using a two-handed technique, the wires are carefully pulled back and forth medially and laterally to free the remaining soft tissues and to allow the wires to be mobilized laterally.

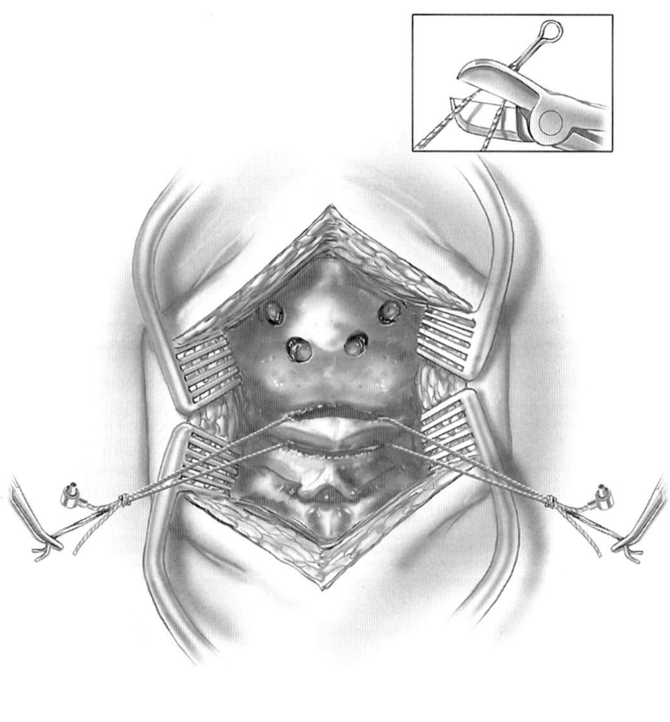

Figure 11-6. The loop at C1 is then cut, and the two wires are passed laterally and loosely tied with a rubber band. These are then snapped and held off to the side. We prefer to use elastic band ties because the wires are fairly flexible and occasionally can flip up, hitting the surgeon's mask and contaminating the field.

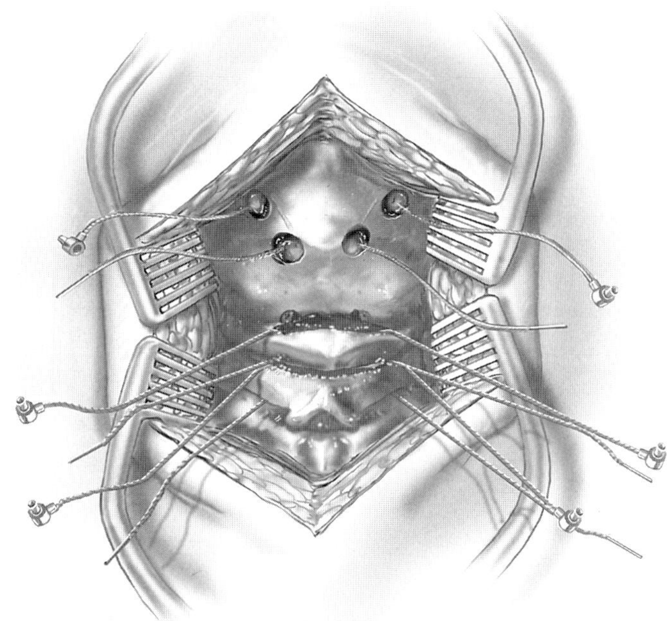

Figure 11-7. A similar technique is used for the C2 lamina as well as the occipital burr holes. Each wire is passed carefully under direct vision. In the occipital region, a single cable is used (as opposed to a "double wire/cable passage" in the cervical spine). The similar loop is created and captured with a right-angle nerve hook, again using the "push me, pull me" technique.

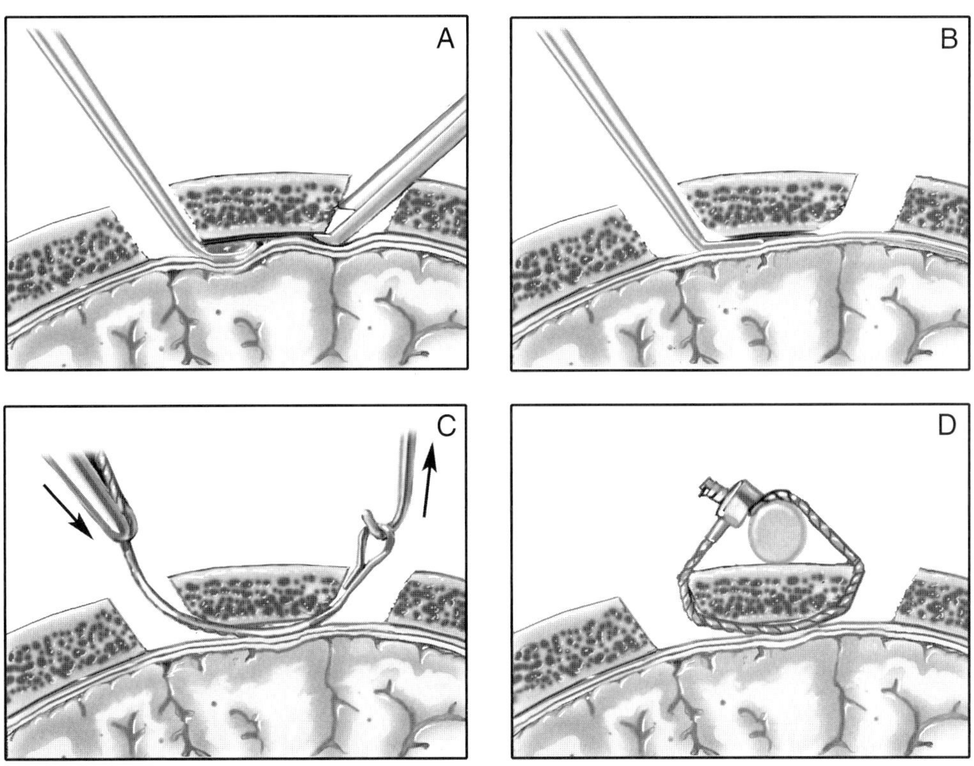

Figure 11-8, A-D. **A,** Burr hole passage of the titanium cable is accomplished using the following steps. Using a forward-angled curette, the dura is dissected from the inner table. A Kerrison rongeur is used to bevel the medial portion of the burr hole to allow for safer passage. **B,** A Woodson dissector is then used to create the potential space for the cable to pass. **C,** The wire leader is passed using a needle driver and a nerve hook. **D,** The cable is fixed into place.

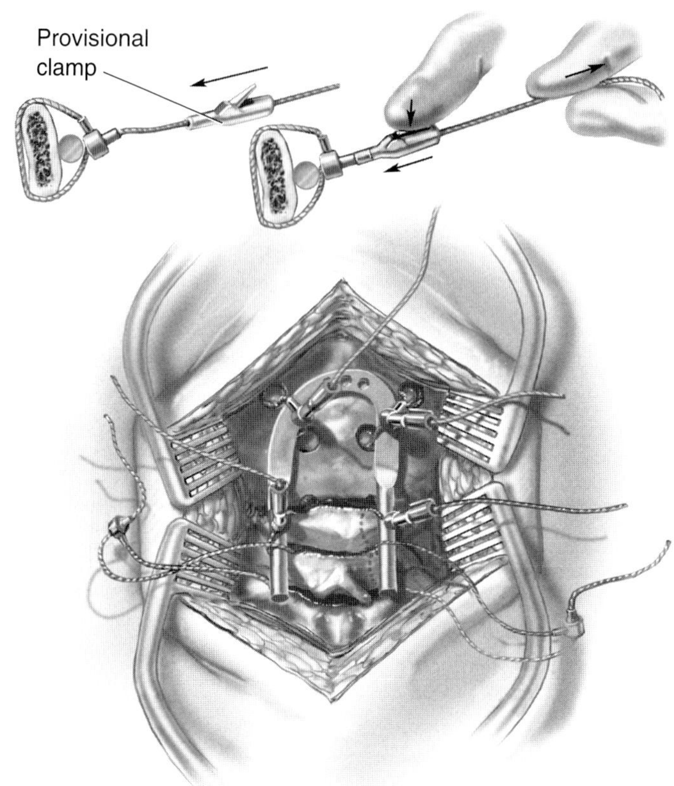

Figure 11-9. Once all the cables have been passed, the titanium loop is cut and contoured to the appropriate length. To prevent any asymmetric movement of the loop, careful attention is made to keep cable placement consistent. In general, we prefer the superior portion of the cable to be placed on the inside of the loop, and the inferior portion of the wire to be placed on the outside of the loop. This is replicated at C1 and C2 bilaterally. This is not relevant with the occipital burr holes. The wires are then sequentially tightened with temporary crimps, with attention paid to maintaining the loop in the proper position. Each wire is sequentially tightened in a fashion similar to tightening the bolts on a car tire. Once each wire is tightened to the appropriate tension, the loop is checked for any mobility. We typically tighten from a cephalad to caudal direction, beginning with the occiput.

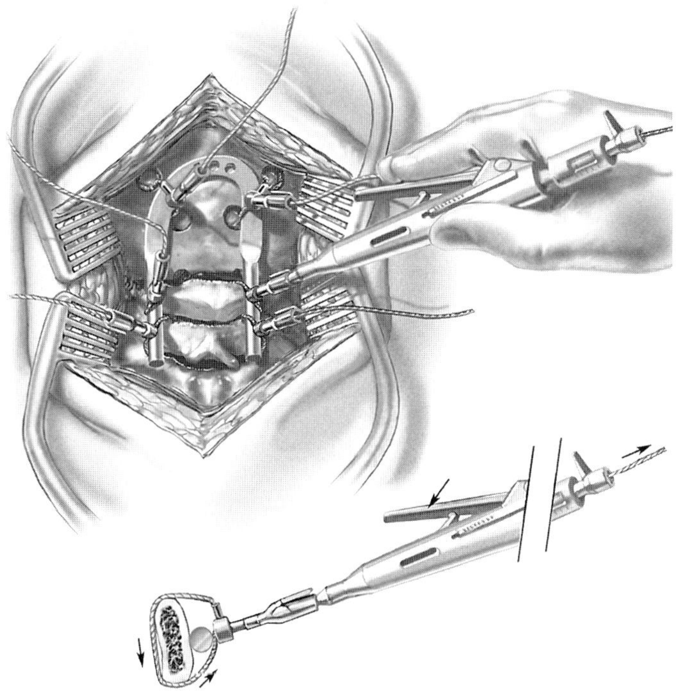

Figure 11-10. Although the tensioner has foot-pound measurements, it is our philosophy to use touch and feel to judge when a cable is adequately tightened. Occasionally, a low foot-pound pressure can still be enough to cut the bone. As the temporary crimp is tightened, the surgeon must carefully look at the way the wire is incorporating the loop-bone interface. Once the loop is in proper position and there is significant spring to the tensioner, the hat can be crimped and permanently locked.

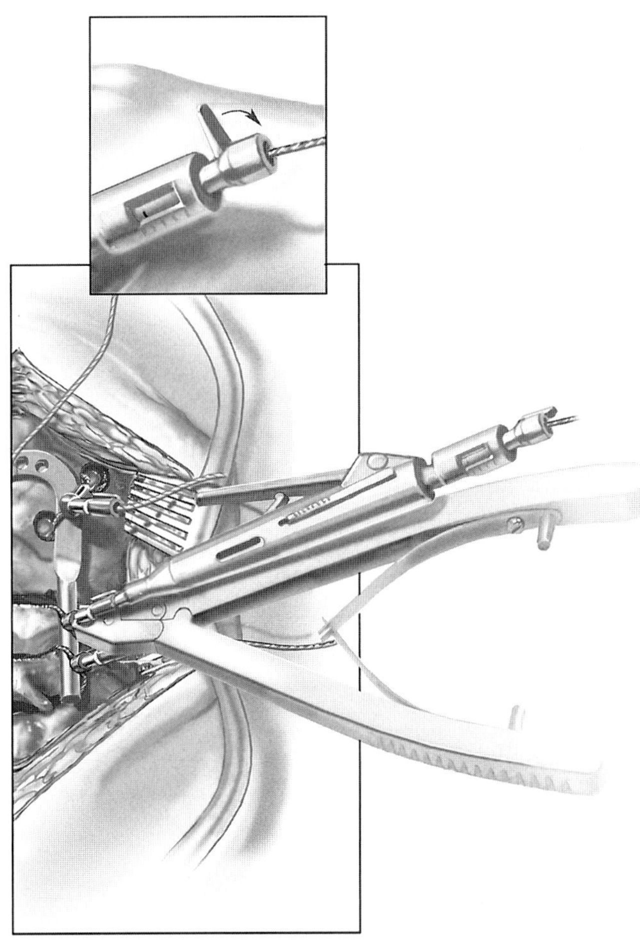

Figure 11-11. Once the tensioner is at an adequate tension, the crimper is placed on the hat and tightened. It is important that the surgeon can see the hat while tensioning; occasionally, the hat will slide laterally and make it very difficult for the crimper to be put into position. The surgeon should carefully monitor the hat as the wire is being tensioned and guide the hat to an upright position for easy crimping.

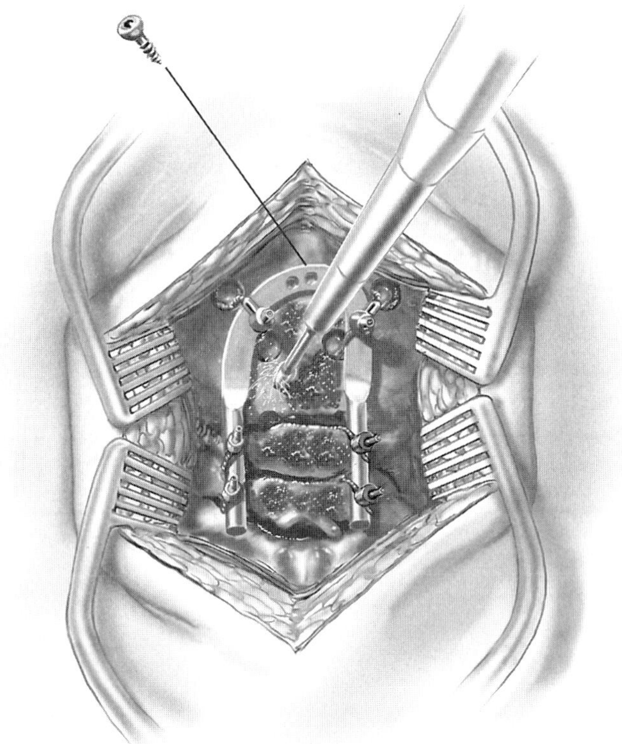

Figure 11-12. Once each hat is crimped, the wires are cut, and the remaining bone surface is decorticated with a high-speed drill down to bleeding bone. The surgeon may choose to use a cancellous bone screw on the midline of the occipital region. This will add stability to the construct but is not absolutely necessary.

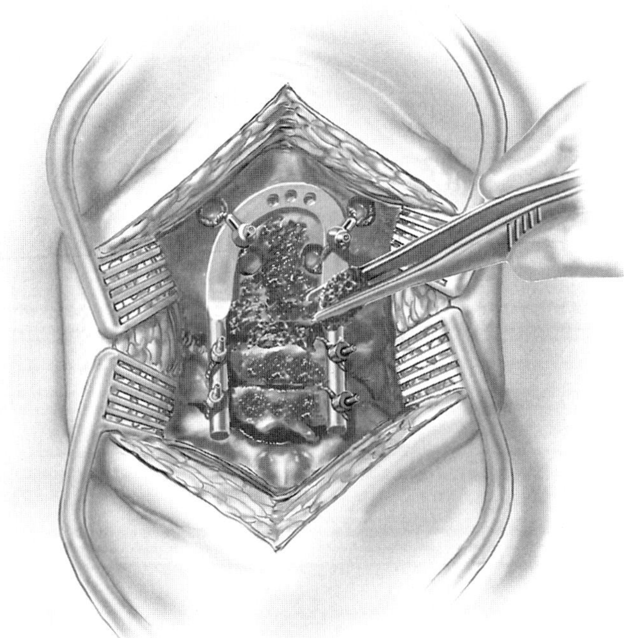

Figure 11-13. Once the bony surface has been adequately decorticated, the autologous bone that was morselized and harvested earlier in the procedure is then packed over the bone surfaces. Options for autologous bone graft include rib harvested through a small thoracic incision or the corticocancellous iliac crest (see Chapter 1).

As an alternative to the precontoured titanium loop, a titanium rod can be customized to contour the occipital-cervical region. Although this may be difficult, we prefer the use of the BendMeister rod (Medtronic Sofamor Danek, Memphis, TN). We typically choose a template (endotracheal tube stylet) to premeasure the appropriate length and contour. The contouring of the rods involves two steps. First, the closed loop is created. Next, the craniocervical angle is contoured.

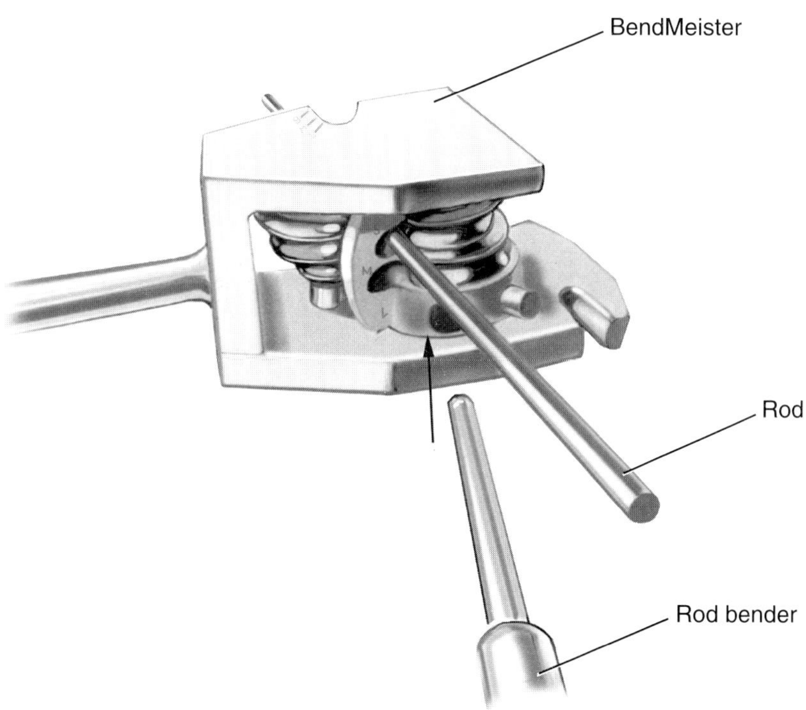

A

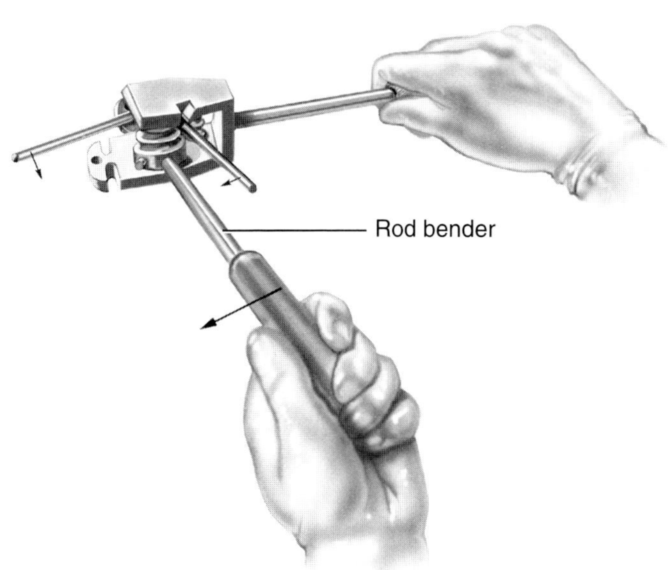

B

Figure 11-14, A and B. Creation of the closed loop. **A,** The straight rod can be contoured into one of three sizes (loop width). The rod is inserted into the appropriate roller of the BendMeister. **B,** A rod bender is inserted, and the appropriate loop is contoured.

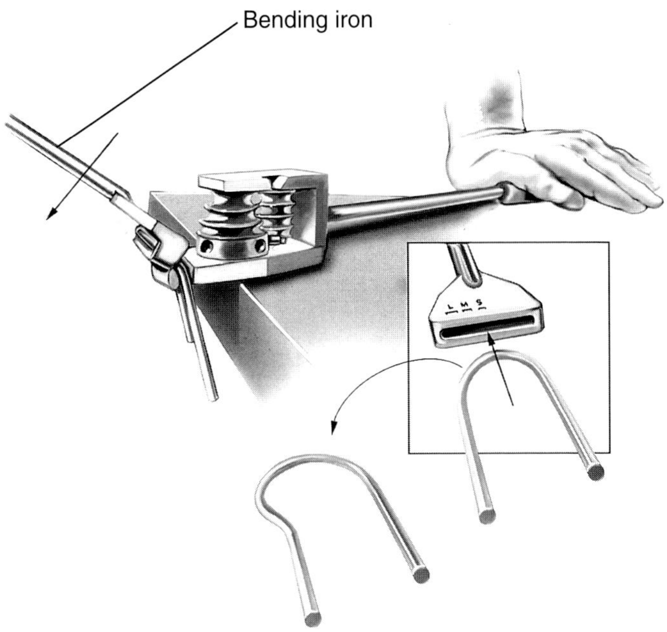

Figure 11-15. Craniocervical contouring. The occipital-cervical bend is last. The closed portion of the loop is placed into the bending iron and the open portion into the BendMeister, held firmly on a sterile table. The bend is created, usually at approximately 120 degrees. It is critical to match the contouring of the loop with the craniocervical angle. The closed portion of the loop must lie below the inion. Also, the length of the rod must match the length of the instrumented segment. Lastly, the metal must be contoured to contact all bone surfaces being fused. The metal must be brought to the bone.

COMMON PITFALLS

- A common pitfall in creating the burr holes for wire passage in occipital-cervical fusion is to make them either too small, making wire passage difficult, or too close together, which potentially weakens the construct because the wire can pull out more easily.
- Another common pitfall is to tighten and lock each loop completely instead of gradually and sequentially tightening them. If the loops are tightened and locked individually, the loop can migrate to one side and become eccentrically placed.

POSTOPERATIVE RESULTS

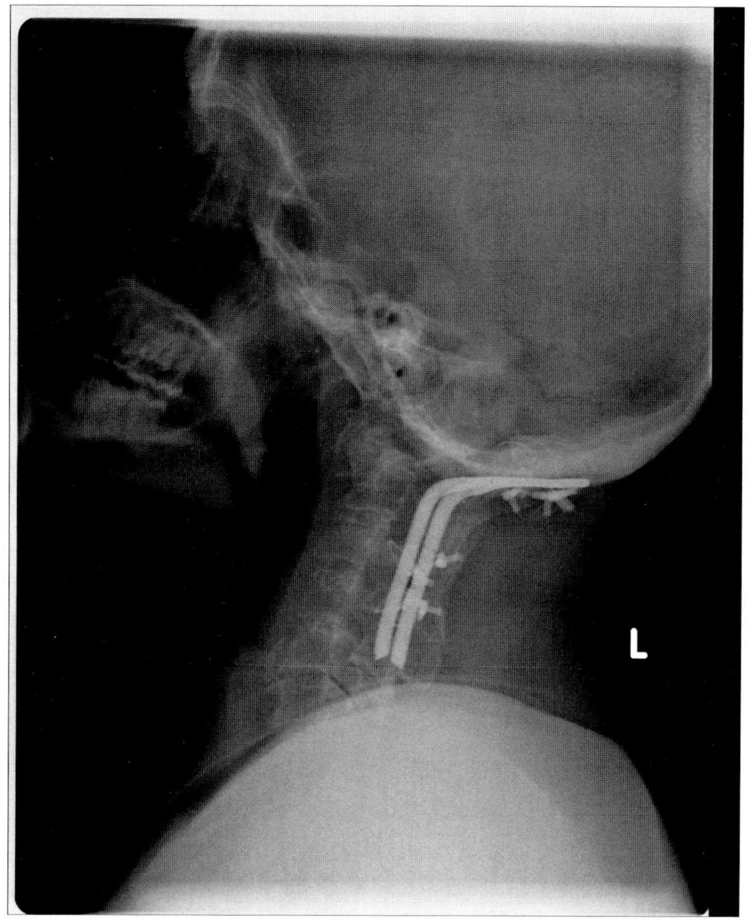

Figure 11-16. Occipital-cervical loop fixation with occipital titanium cable and sublaminar cable fixation, rib graft, and autologous iliac crest (with solid arthrodesis).

CHAPTER XII

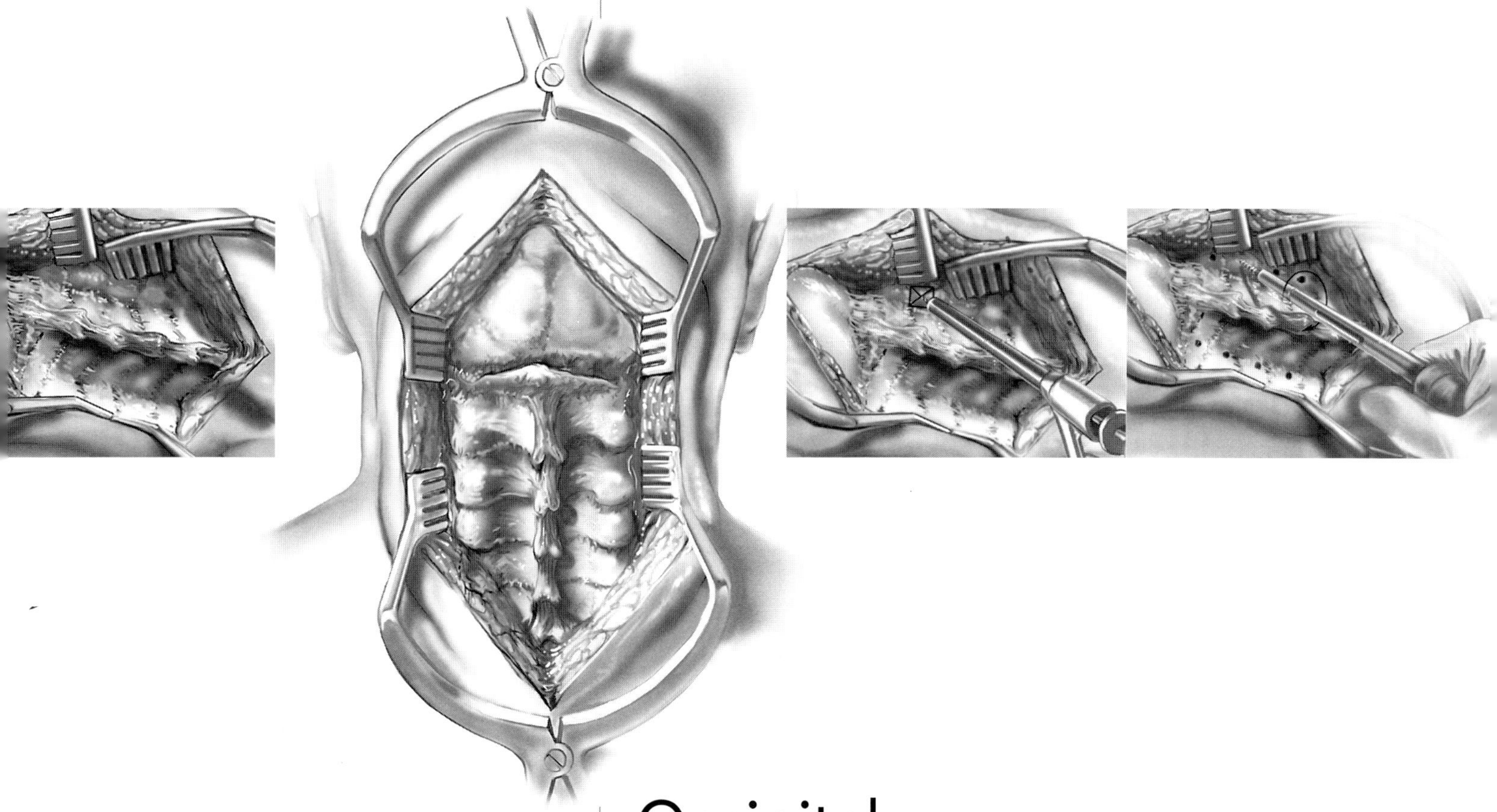

Occipital-Cervical Fusion: Screw and Rod Technique

The technique we most commonly use employs screw fixation (anchor) coupled with a rod (longitudinal member). The advantage of this technique is the ability to secure the spine to the occiput with rigid screws. These screws may be anchored at various points, including the C1 lateral masses, C2 pars, C2 pedicle, cervical lateral masses, and cervical pedicles. This may also be coupled with a screw placed across the C1-C2 articular joint. Furthermore, when deemed appropriate, occipital-cervical-thoracic constructs may be secured with thoracic pedicle screws.

Although numerous systems are currently available, we prefer the Vertex System, which allows placement of a polyaxial screw with a saddle that permits a rod-screw interface. Offset connectors are available for disparities in mediolateral screw head alignments. The advantages of this system over plate fixation systems include optimal placement of screws in the desired anatomy, screw fixation of the occiput, and lack of settling in occipital-cervical fusions.

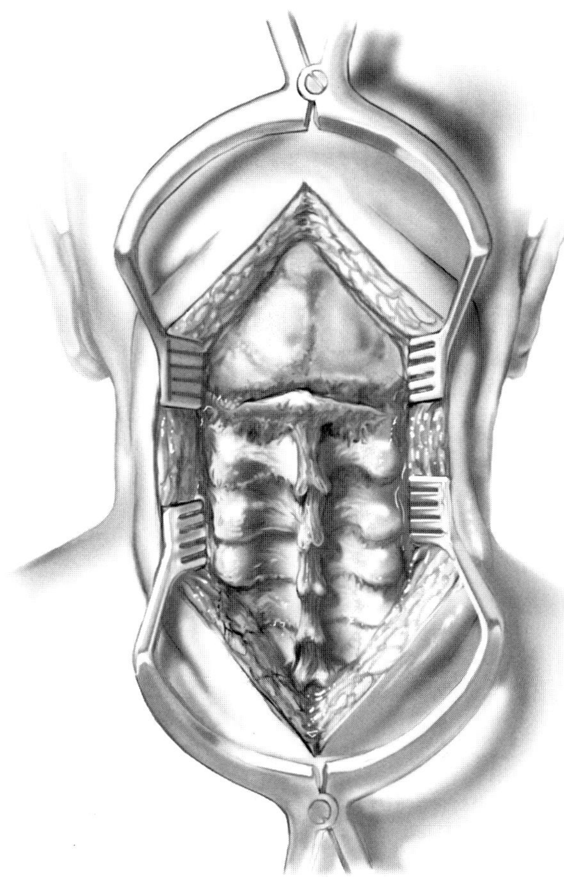

Figure 12-1. Exposure is carried as caudal as necessary, allowing visualization of the occipital bone and C1 through C5. A subperiosteal technique is used, and all soft tissue is removed. We have used this technique in longer constructs to fuse the occiput to the thoracic spine if necessary, but for illustrative purposes we are demonstrating exposure necessary for an occipital-to-C5 fusion.

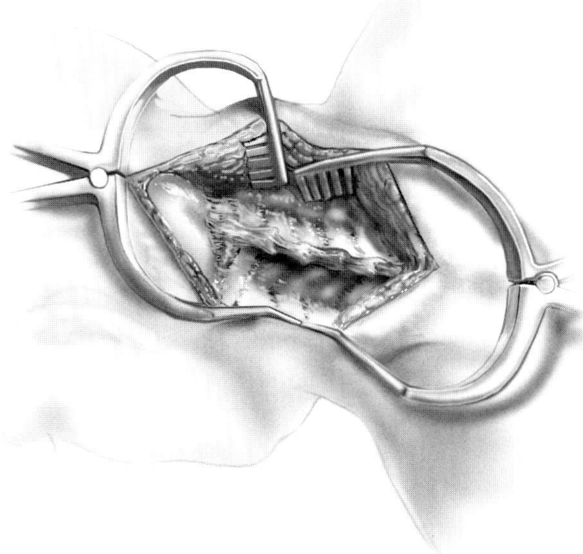

Figure 12-2. Lateral view of Figure 12-1.

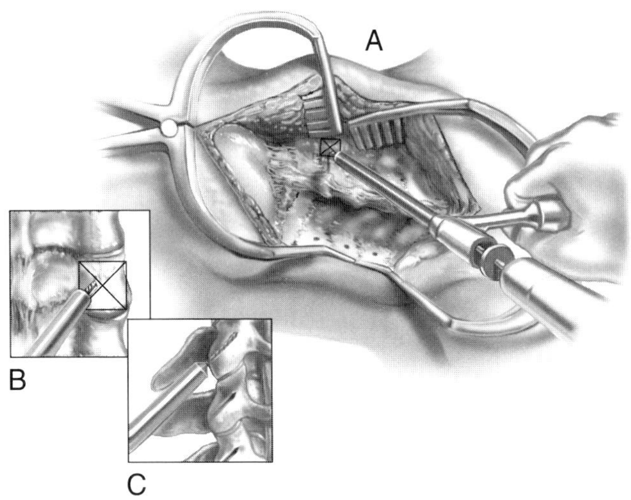

Figure 12-3, A–C. **A,** The lateral mass screw entry point is approximately 1 mm medial to the midpoint of the central portion of the lateral mass. (Refer to Chapter 14 for anatomical discussion of the cervical lateral mass.) The cortex is pierced with either an awl or a high-speed drill, and holes are drilled in a standard fashion. **B** and **C,** The holes are tapped.

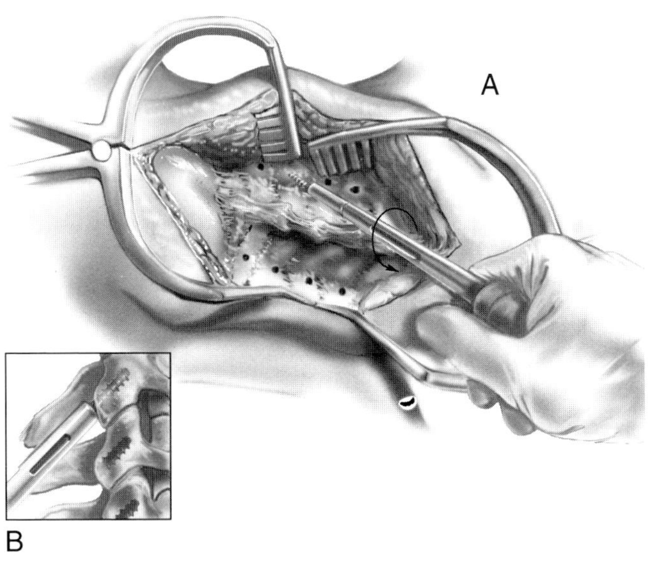

Figure 12-4, A and B. Subaxial cervical polyaxial lateral mass screws of appropriate length (Table 12-1) are then placed using the approximate trajectory of 30 degrees lateral and 20 degrees cephalad into C3-C7 lateral masses. Placement of either C2 pars or pedicle screws and thoracic pedicle screws will be discussed in Chapter 17.

Table 12-1 **Commonly Used Screw Lengths**

Level	Diameter × Length
C2 pars	4.0 × 16 mm
C3-C7 lateral mass	3.5 × 14 mm (small patients) 3.5 × 16 mm (large patients)
T1 pedicle	4.0 × 18–24 mm
Occipital	4.0 × 10–12 mm

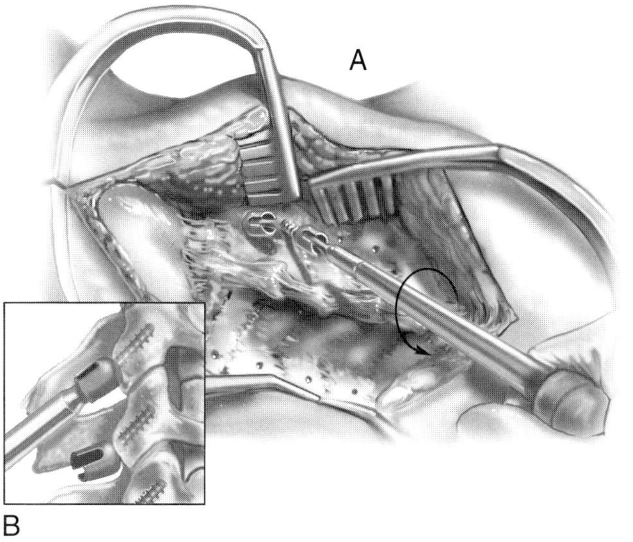

Figure 12-5, A and B. Screws are placed at each level, and a template is shaped to fit the saddles of each polyaxial screw. Before the rod is contoured, we usually shorten the superior plate by one hole segment. It has been our experience that a four-holed occipital segment is too long and will ride too superiorly over the level of the inion. We usually attempt to place six screws into the occiput when the anatomy allows. These screws are directed medially toward the occipital keel. A rod is then contoured to the appropriate shape to allow for a good bone-metal interface and to minimize any stress risers.

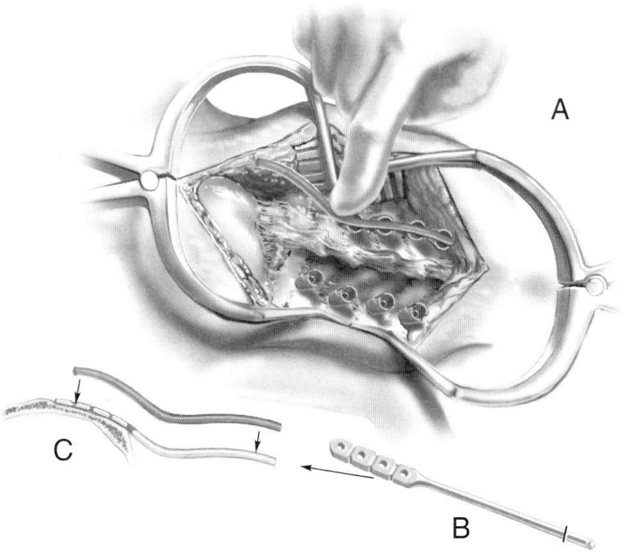

Figure 12-6, A–C. After the sagittal bend is placed (matching the occipital kyphotic contour and the occipital-cervical lordotic bend), the plates can be rotated medially to approximate the occipital bone midline. This allows for placement of convergent screws into the occipital keel for optimal bone purchase. We usually place 10- to 12-mm occipital screws (see Table 12-1). The customized rods are then placed bilaterally, and occipital screw holes are drilled, tapped, and screwed. As discussed above, we usually cut off the distal plate segment.

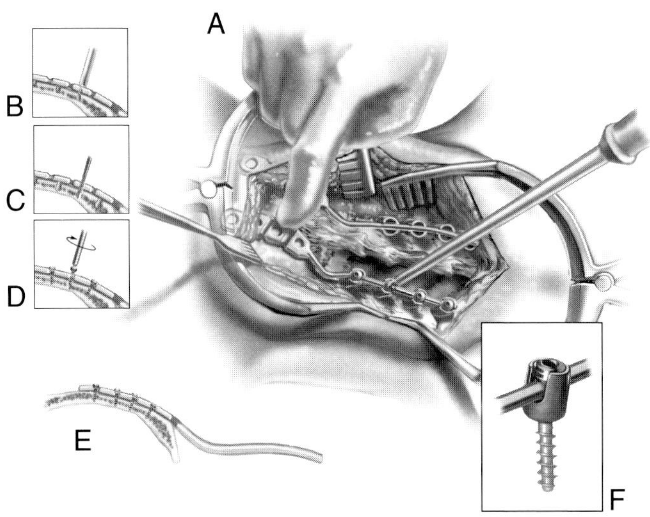

Figure 12-7, A–F. Once the rods have been adequately fastened with top-loading screws, they are tightened sequentially in alternating order.

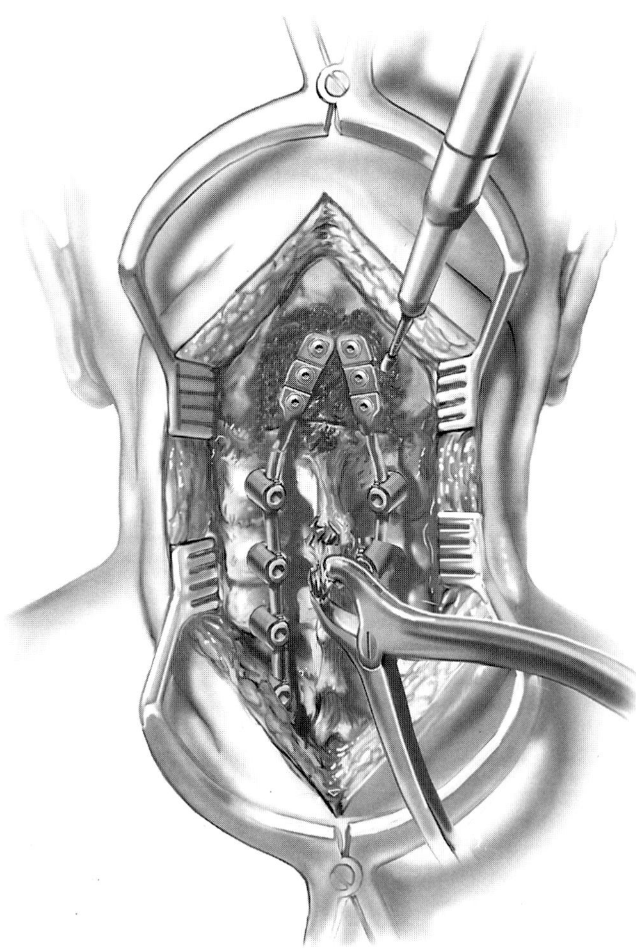

Figure 12-8. The occipital bone and lamina are then decorticated with a high-speed drill, and the spinous processes are greenstick fractured.

COMMON PITFALLS

- A potential pitfall of any occipital-cervical fusion is fusing the patient in suboptimal sagittal balance or with a coronal tilt. When positioning the patient before prepping, the surgeon must carefully assess the patient's head position in which in all planes to verify the optimal position to fuse the patient. Sometimes it is helpful to obtain a lateral cervical spine radiograph to get a good idea of the sagittal position. To assess the coronal position, the surgeon places the fifth digit into the patient's external auditory meatus bilaterally. With a hitchhiker position of the thumb on each side, the surgeon can get a good assessment of the coronal plane.

POSTOPERATIVE RESULTS

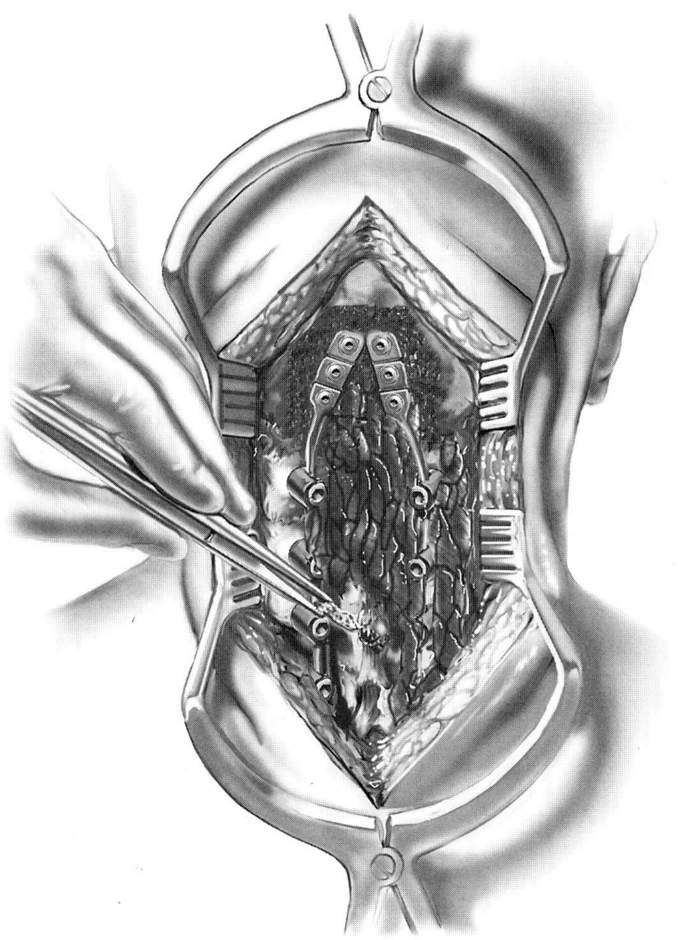

A

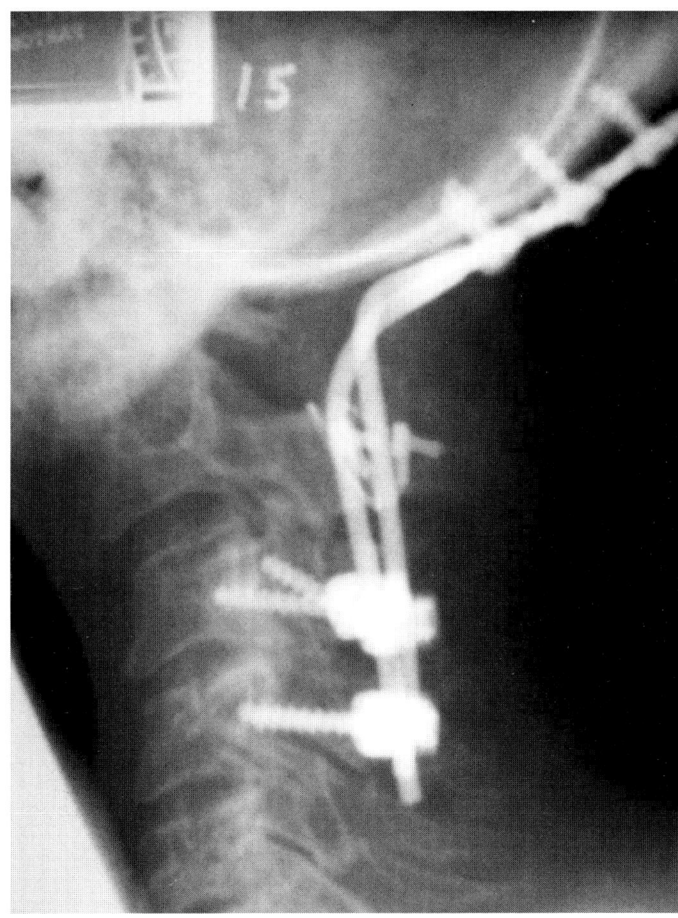

B

Figure 12-9, A. Morselized autologous iliac crest bone is then added to the decorticated area (including facet joints) in a standard fashion.

Figure 12-9, B. Lateral cervical spine radiograph demonstrating occiput-to-C4 fixation.

CHAPTER

XIII

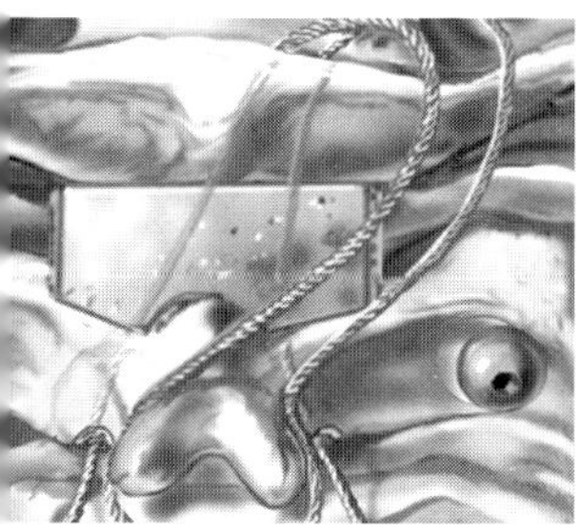

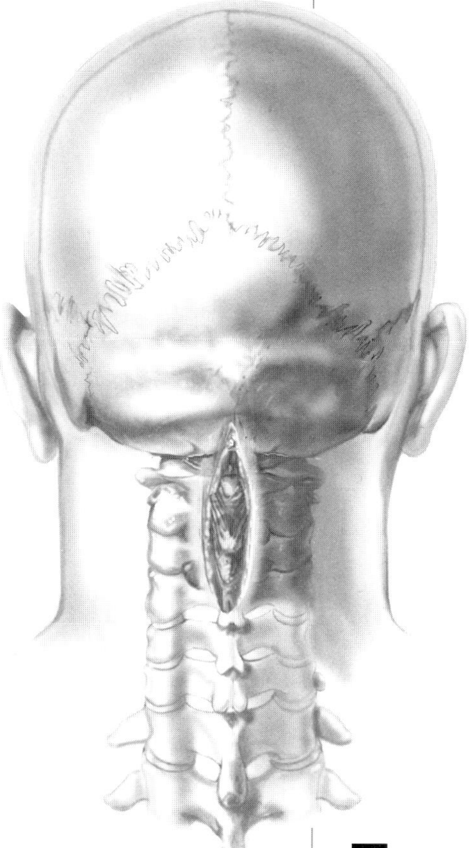

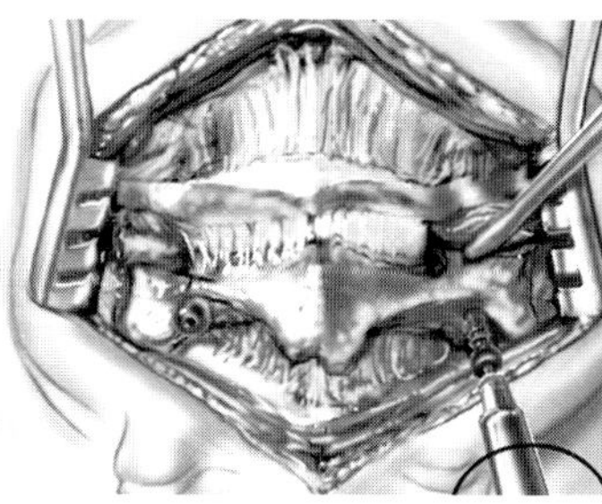

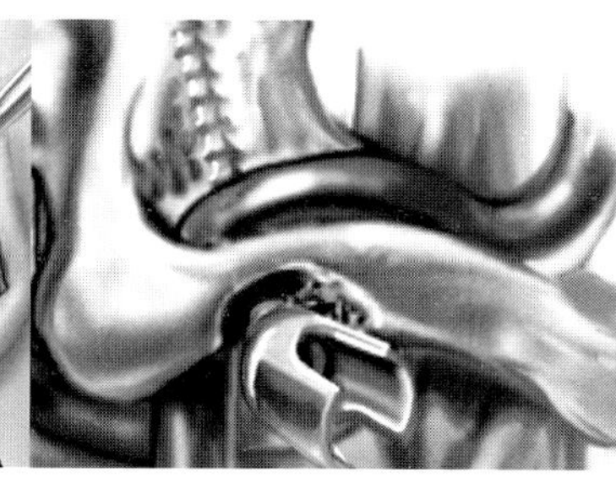

Transarticular Screw Fixation

C1-C2 transarticular screw fixation has been shown to be an extremely effective method of stabilization for C1-C2 instability. The fusion rates for this technique are in the 90% to 95% range, which are significantly higher than older posterior wiring techniques. Preoperative planning with thin-cut computed tomography (CT) scan images with sagittal reconstructions are key to this procedure. More recently, we use computer-assisted three-dimensional modeling to check screw trajectories and the path of the vertebral artery. Approximately 20% of patients may not be candidates for bilateral fixation due to an aberrant vertebral artery loop that indents or grooves the C2 pars intraarticularis. This must be identified preoperatively to determine whether a single screw can still be safely placed; this technique still confers a strong biomechanical advantage over wire fixation alone.

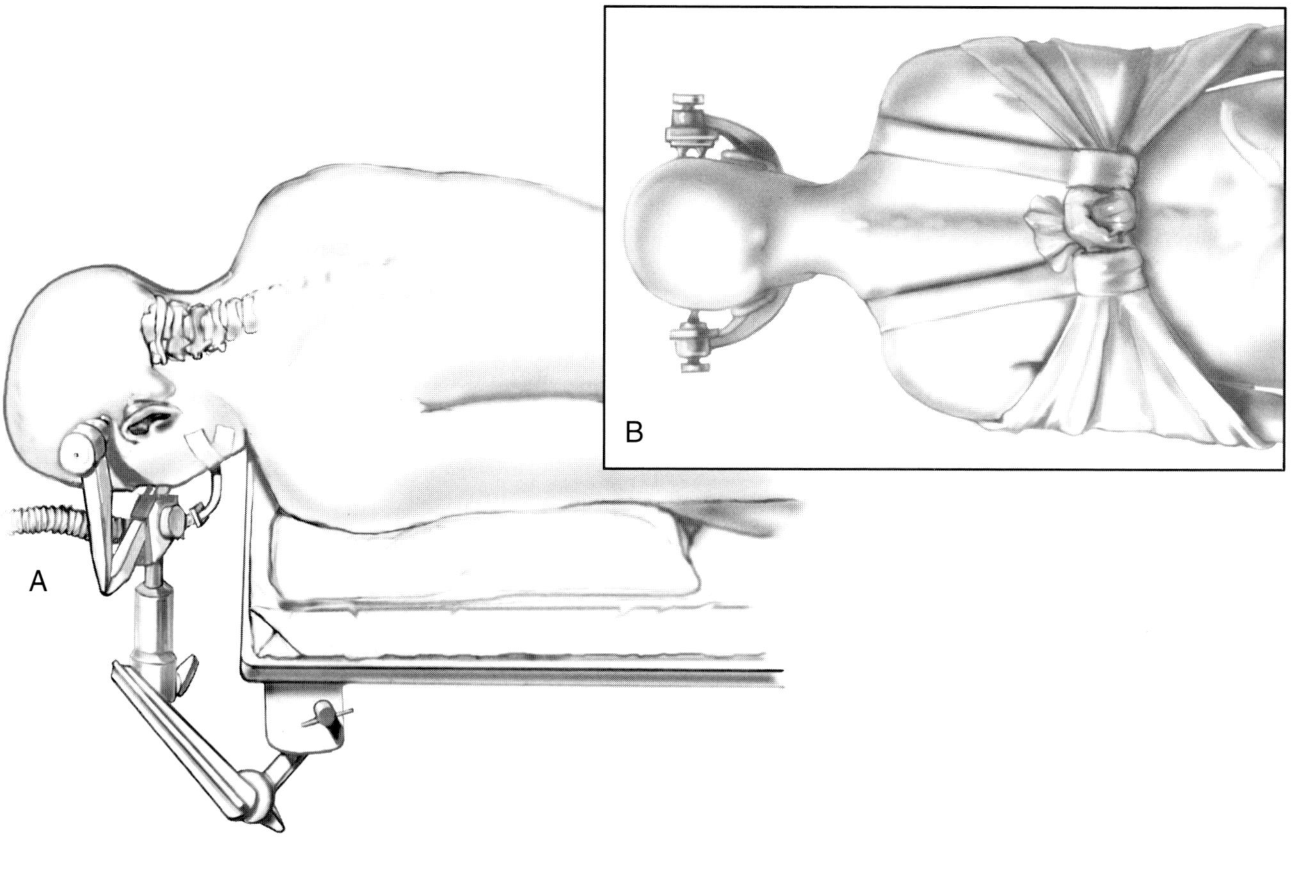

Figure 13-1, A and B. A, After intubation, the patient is placed in the prone, military tuck position with skeletal three-point fixation. Chest rolls are used as bolsters, and the patient's arms are tucked at the side with a long sheet that is secured with towel clamps posteriorly. **B,** The towel is secured in such a way that the posterior iliac crest is left uncovered for a separately prepared graft area for autograft harvest. Lateral fluoroscopy or plain x-rays can be obtained to verify proper alignment when appropriate (i.e., fracture dislocations). Flexing the knees and dialing in a reverse Trendelenburg position optimizes the bed position for surgeon comfort. A Mayo stand is positioned between anesthesia and the patient and draped into the field. This allows anesthesia access to the patient's head and prevents the surgeon from placing undue stress on the head.

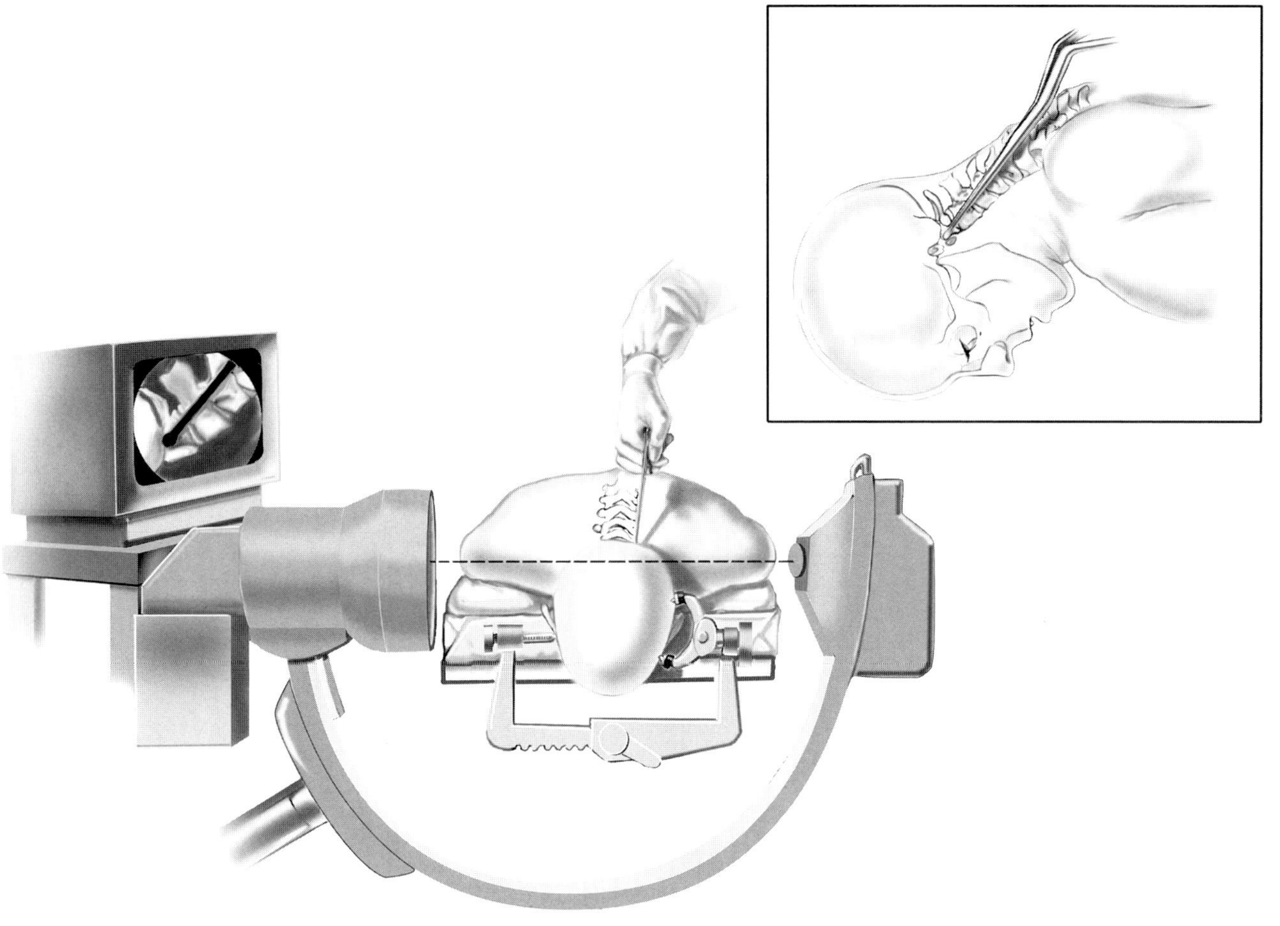

Figure 13-2. The military tuck position is particularly important for C1-C2 transarticular screw fixation. This allows the proper trajectory into the C2 pars. Using an external instrument, a fluoroscopic image can be checked to predict the feasibility of achieving the appropriate drill trajectory for C1-C2 transarticular screw fixation. Before any skin preparation or draping, the appropriate trajectory can be gauged with a surgical instrument on the lateral aspect of the patient's neck (see *inset*). This allows any appropriate adjustments to be made before having the patient prepared and draped.

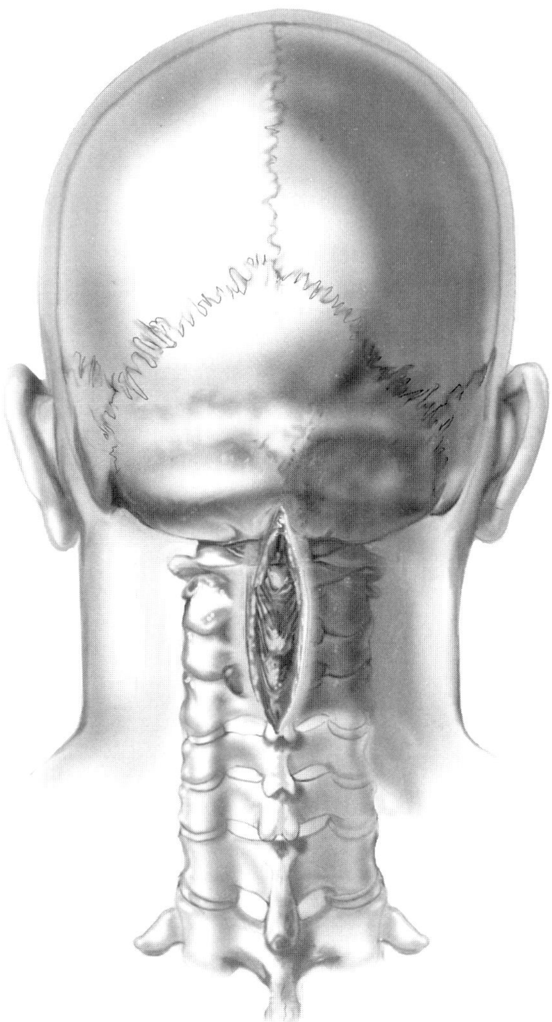

Figure 13-3. The incision for C1-C2 transarticular screw fixation should extend from C1 to the superior portion of C3. The C2-C3 facet joint must be exposed completely with preservation of the synovium. This joint is an important landmark for screw entry. Also, the surgical area should be prepared down to include the T1-T2 area. This area will serve as the percutaneous entry point for the drill guide.

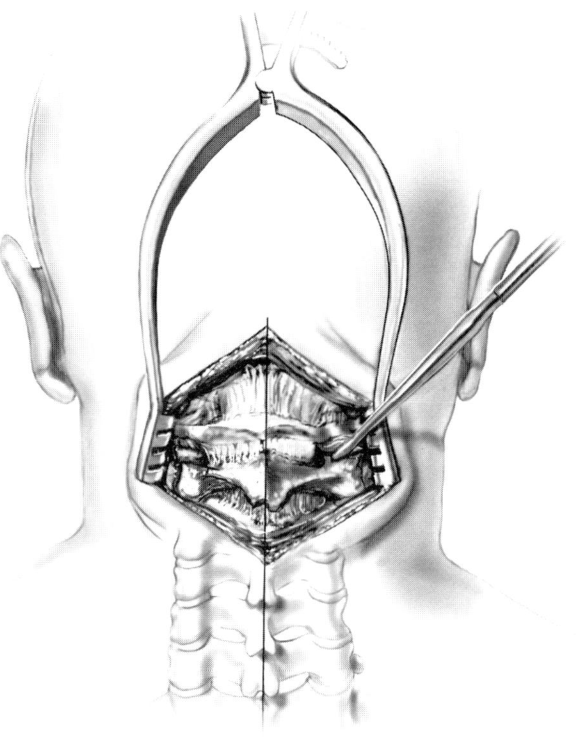

Figure 13-4. The upper cervical dissection is carried down to expose the C1 ring and the entire superior and medial aspect of the lateral mass of C2 with careful preservation of the C2-C3 joint. The C2 pars should be carefully dissected with bipolar cautery and a Penfield dissector or straight curette to clearly visualize the medial pars up to the C1-C2 joint. Significant venous bleeding can be encountered at times, and this is usually controlled with absorbable gelatin sponge (Gel Foam). With careful dissection, and staying close to the cortical bone of the medial C2 pars, bleeding can often be minimized. Avoid dissection of the lateral border of the C2 pars because this usually results in venous bleeding, puts the vertebral artery at risk, and is not necessary for the exposure.

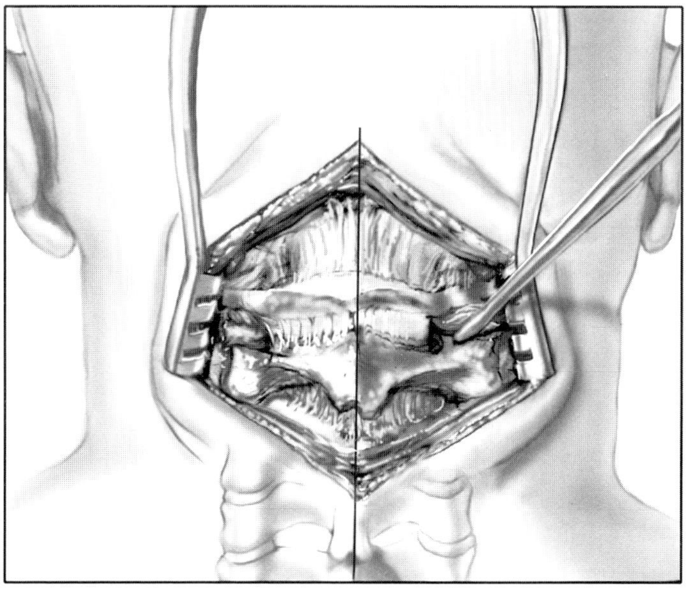

Figure 13-5. Close-up view of dissection of C2 pars.

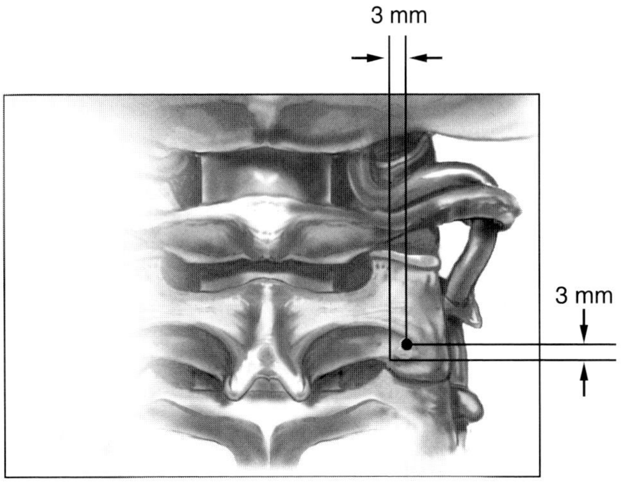

Figure 13-6. The C2 pars entry site for screw trajectory is 3 mm superior to and 3 mm lateral to the medial inferior C2-C3 facet joint. This landmark is usually highlighted by a ridge of bone that extends laterally on the C2 lamina. This ridge can usually be followed to its lateral terminus, which marks the roof of the pars and the entry site 3 mm up and 3 mm lateral to the medial inferior C2-C3 facet joint. Three-dimensional imaging (e.g., Stealth system, Medtronic) is also helpful for determining the entry point for a transarticular screw.

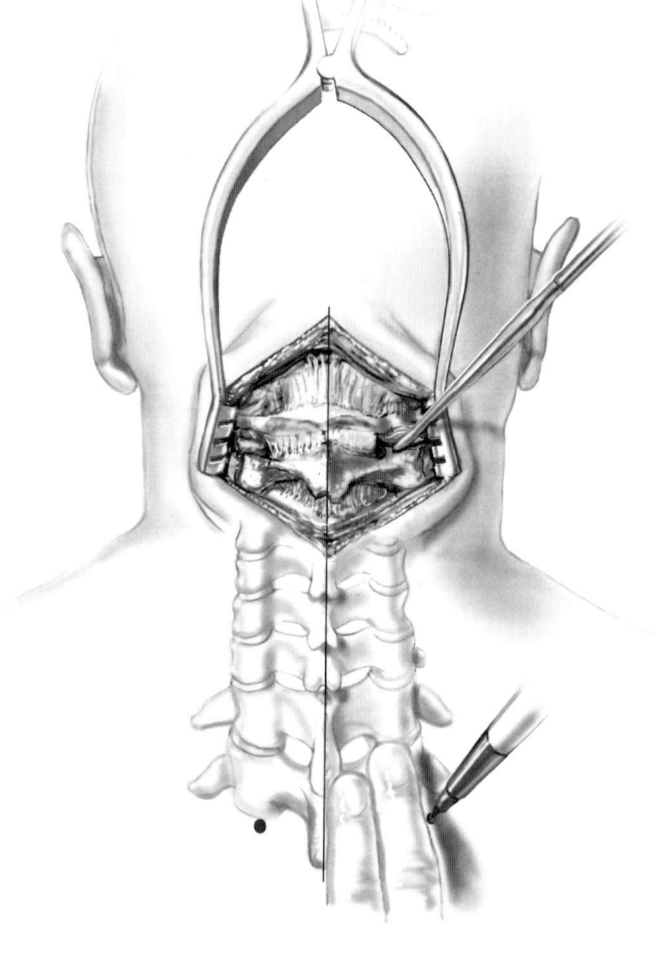

Figure 13-7. Once the upper cervical exposure is complete, the percutaneous drill guide entry site is identified two fingerbreadths lateral to the midline at the level of approximately T1.

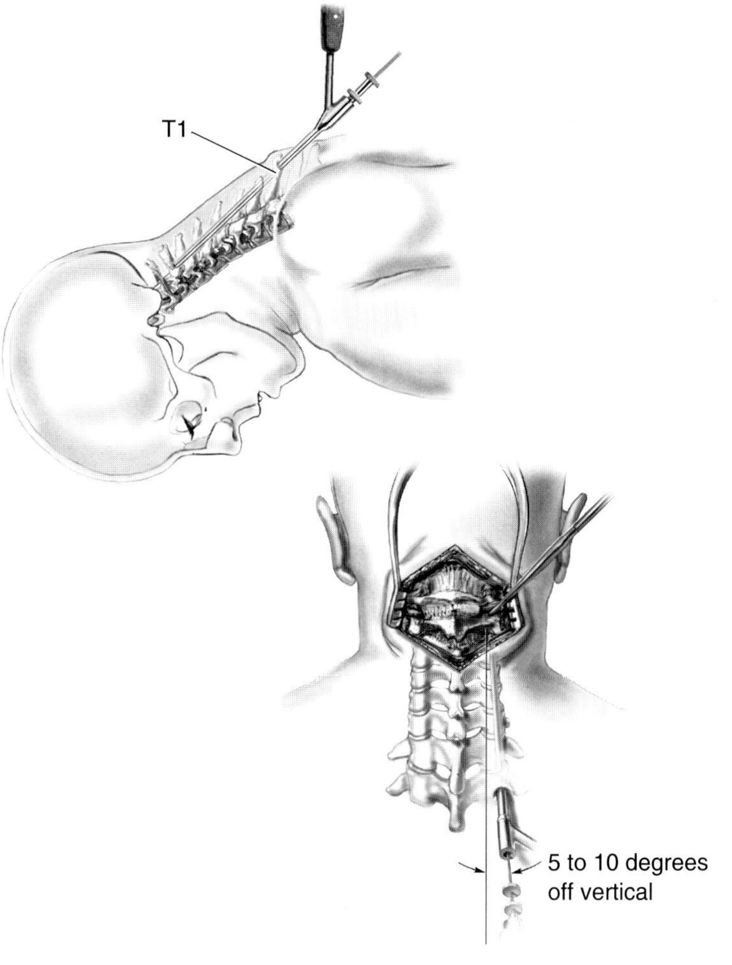

Figure 13-8. A small stab incision is made at the drill guide entry site, and the drill guide is advanced from the thoracic area into the upper cervical exposure.

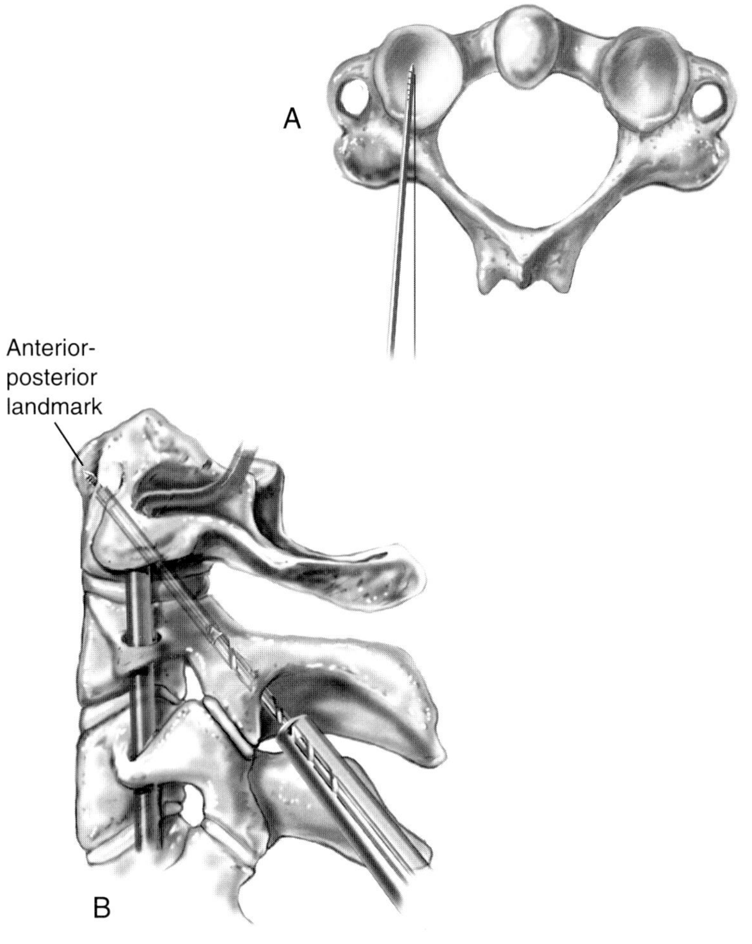

Figure 13-9, A and B. **A,** The drill is angled 5 to 15 degrees medially, and a K-wire is passed under direct lateral fluoroscopy or image guidance. **B,** Under direct vision, the K-wire is passed toward the anterior tubercle of C1 in the anterior-posterior dimension and 5 to 15 degrees in a lateral-to-medial direction. As the C1-C2 joint is crossed, a gentle resistance is usually felt with the drill. We prefer to use an "on-off-on" drill technique with short bursts of power to avoid overpenetration.

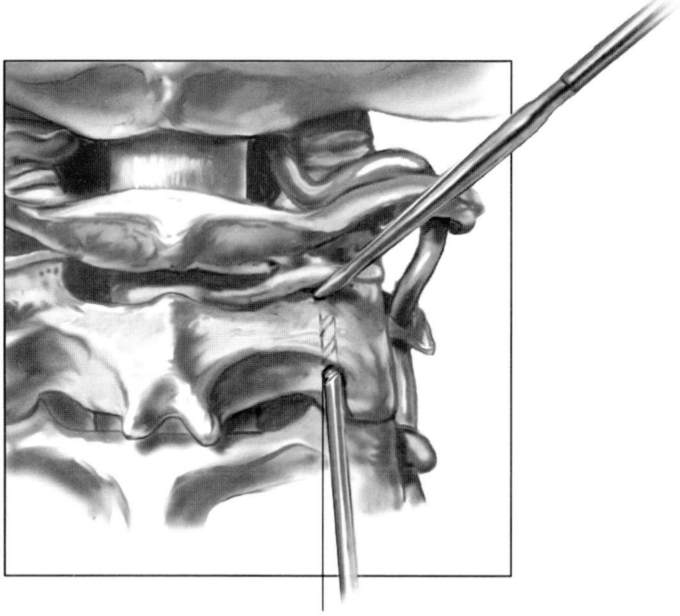

Figure 13-10. As the K-wire is passed, the C2 nerve root is gently elevated to make visible the roof of the C2 pars and the C1-C2 joint space. Often the surgeon can see or feel the K-wire in the joint space once it has been passed. This direct vision ensures that the K-wire is not too shallow in the C2 pars, a circumstance that might weaken the screw purchase.

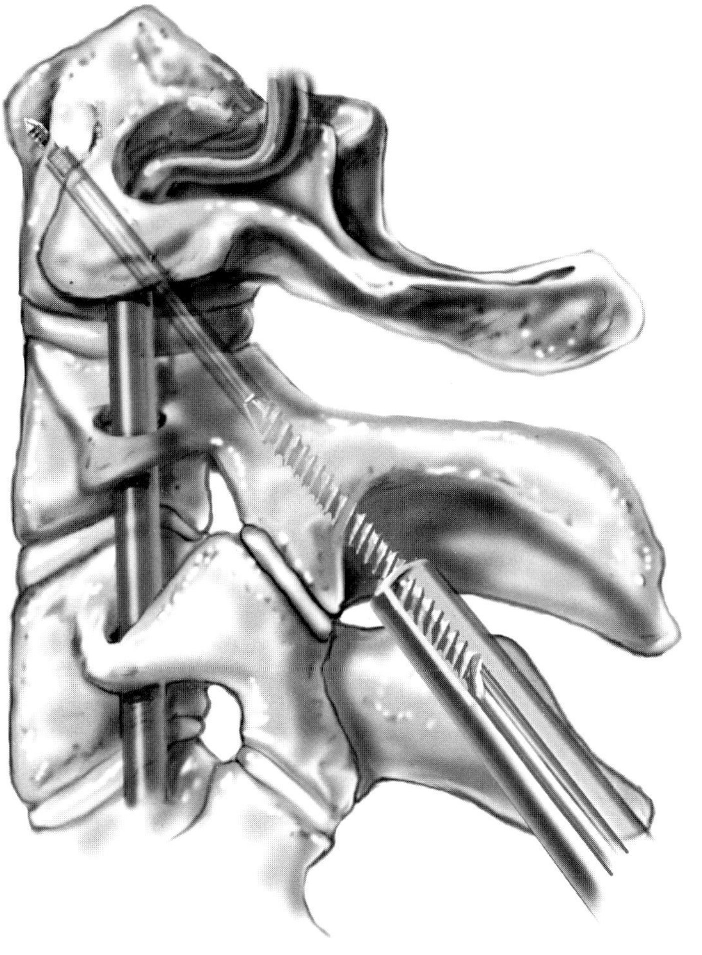

Figure 13-11. After the K-wire has been placed and verified to be in good position, the cannulated drill is passed over the K-wire. In patients with osteoporosis, sometimes drilling is not necessary, and the cannulated tap can be passed directly over the K-wire.

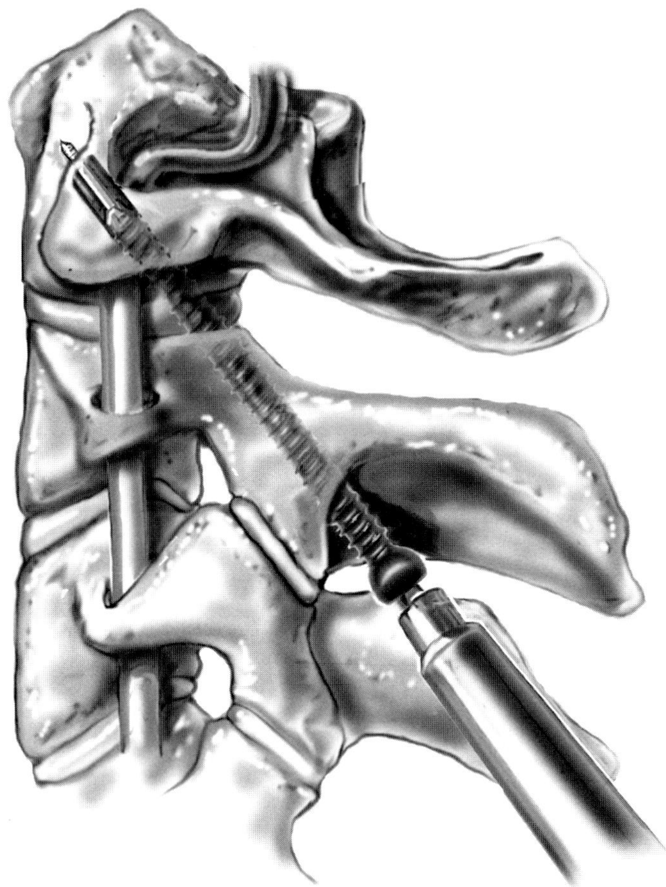

Figure 13-12. Once the drilling and tapping are complete, the cannulated screw is passed over the K-wire. After the screw enters the C1 lateral mass, the K-wire can be removed to prevent inadvertent advancement of the K-wire beyond the C1 lateral mass.

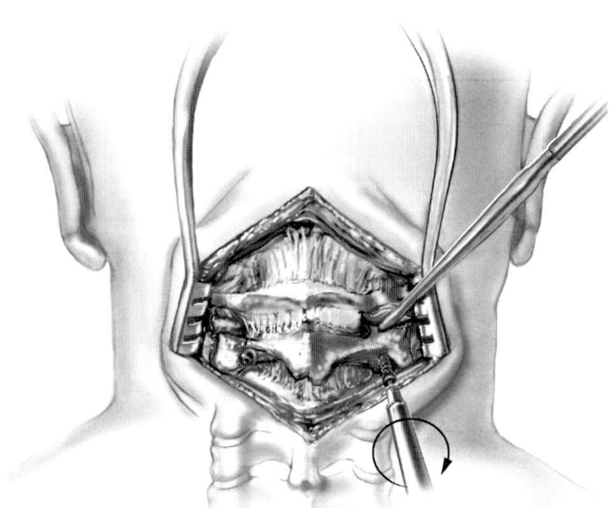

Figure 13-13. Posterior view of screw placement.

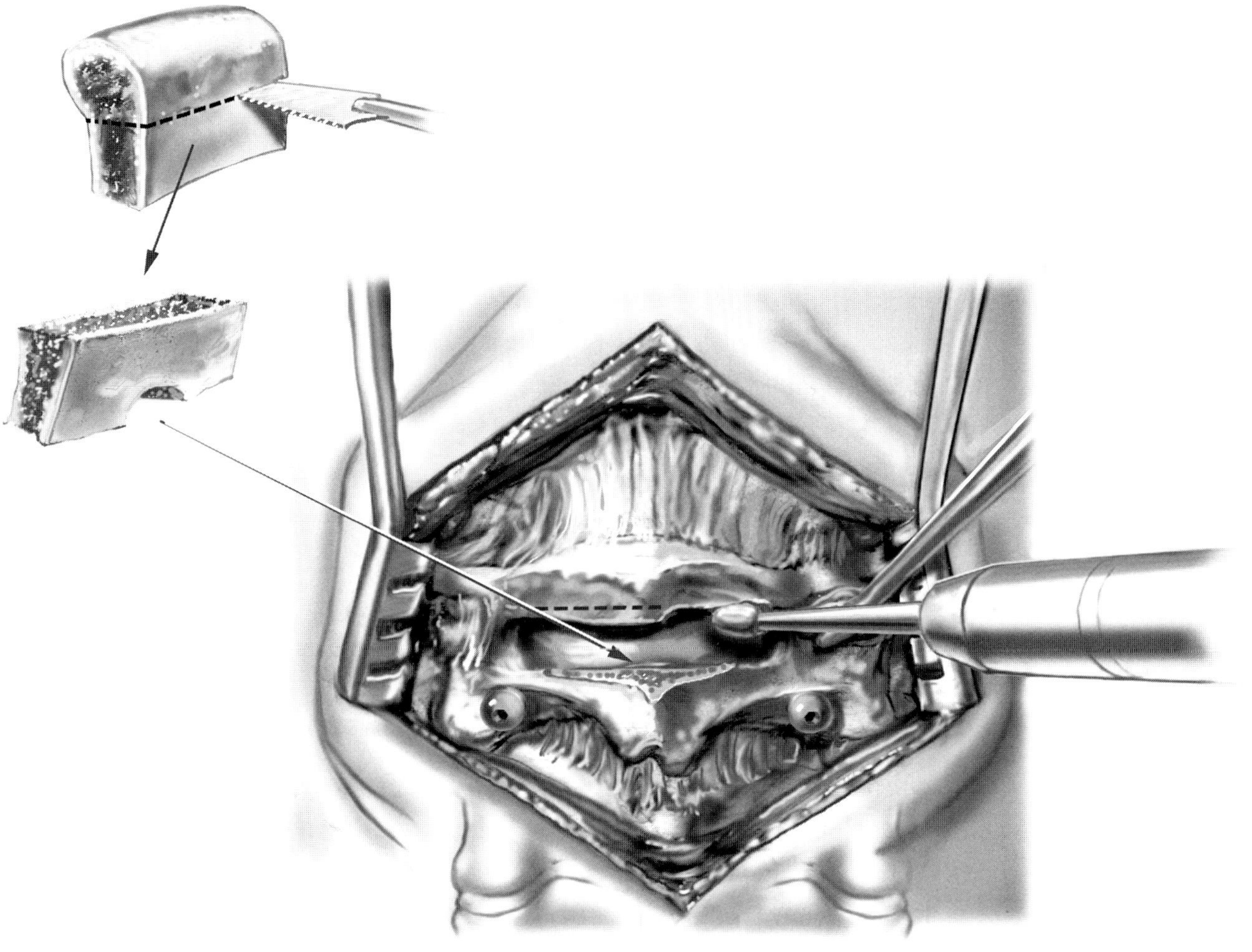

Figure 13-14. Once the transarticular screw fixation has been accomplished, we apply a posterior tension band construct with autograft using a Sonntag loop wiring technique. This provides three-point fixation, adds little time to the case, and augments the construct with structural autograft. It is important to decorticate the inferior surface of the C1 ring and the superior surface of C2 so that there will be a cancellous bone–on–cancellous bone interface, increasing the fusion rate. We will harvest a tricortical graft from the iliac crest and then cut off the superior surface to customize the graft.

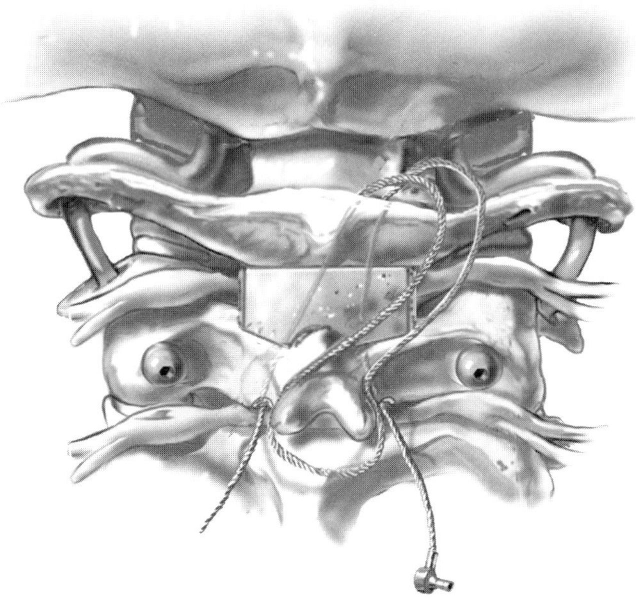

Figure 13-15. The loop is then placed under the C1 ring, and the graft is sunk into position. The loop is brought around the C2 spinous process to lasso the bone tightly. The cable is then tightened and secured into position.

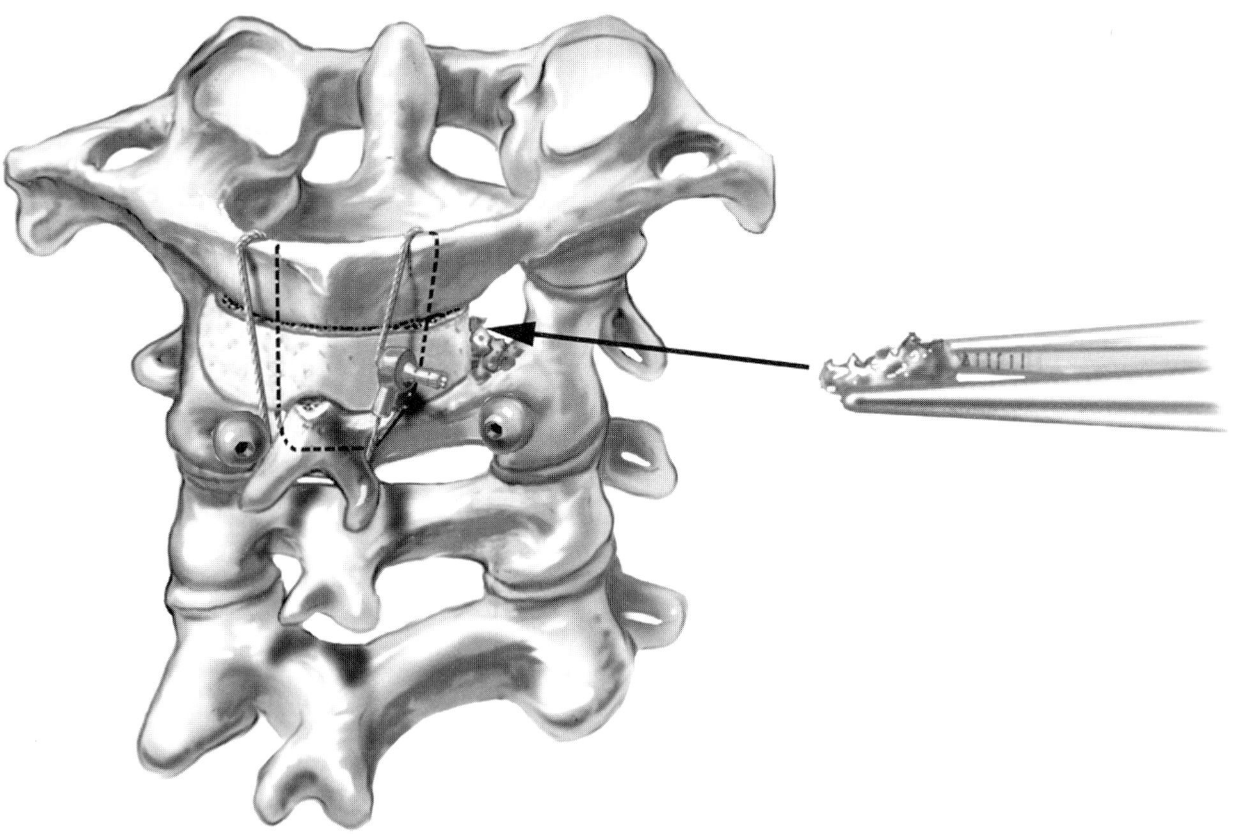

Figure 13-16. Morselized bone is then placed lateral to the autograft to augment the fusion. The wound is closed in multiple layers.

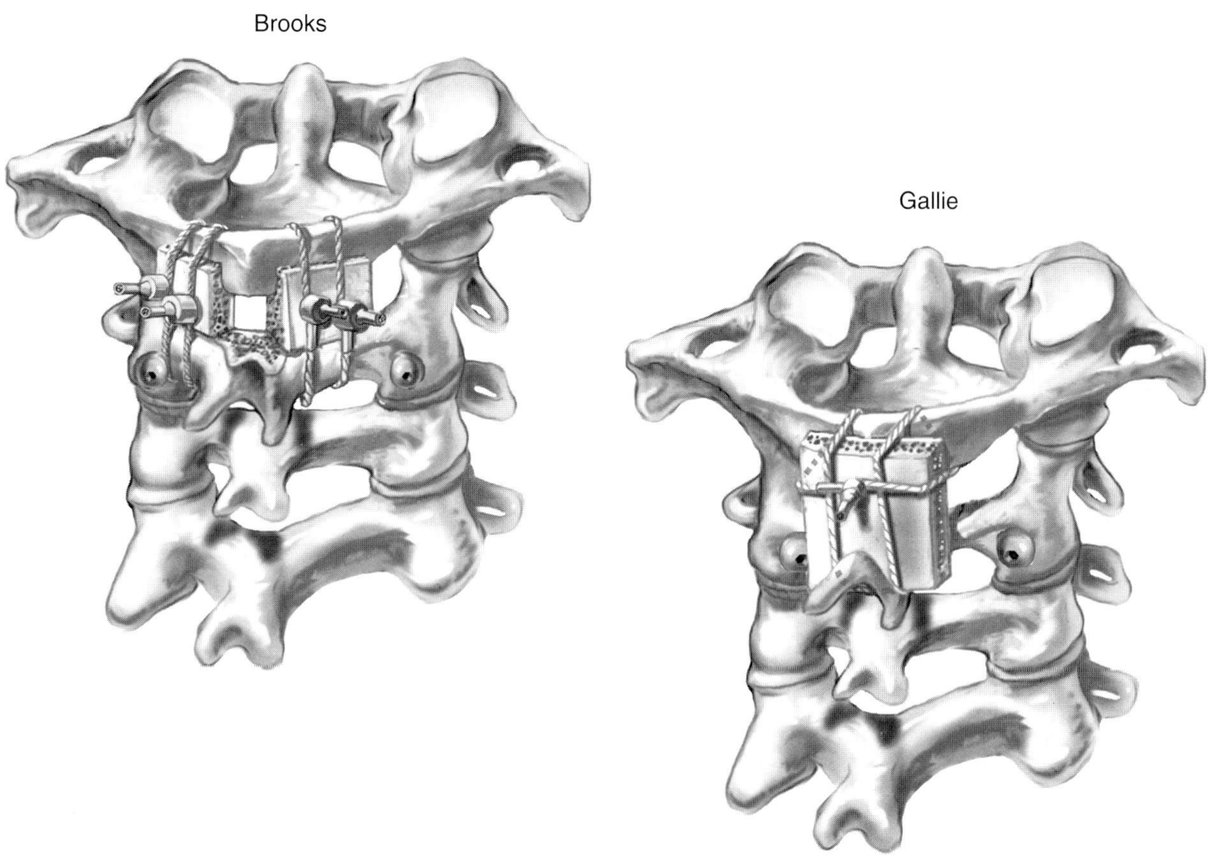

Figure 13-17. Traditional wiring techniques have included the Brooks and Gallie types of fusions. These techniques yielded a fusion rate that approximated 80%. With C1-C2 transarticular screw fixation in addition to posterior wiring techniques, the fusion rates are approximately 95%. There are biomechanical advantages to the Sonntag wiring technique compared with Brooks and Gallie. There are also biomechanical advantages to the C1-C2 screw technique over other wiring techniques.

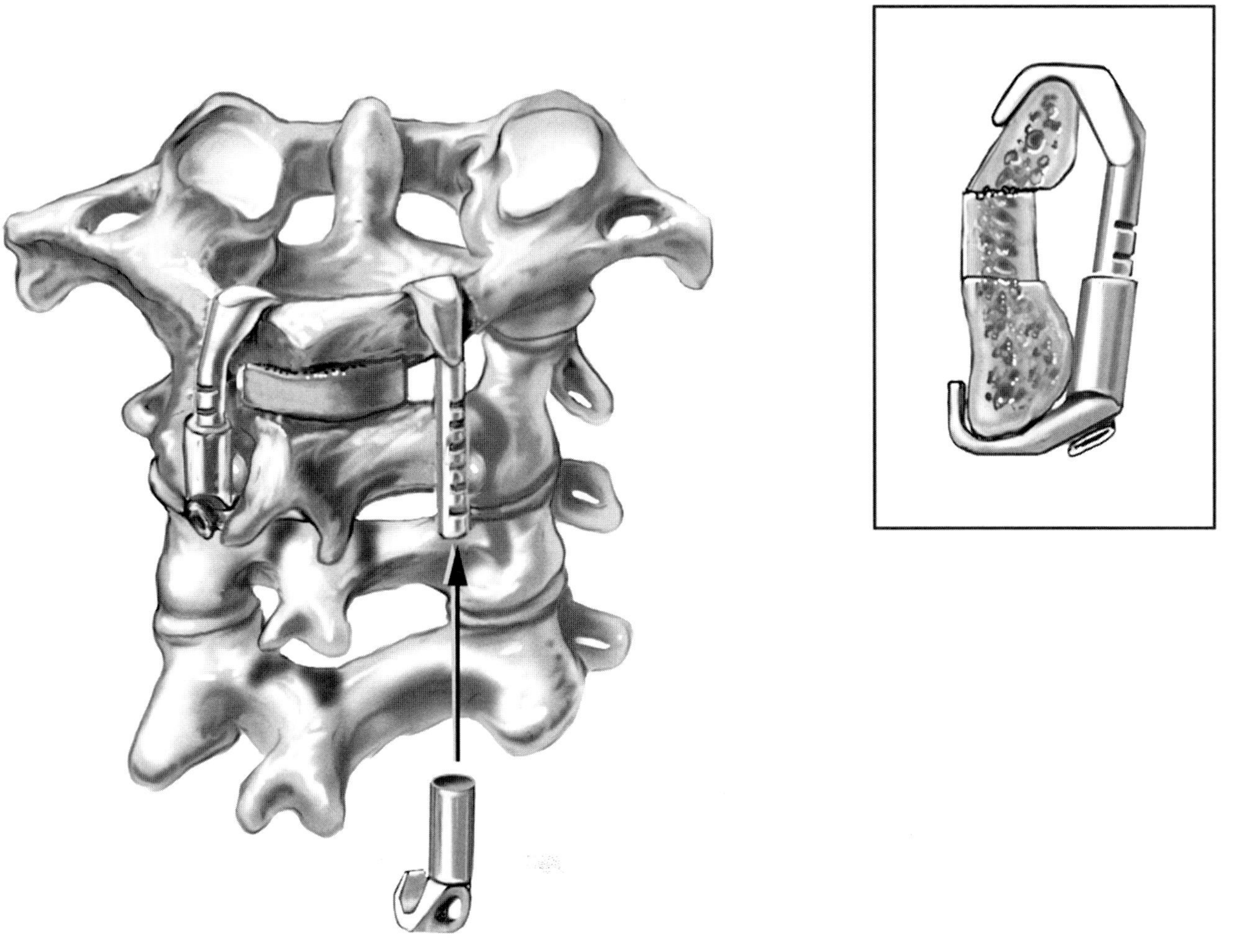

Figure 13-18. Posterior C1-C2 clamp fixation is another option for posterior tension reconstruction. When using clamps, a narrower autograft must be used to allow the hook seating.

COMMON PITFALLS

Figure 13-19, A and B. **A,** Positioning. There is a natural tendency for the surgeon to place a patient in proper cervical lordosis when performing a posterior arthrodesis. Although this is the case for posterior cervical fixation of the subaxial cervical spine, it is not the case for C1-C2 transarticular screws. **B,** To obtain the proper trajectory to place a transarticular screw, the head must be kept in a military tuck position. In addition, the head can be positioned with C-arm assistance to verify that the trajectory is amenable to screw fixation. Although we have not had this problem, there is the potential that the malalignment or displaced fracture may not be reducible with positioning, which would therefore require a posterior cervical tension band instead of a transarticular screw.

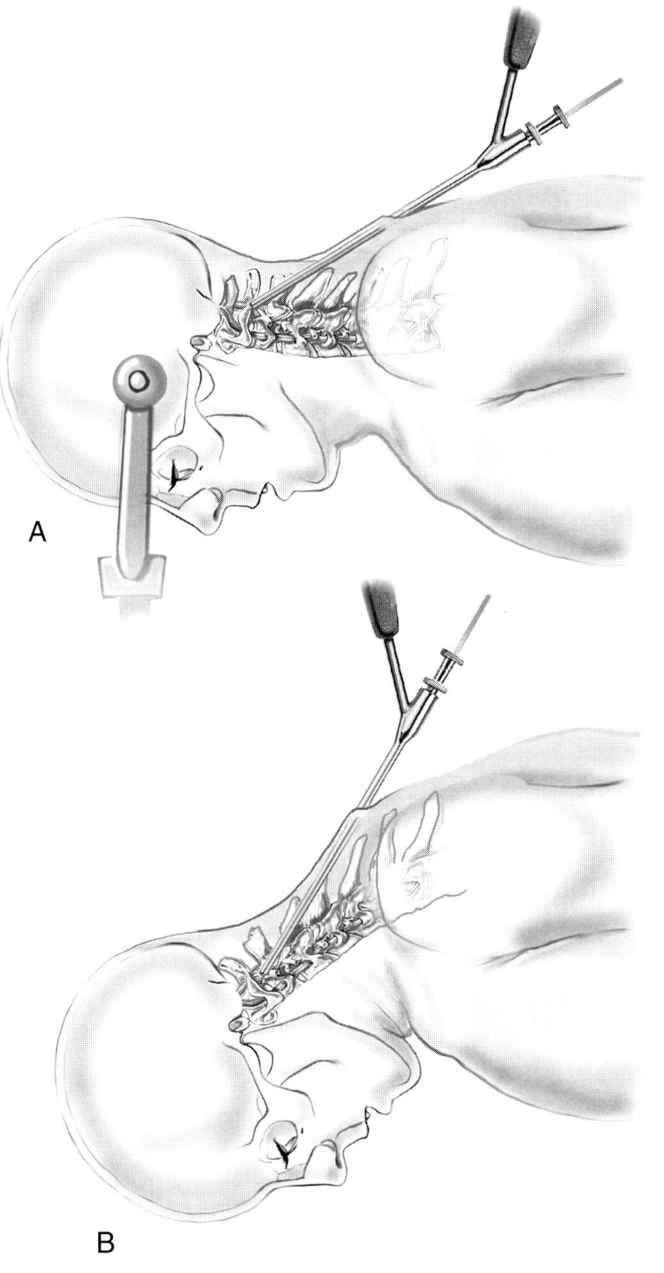

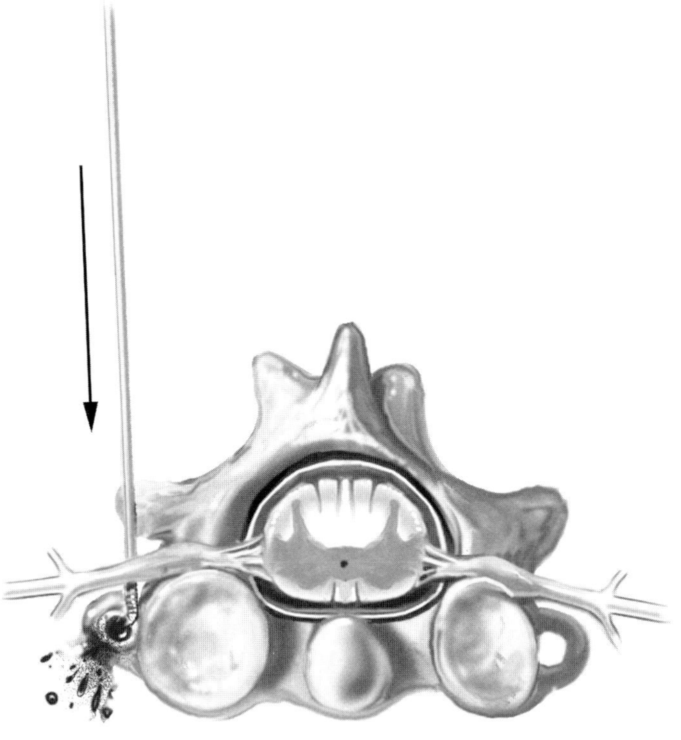

Figure 13-20. If a medial trajectory is not used, the K-wire can migrate laterally, putting the vertebral artery at risk. In addition, if proper preoperative evaluation with thin-cut CT scanning is not performed, the vertebral artery loop may jut into the pars. Some patients have an aberrant vertebral artery loop that puts the vertebral artery at risk. If the vertebral artery is inadvertently injured during the first screw placement, **do not** place a second screw on the contralateral side. This is critical because most unilateral vertebral artery injuries do not result in any cerebrovascular event. If, however, the second opposite artery is also injured, the patient has a high risk for brain stem infarct.

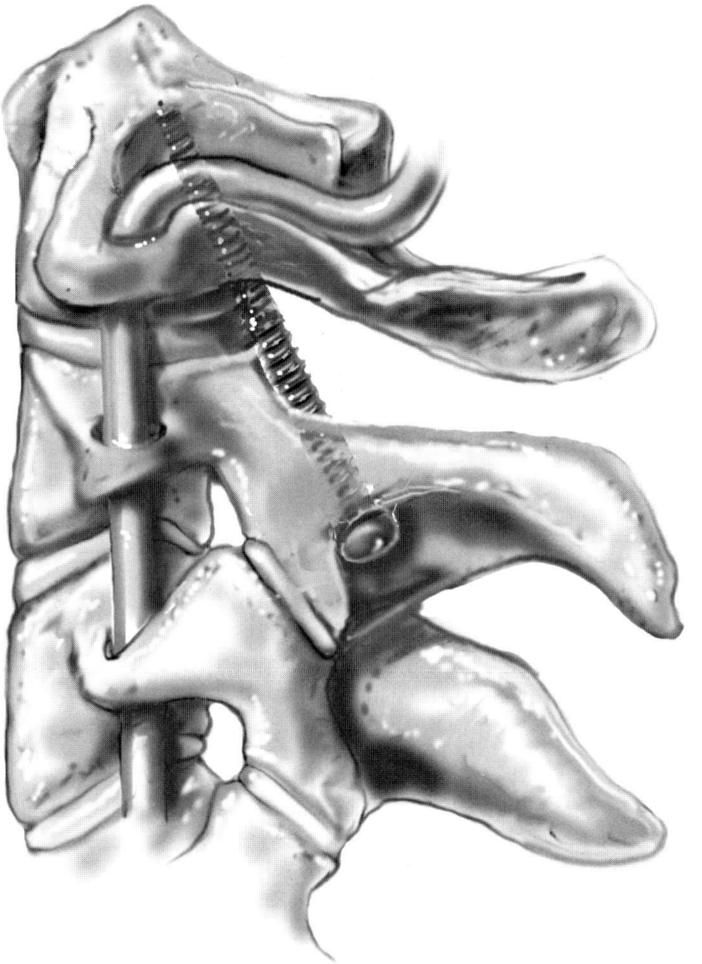

Figure 13-21. An inappropriate caudal-rostral trajectory causes a shallow purchase of the C2 pars and posterior breakout of the screw.

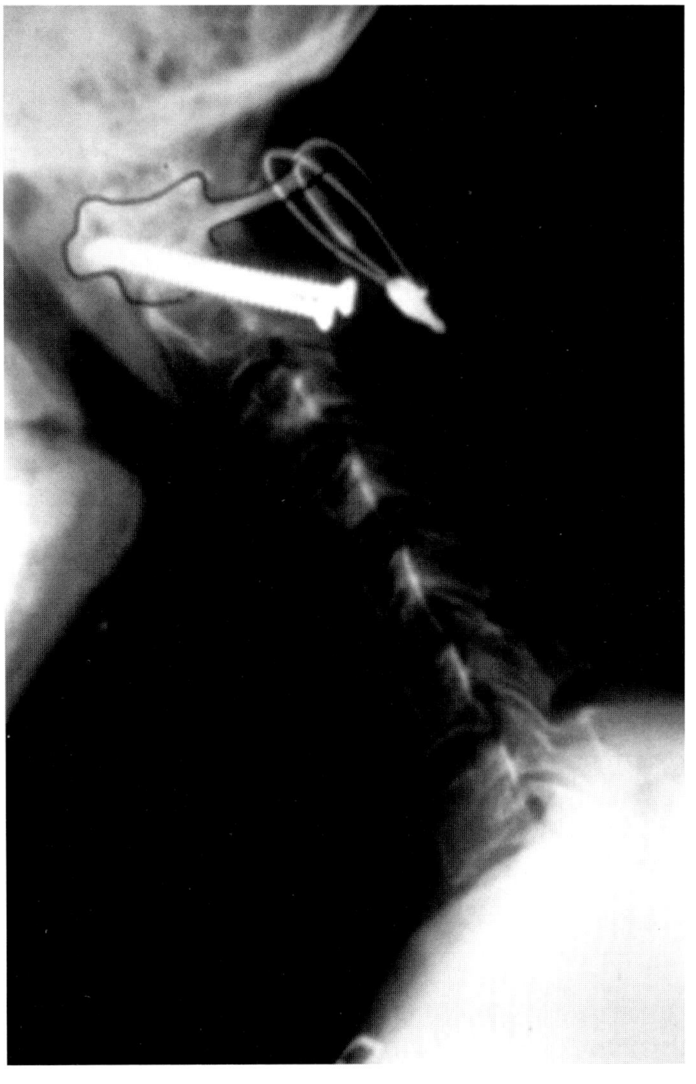

POSTOPERATIVE RESULTS

Figure 13-22. Lateral cervical spine x-ray demonstrating good position of the C1-C2 transarticular screws and posterior tension band fixation.

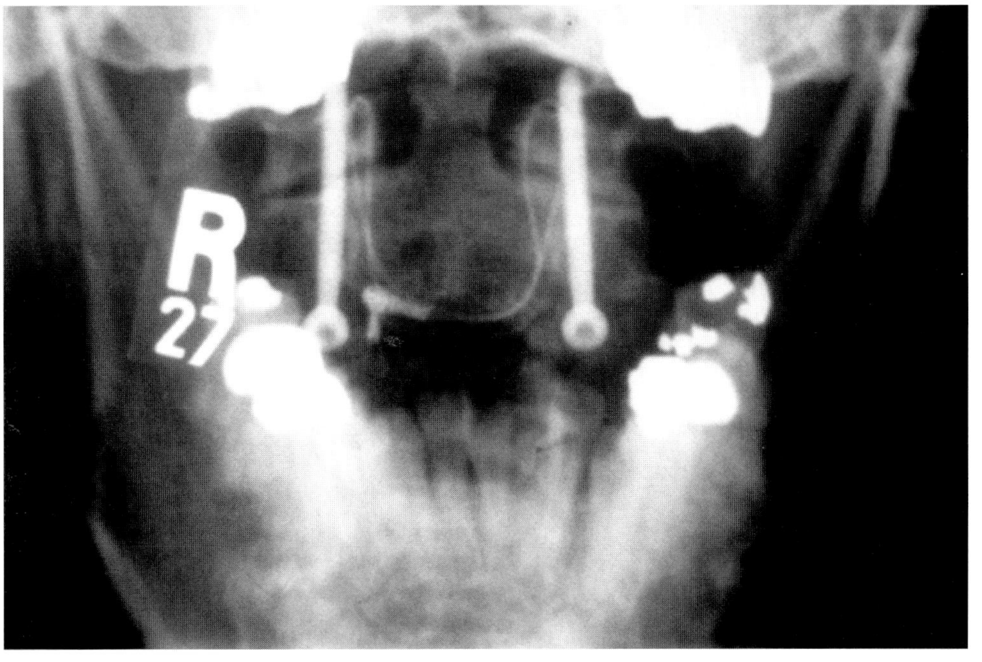

Figure 13-23. Anterior-posterior cervical spine radiograph demonstrating C1-C2 screws crossing the C1-C2 joint space with a very slight lateral-to-medial trajectory. Also, there is a posterior tension band cable fixation.

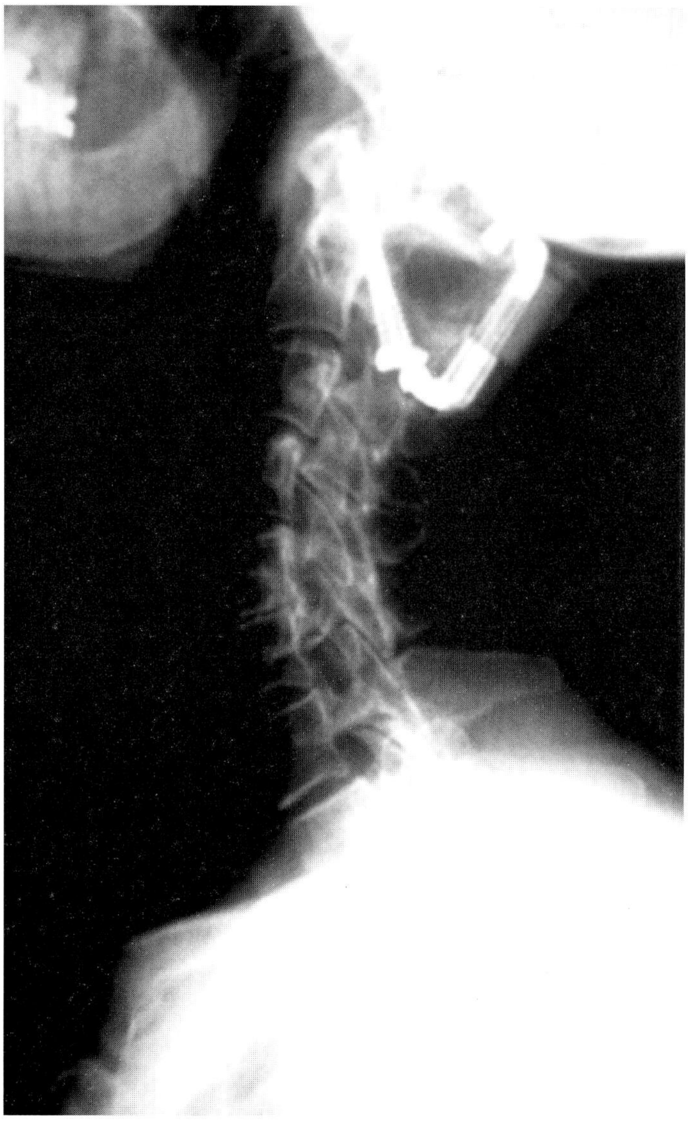

Figure 13-24. Lateral cervical spine radiograph demonstrating C1-C2 transarticular screw fixation and posterior tension band fixation using an Apofix interlaminar clamp technique.

CHAPTER XIV

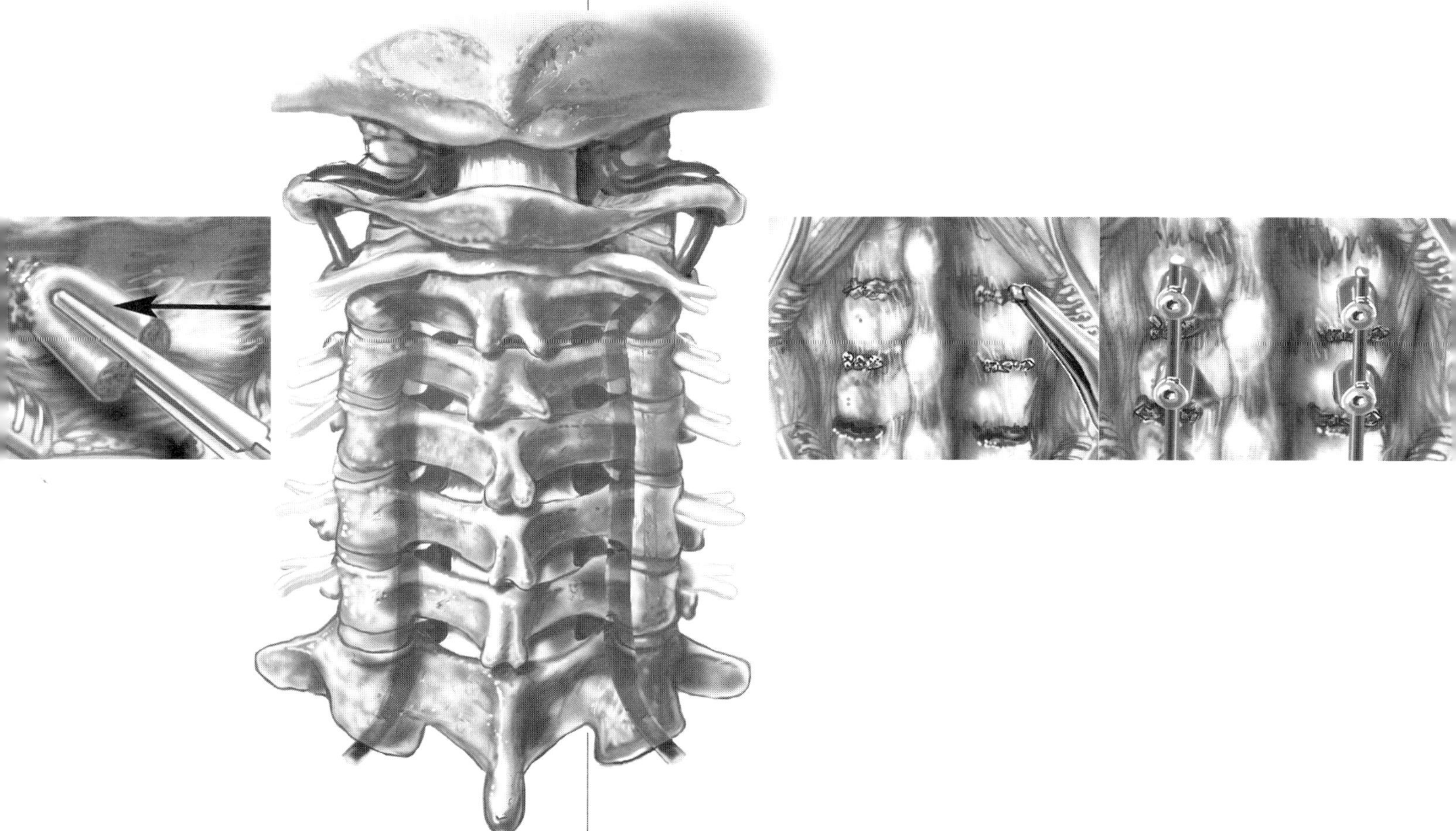

Short- and Long-Segment Lateral Mass Fixation

Lateral mass fixation has become a well-accepted technique to augment fusion and prevent postlaminectomy kyphosis in patients at risk for this problem. The first generation of this technology consisted of fixed plate and screw systems. These devices increased rigidity and promoted fusion but were constrained because of the fixed screw holes. This limitation was a particular problem in long-segment constructs because the surgeon had to place the screws within the confines of the plate. This led to the development of polyaxial screw rod constructs that allowed the surgeon to place the screws first and precisely where he or she wanted. The screws could then be connected to a rod for fixation. The polyaxial design and offset connectors and hooks allowed significant flexibility and ease to affix the rod to the screws.

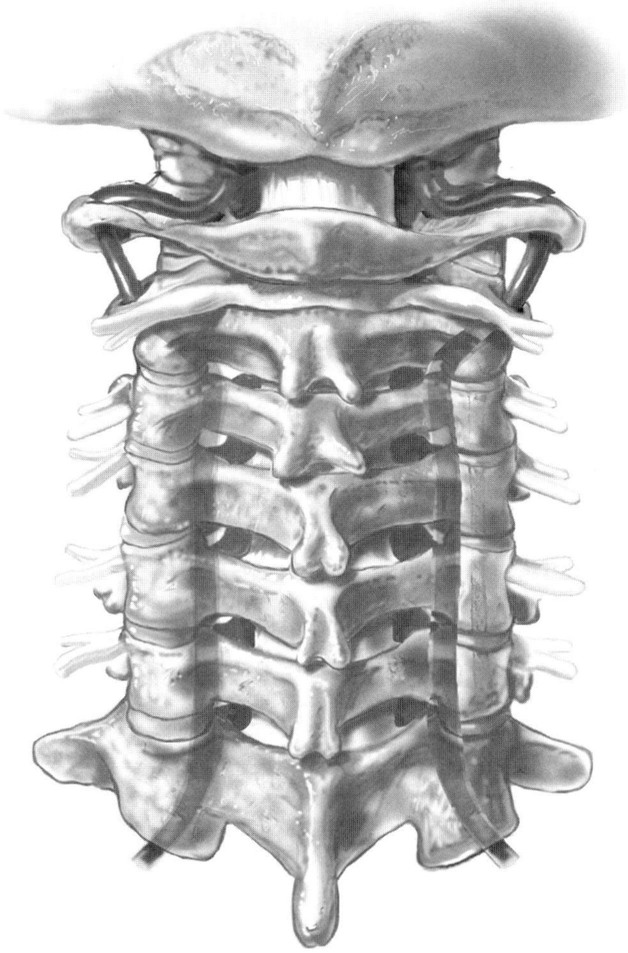

Figure 14-1. The figure demonstrates the pertinent anatomy to be considered during placement of lateral mass screws in the cervical region. The vertebral artery lies anterior to the cervical nerve roots and at the medial border of the facet line. The cervical nerve roots exit horizontally at the level of the facet joint. When placing lateral mass screws, it has been our habit to stand on the opposite side of the patient so that adequate screw trajectory can be obtained. We have found that the normal tendency to skive laterally opposite the surgeon's side actually helps in placing screws at the appropriate medial-to-lateral trajectory. After the contralateral lateral mass screws have been placed, we have made a habit of switching sides to place the other screws so that each is placed with the surgeon standing on the contralateral side. The exception to this rule is the placement of C2 pars or cervical and thoracic pedicle screws, which should be passed from the ipsilateral side.

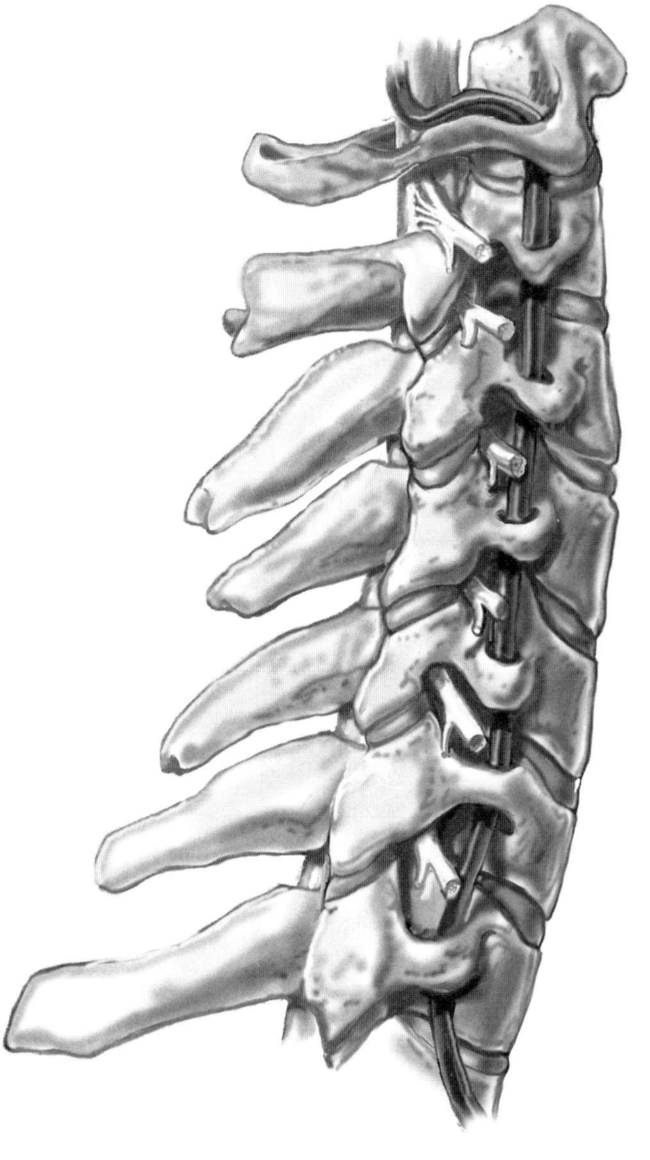

Figure 14-2. Lateral anatomical view of the cervical spine, demonstrating the relationship of the nerve roots and vertebral artery with regard to the facet joint. The angle of the facet joint, which determines the superior/inferior trajectory for screw placement, should be noted.

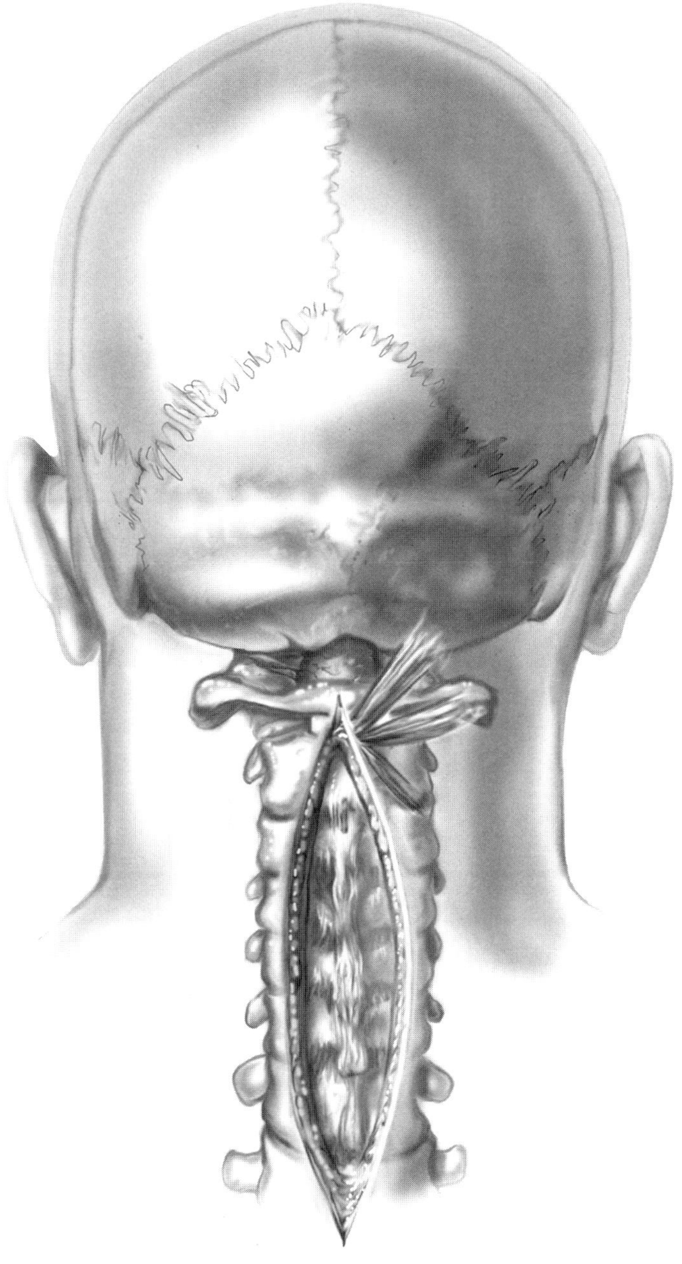

Figure 14-3. Exposure for short- and long-segment cervical lateral mass fixation consists of a midline incision with exposure of the appropriate level spinous processes, lamina and lateral mass, and facet joints. An x-ray can be used to localize the appropriate levels.

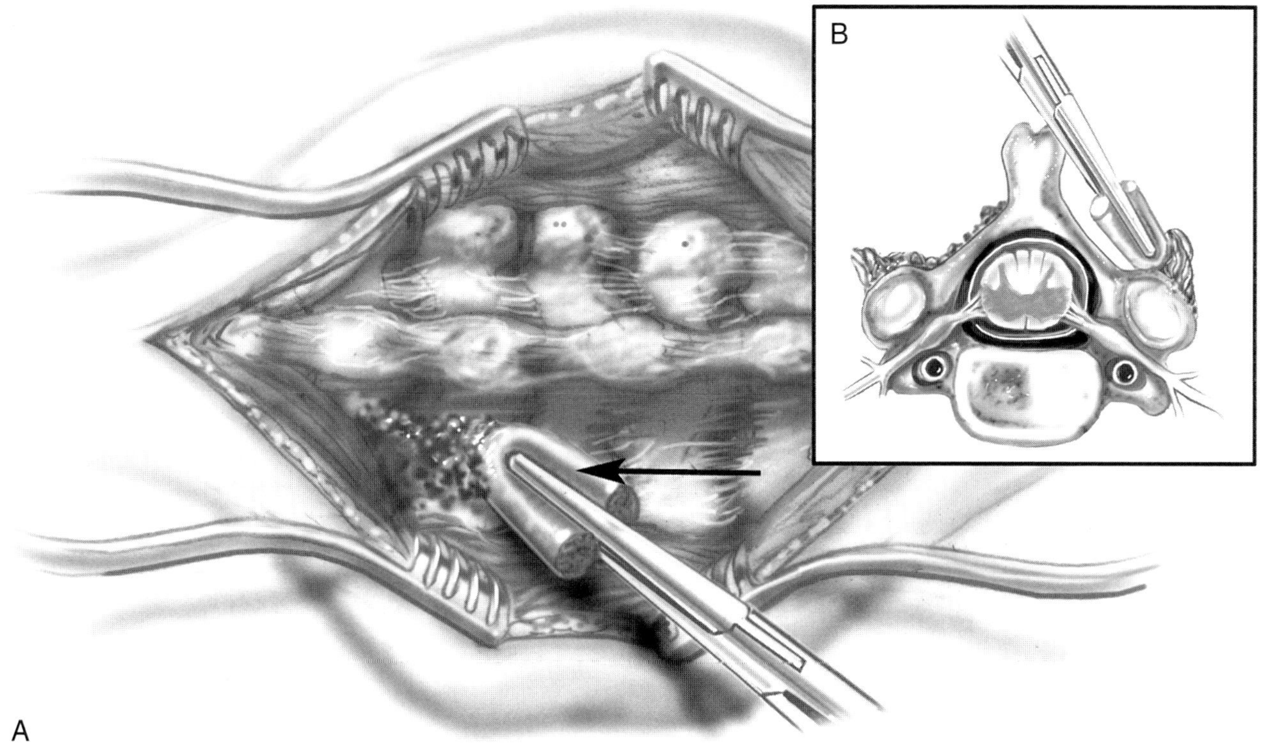

Figure 14-4, A and B. Once the appropriate levels are identified and exposed, the bone is cleaned of any soft tissue or charr with a Kittner dissector or sponge with a periosteal elevator. This technique allows for a clean cortical surface and helps in the orientation of the landmarks of the lateral mass. In patients with significant instability, great care must be maintained to not exert too much pressure on the spine during dissection because this might result in inadvertent movement of the unstable spine and poses the potential for spinal cord injury. The entire lateral mass, including the lateral border, must be exposed so that the landmark can be visualized and scored.

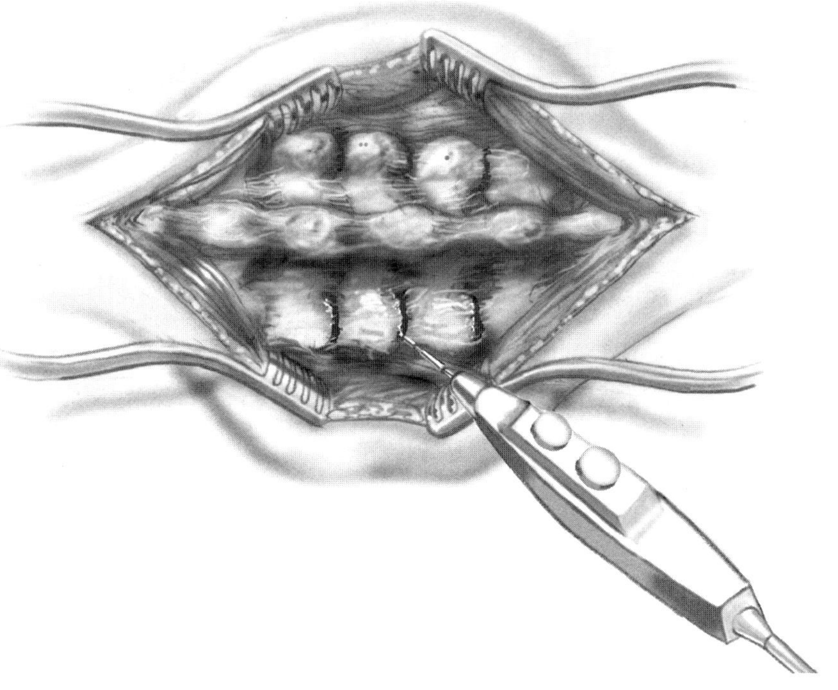

Figure 14-5. Once the bone has been cleaned, a monopolar device is used to cauterize and score the facet joints intended for fusing. This will also help the surgeon outline the borders of the lateral mass.

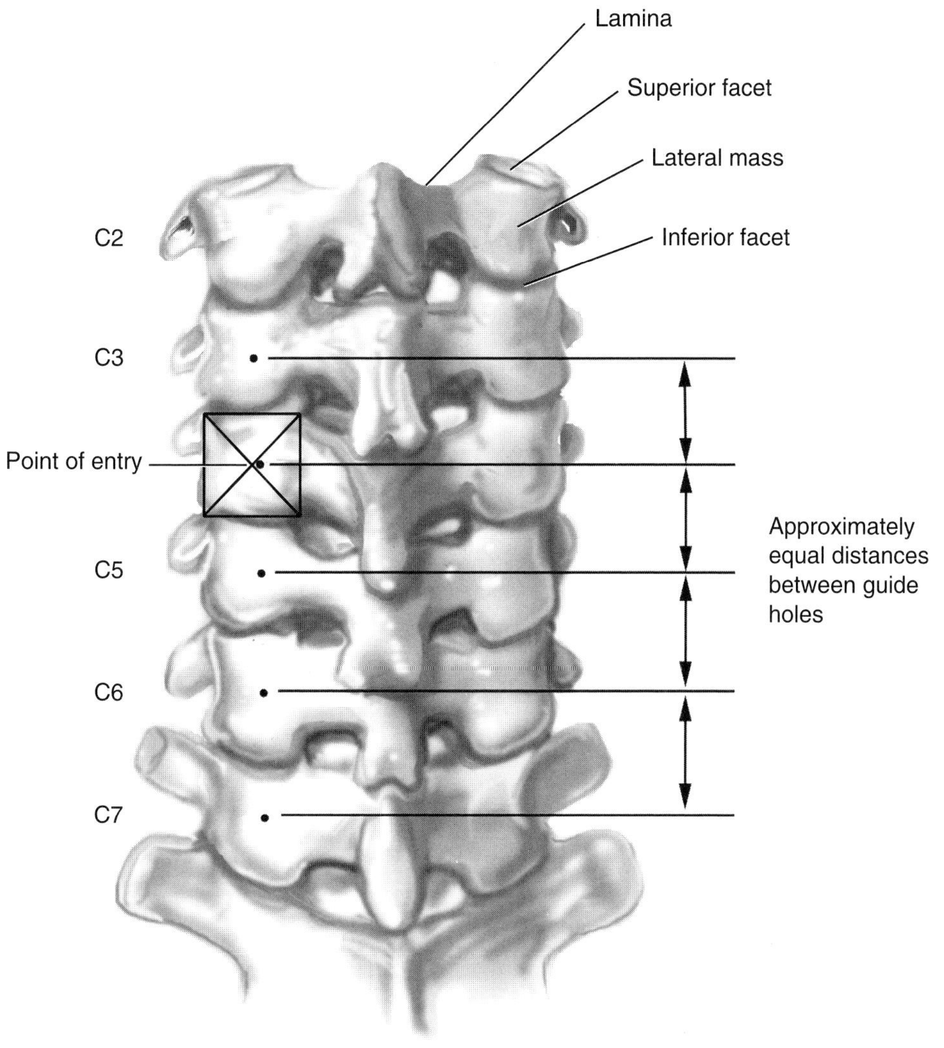

Figure 14-6. Appropriate entry site lateral mass screw fixation. If the lateral mass is considered a box of bone, one can create an imaginary "X" in the center of the box to help identify the screw entry site. The superior and inferior borders of the box are outlined by the facet joints. Diagonals are then drawn across the box. The lateral mass entry site is 1 mm medial to the intersection of the diagonals.

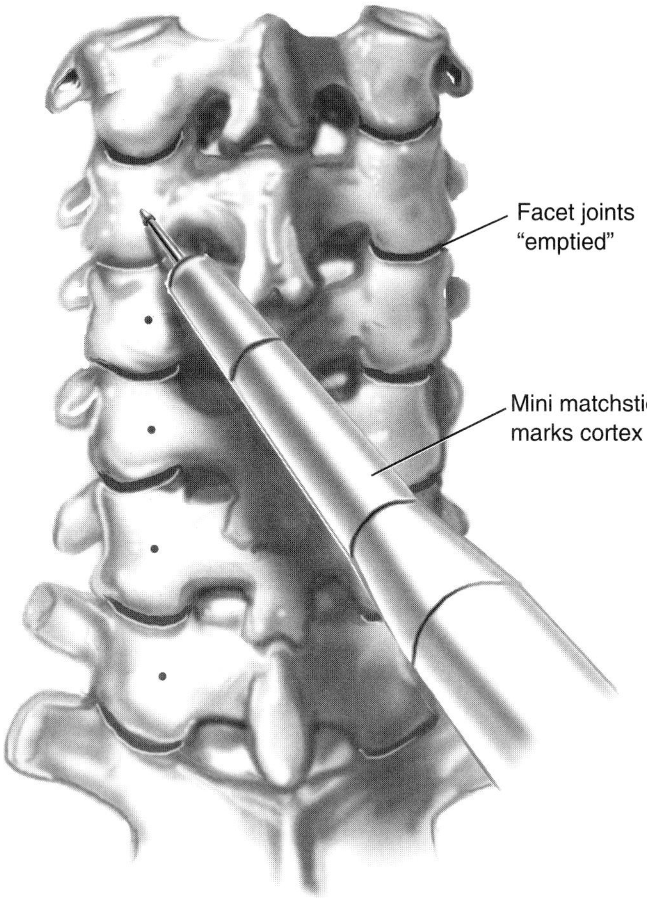

Figure 14-7. The appropriate entry points are scored with a mini matchstick drill. The cortex should be punctured with the mini matchstick burr to allow for adequate anchoring of the mini driver drill when the pilot hole is drilled.

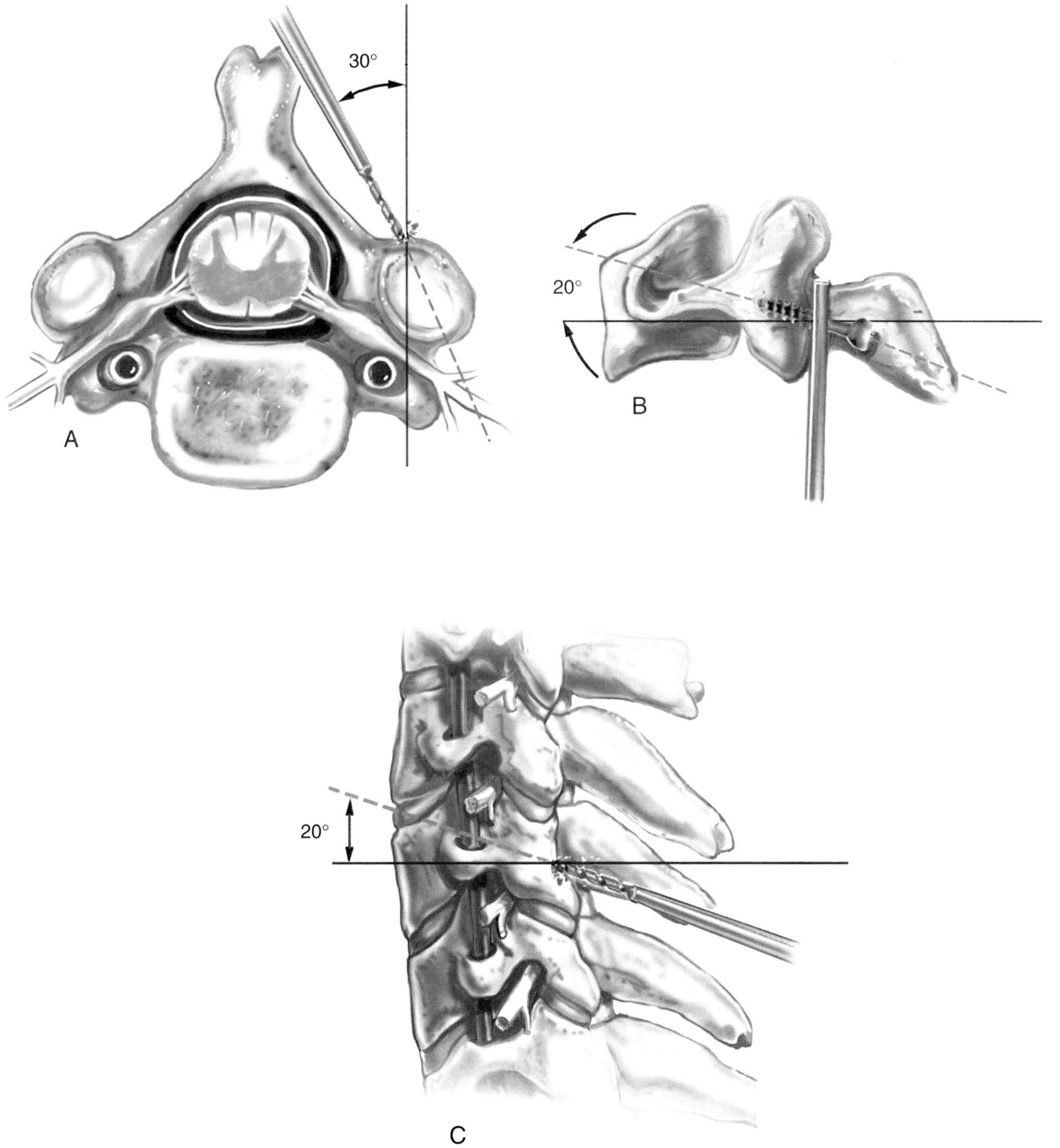

Figure 14-8, A–C. **A,** Axial schematic demonstrating appropriate medial-to-lateral angulation of 30 degrees with the drill bit aiming laterally to avoid the foramen transversarium housing the vertebral artery. **B,** Schematic demonstrating the cephalad-caudal trajectory of 20 degrees. This angulation directs the drill bit rostrally above the exiting nerve root. **C,** Lateral schematic of the appropriate drill entry site trajectory.

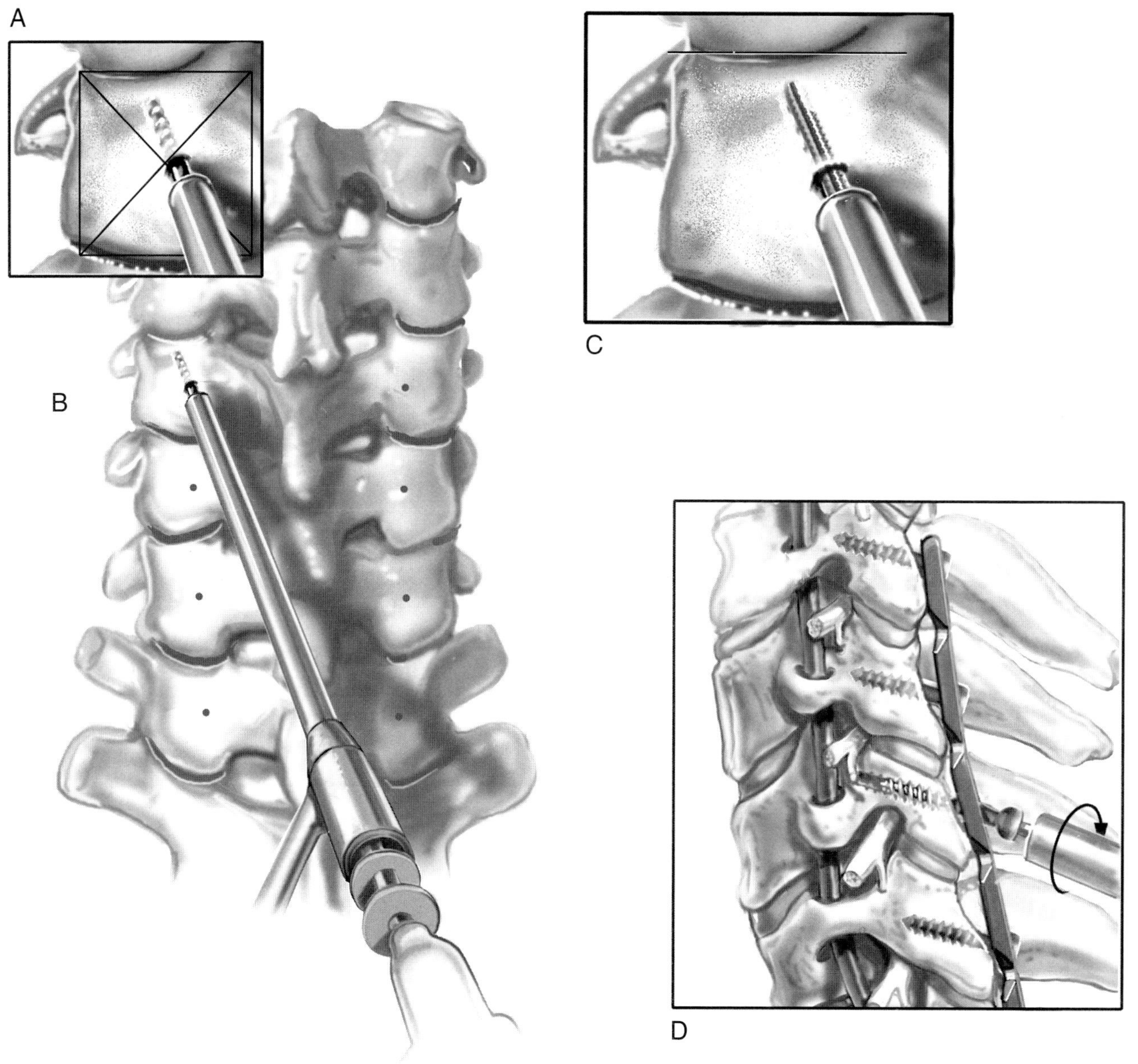

Figure 14-9, A–D. **A,** The sequence of placement of lateral mass screws includes puncturing the cortex at the appropriate entry site. **B,** This is followed by the use of a mini driver drill, drilling in a direction 30 degrees medial to lateral and 20 degrees caudal to cephalad. The depth of the mini driver drill bit should not exceed 14 to 16 mm. **C,** Once the adequate pilot hole has been drilled, a tap is used to enlarge the screw entry site. **D,** This is followed by placement of a lateral mass screw of appropriate length, usually 14 to 16 mm long from C3 to C7.

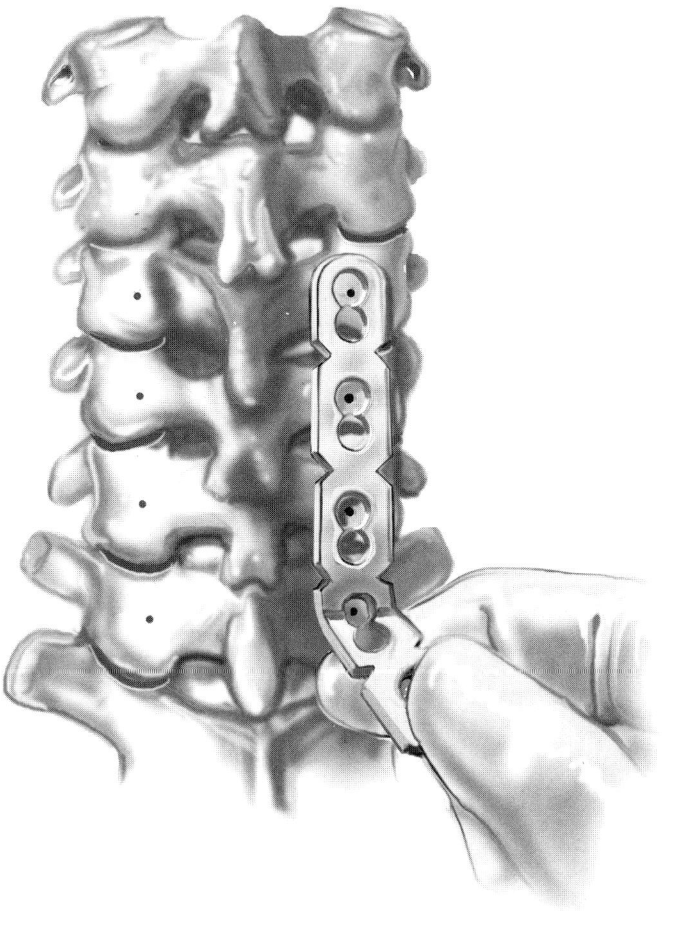

Figure 14-10. Templating is helpful for affixing the appropriately sized plate onto the lateral masses. Rather than placing screws that are dictated by prefixed plate holes, we prefer to drill and tap pilot holes before affixing the plate. Various templates are then tried that best fit the predrilled holes for the appropriately sized plate. Once the plate size has been appropriately templated, it is ready to be affixed.

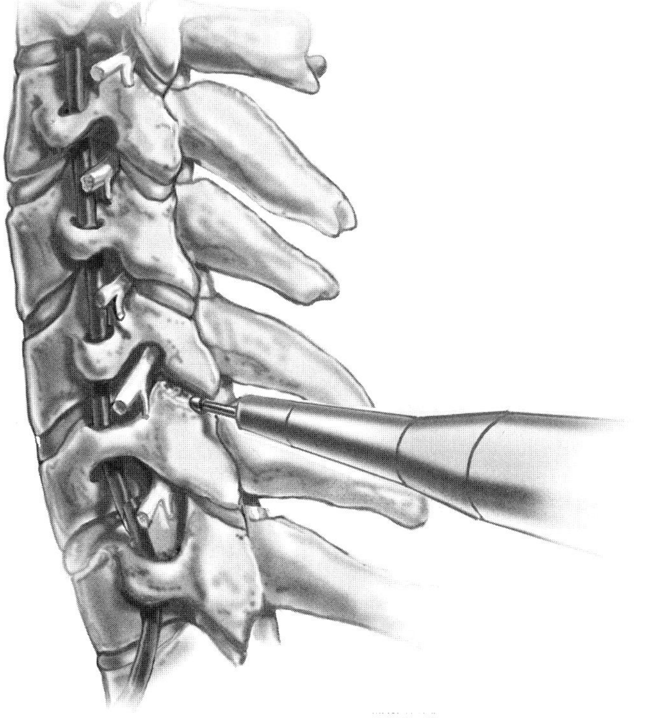

Figure 14-11. Before placing the lateral mass plate, the facet joints are decorticated. The cartilaginous end plate is removed with the use of a mini matchstick drill bit.

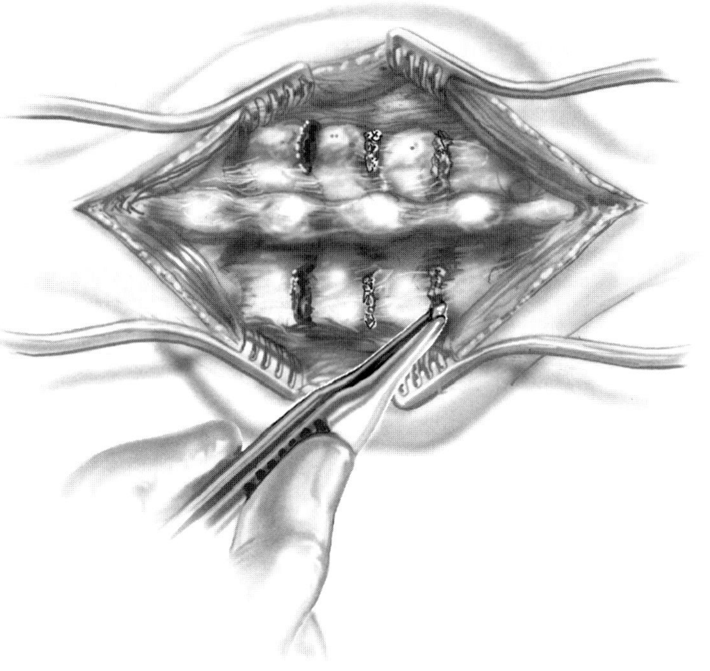

Figure 14-12. The decorticated facet joints are then packed with small bits of morselized bone graft obtained from either products of decompression or by harvest of autograft iliac crest bone graft.

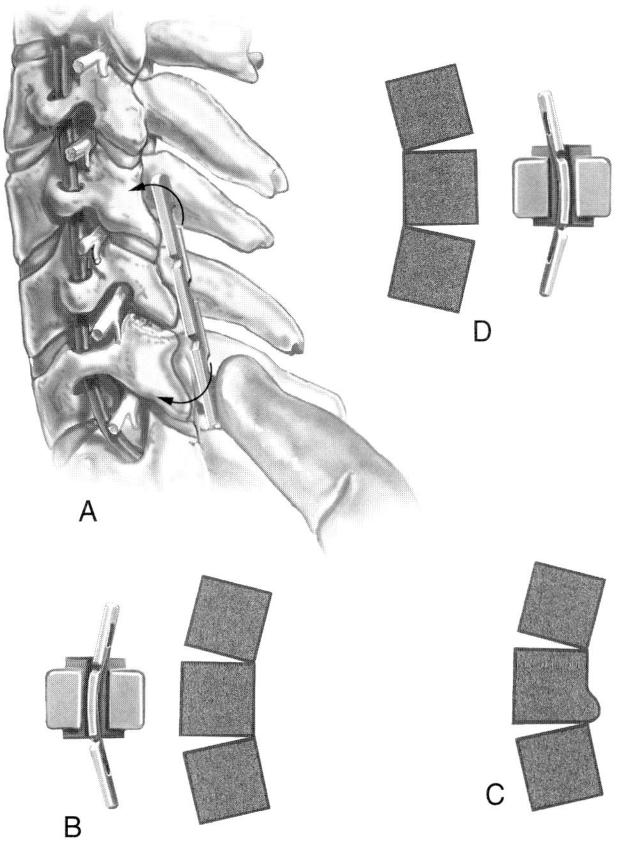

Figure 14-13, A–D. The cervical contours of the lateral masses must be taken into consideration before placement of the lateral mass plate. Appropriate gardening of osteophytes should be performed to avoid any possible pivot points that may create stress risers. The lateral mass plate can be bent to approximate the cervical lordosis or kyphosis, as needed.

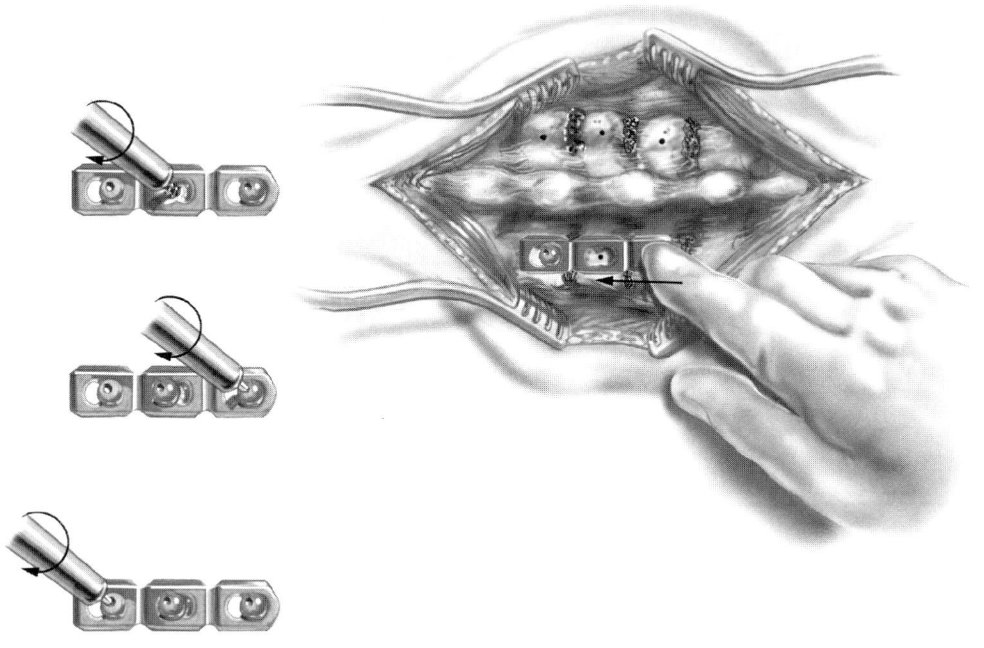

Figure 14-14. The plate is then fixed onto the spine and secured for placement of the final screws. The first screw is placed shallowly and then the plate is adjusted by shifting it either rostrally or caudally so that the tapped holes can match with the plate apertures. Screw tightening should be performed in a sequential fashion, alternating until firm purchase is obtained at each level. If a screw is initially tightened too much at one level, it may prevent the plate from laying flush against the bone.

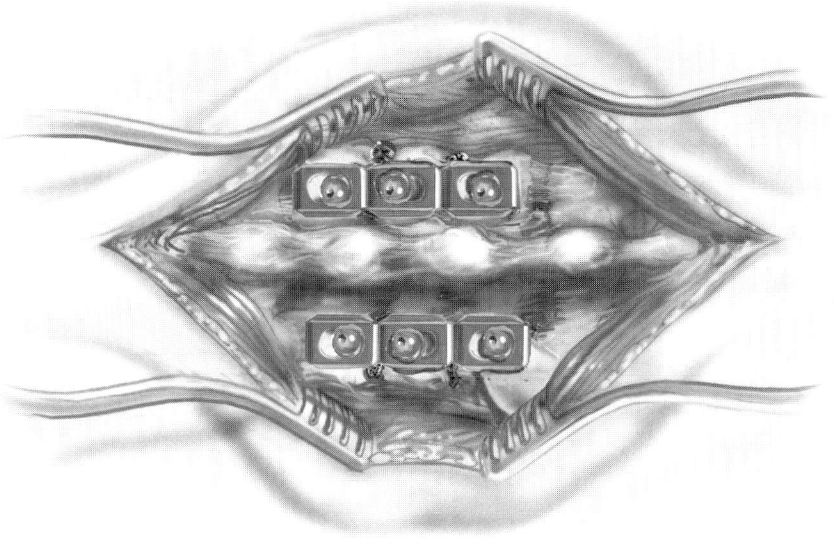

Figure 14-15. Posterior view of a completed short-segment lateral mass fixation. After the plate is securely tightened, the exposed lateral portion of the lateral mass, medial lamina, and spinous process can be decorticated with a mini matchstick drill bit. Morselized bone can be laid over this area. If a decompression is necessary, it can be performed either before or after plate fixation. The screw entry sites should still be predrilled and tapped before the decompression is performed. Predrilling before decompression preserves the anatomical landmarks for proper screw placement, and the dura and spinal cord have some additional protection during the procedure.

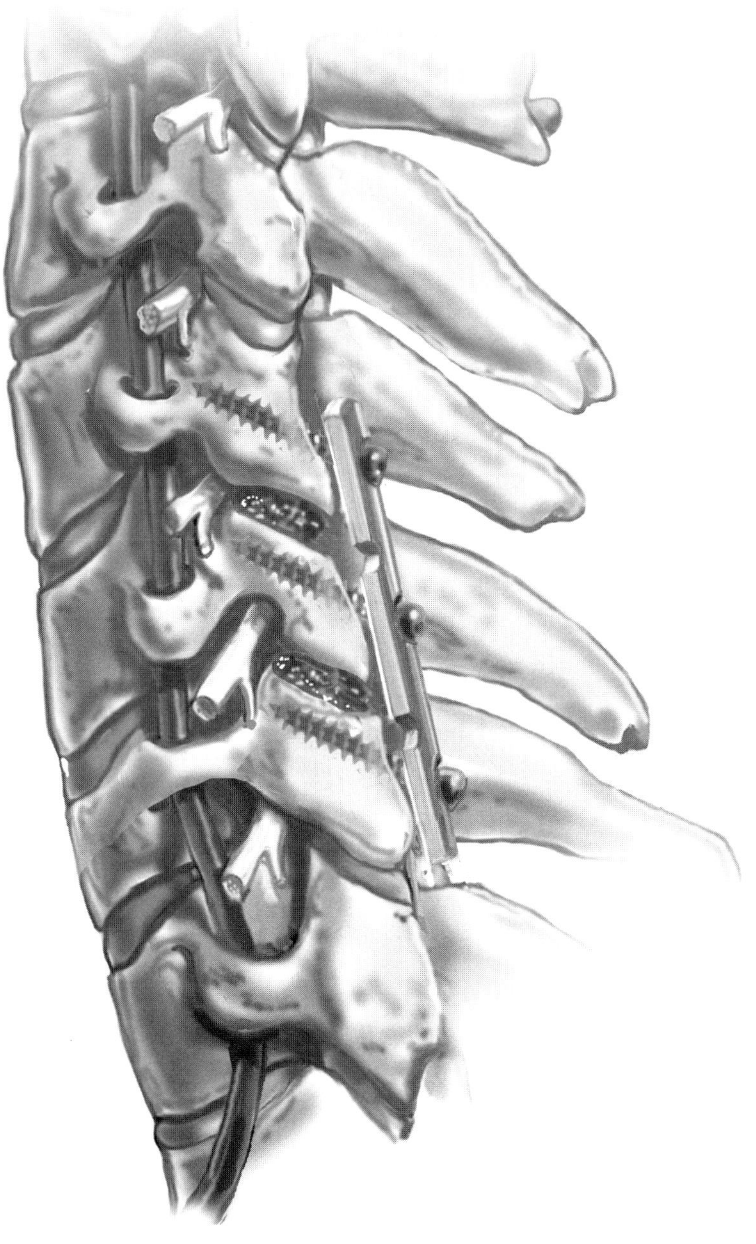

Figure 14-16. Lateral view of a short-segment lateral mass fixation. Length should be determined by patient size, but in general, 14-mm screws are used for women, and 16-mm screws are used for men. In patients with osteoporosis, bicortical purchase should be considered, and screw length can be premeasured on preoperative CT scan.

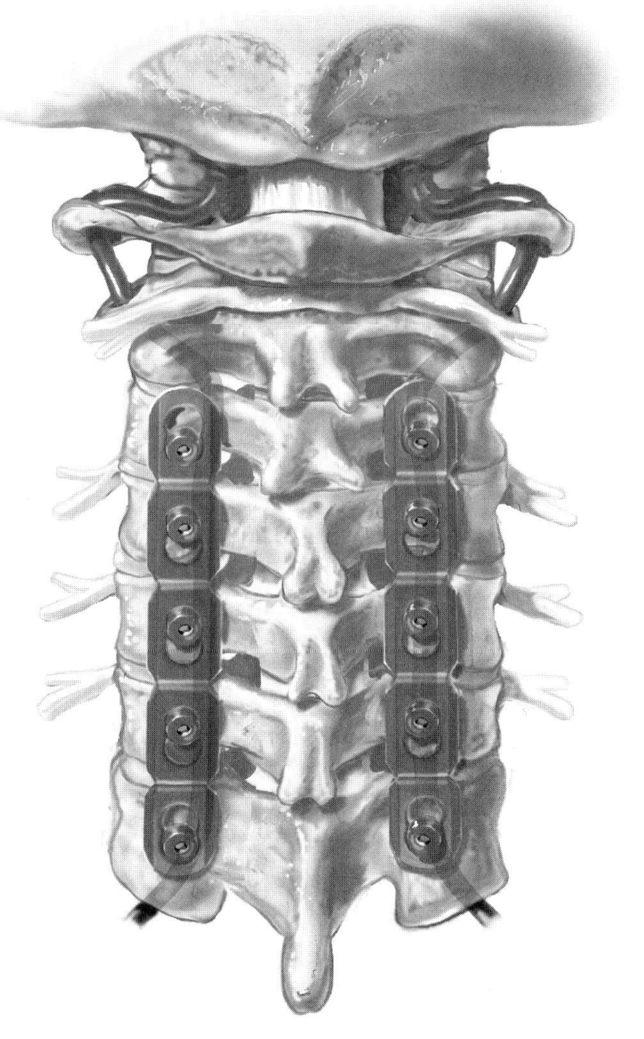

Figure 14-17. Long-segment lateral mass plate fixation is similar to short-segment fixation; however, plate fixation can be more problematic depending on the length of the construct. It has been our philosophy to predrill and tap all lateral mass pilot holes and take the appropriate plate that best suits the lateral mass entry sites. Occasionally, with long-segment fixation, the optimal plate cannot incorporate one of the screw holes due to the slightly varied interval of interjoint spaces caused by spondylosis and collapse of disc space height. If this is the case, we recommend refraining from placing a newly drilled hole and not placing a screw at that level because the hole may be suboptimal and could injure a nerve root. Some flexibility is necessary in long-segment lateral mass plate fixation. This difficulty has been eliminated with polyaxial screw rod systems.

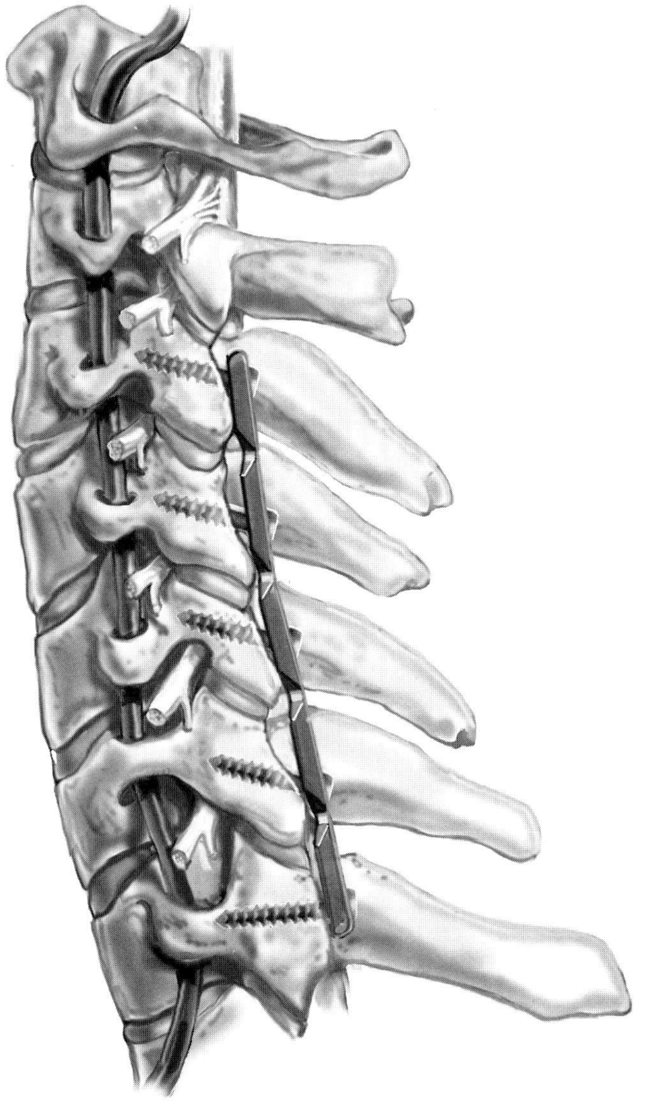

Figure 14-18. Lateral view of a long-segment lateral mass plate fixation, which demonstrates the appropriate trajectory of the lateral mass screw contouring of the plate.

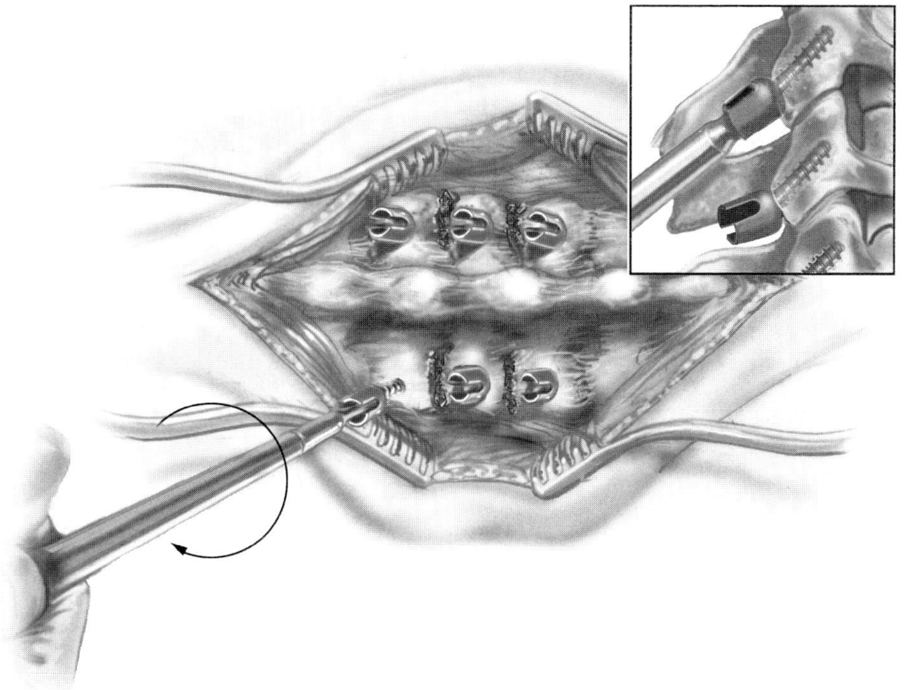

Figure 14-19. The advent of polyaxial screw rod constructs has allowed surgeons to place optimal screws at each level without having to be concerned about a constrained plate dictating ultimate screw placement. Lateral mass polyaxial screws are placed in the same fashion as lateral mass plate screws, with identical screw trajectories and lengths. The only difference is that the screws can be placed immediately after tapping and allow a significant amount of flexibility in affixing the rod.

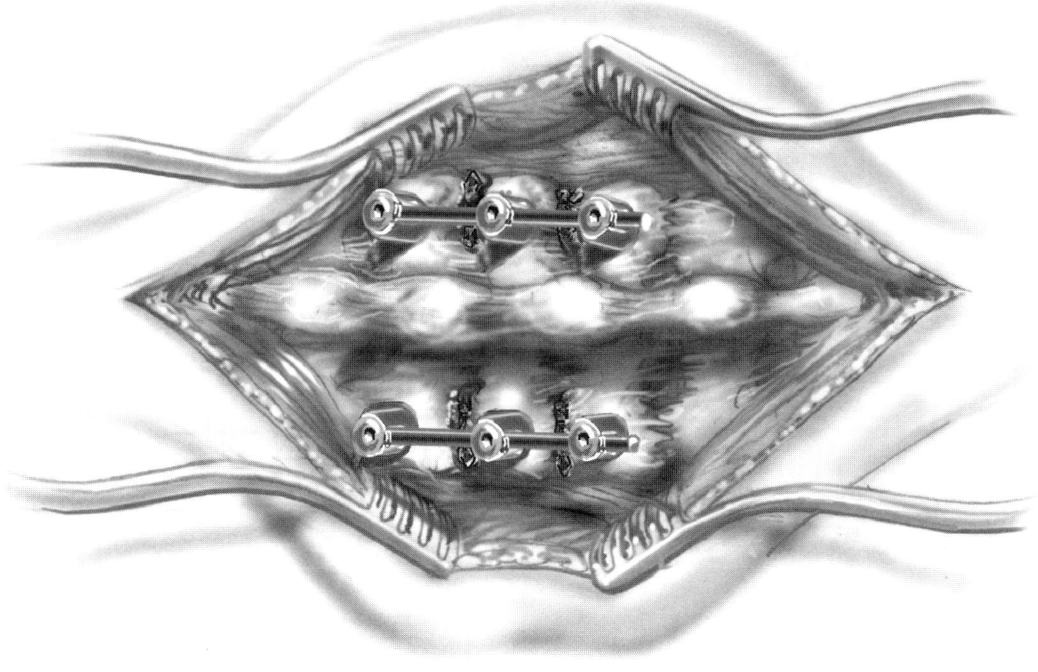

Figure 14-20. The polyaxial screw rod system has been fixed, and top-loading screws have been attached to tighten the rod with the screws.

COMMON PITFALLS

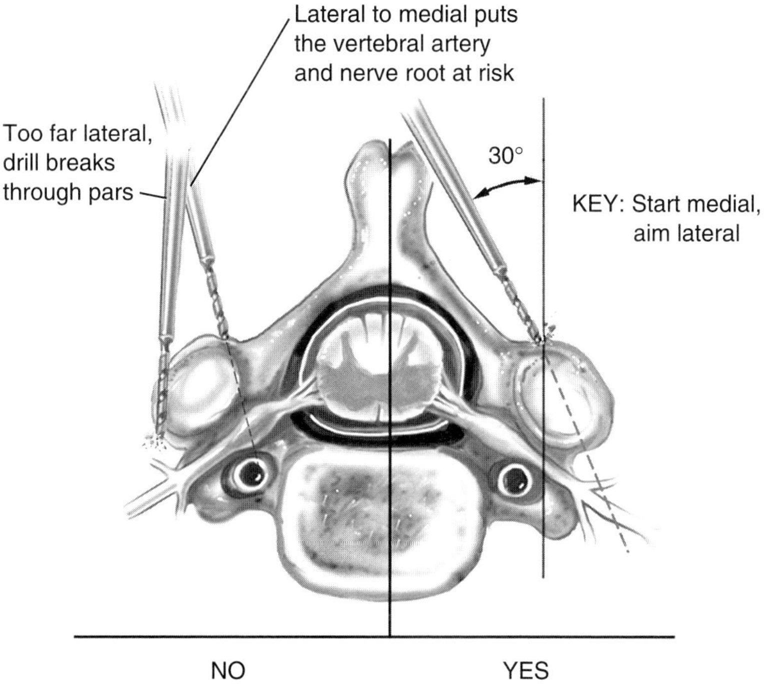

Figure 14-21. Suboptimal lateral mass entry site: Drill trajectory is critical to the safe placement of lateral mass screws. An improperly placed lateral screw entry site can cause the drill to skive off and out of the lateral mass. An entry site or trajectory placed too medially puts the vertebral artery and nerve root at risk. The optimal position for the lateral mass entry site is 1 mm medial to the midpoint in the medial-to-lateral facet line. The trajectory should be 30 degrees lateral and 20 degrees rostral to allow for optimal purchase and avoidance of the vertebral artery and nerve root.

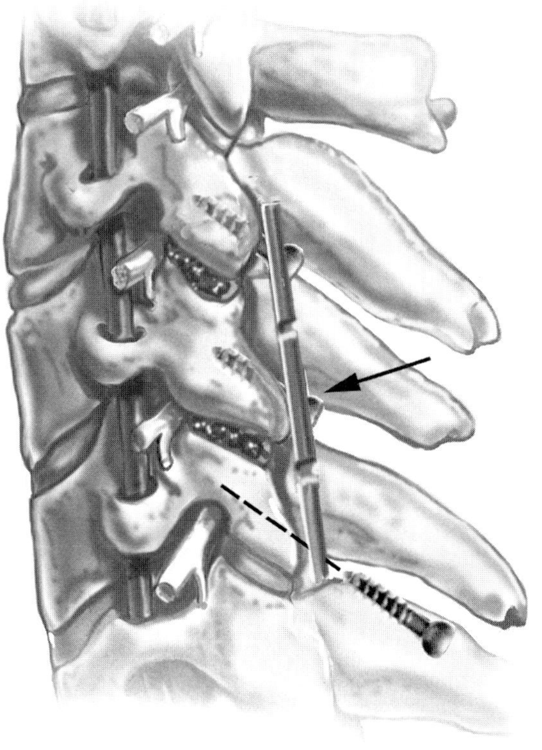

Figure 14-22. Suboptimal gardening of posterior osteophytes can be a problem, particularly with lateral mass plate fixation. An inadequately gardened spine may create a suboptimal screw placement and stress risers within the lateral mass plate. The surgeon should carefully assess the bony contours and create a flat surface on which the plate can lie.

POSTOPERATIVE RESULTS

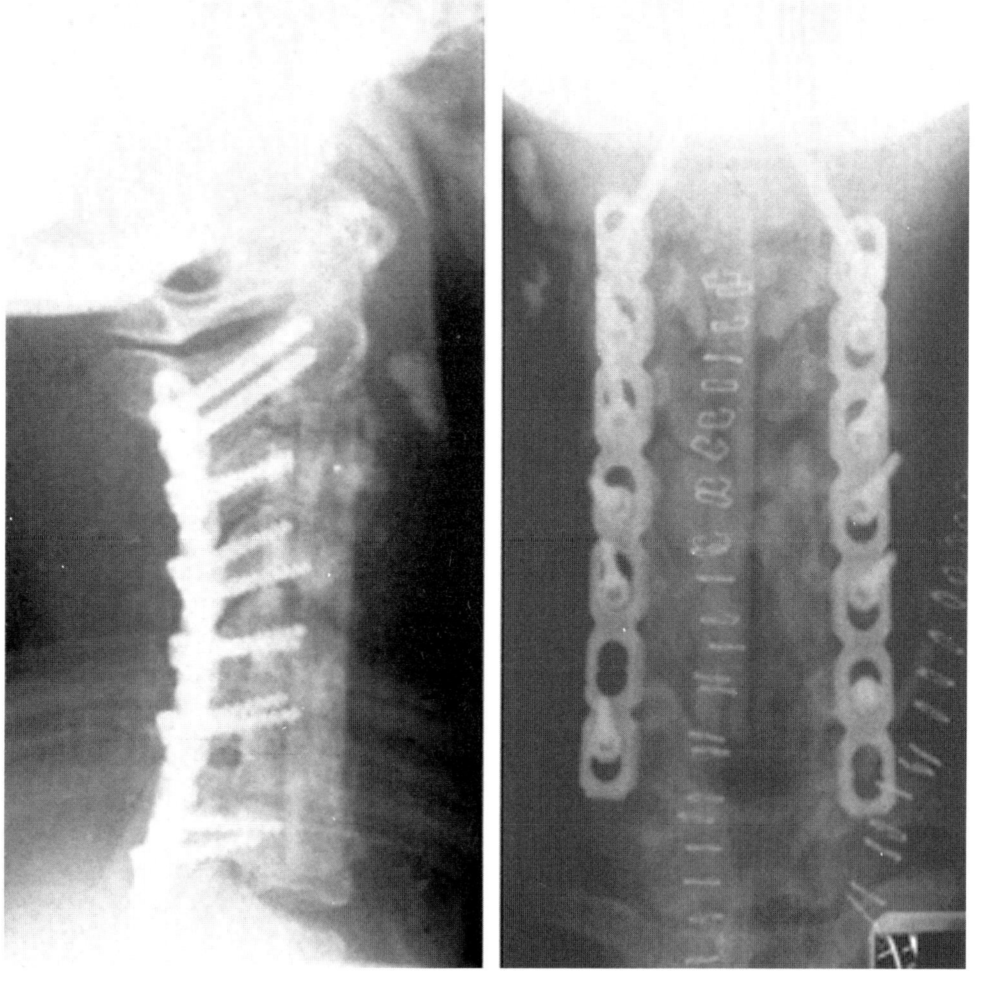

Figure 14-23. Lateral and anterior-posterior views of a long segment lateral mass fixation spanning C2-C7. Note the C2 pedicle screws are best visualized on lateral cervical spine image.

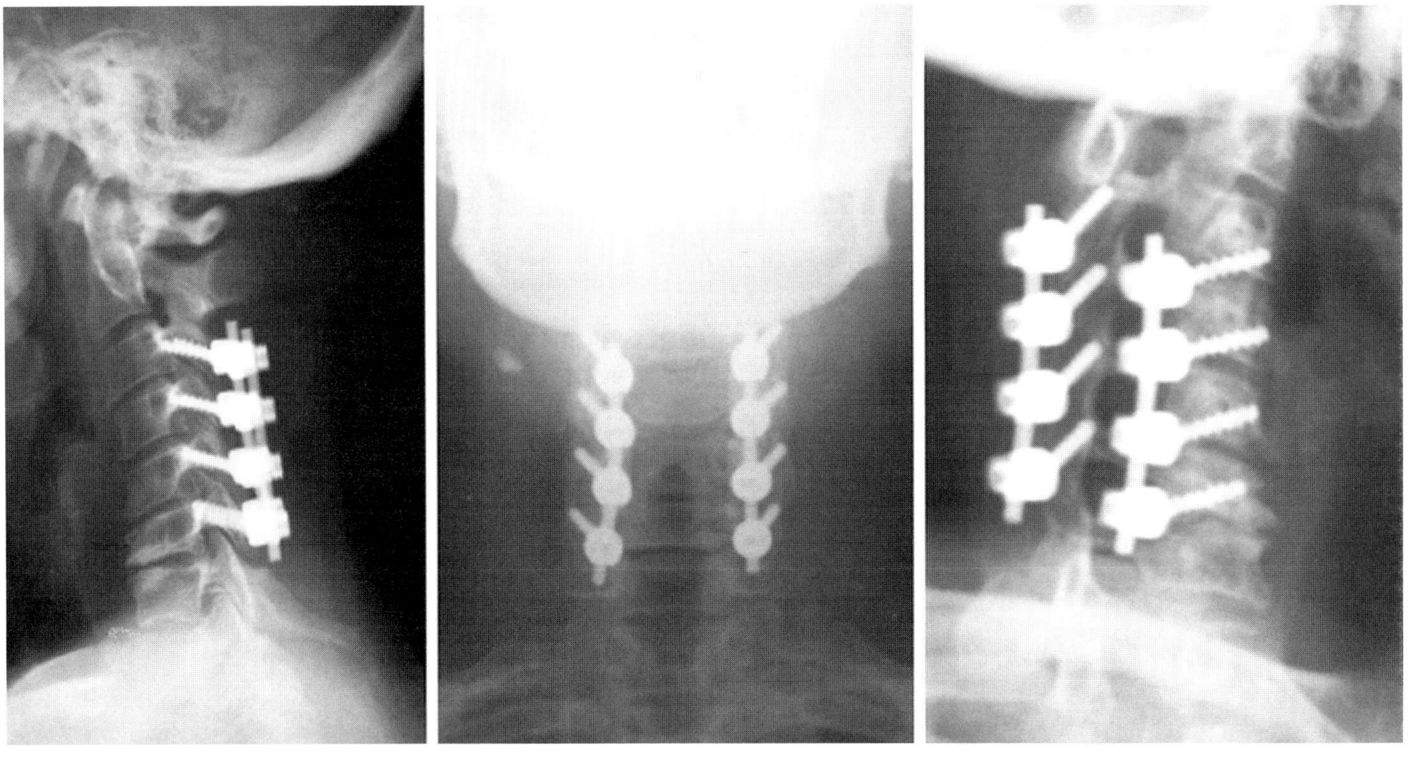

Figure 14-24. Lateral, AP, and oblique views of a C3-C6 posterior-cervical fusion using a polyaxial screw design coupled with rod fixation.

CHAPTER XV

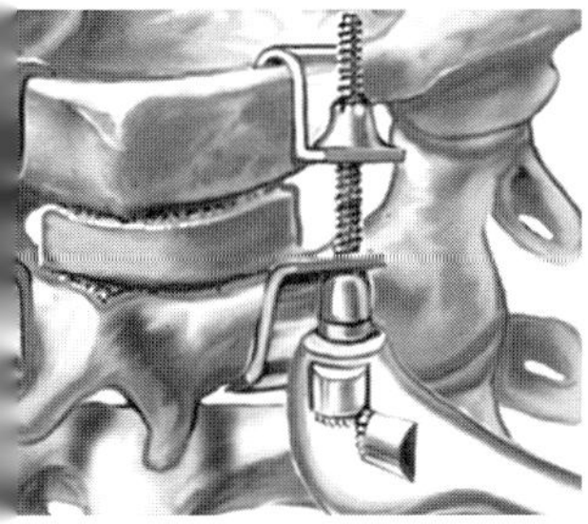

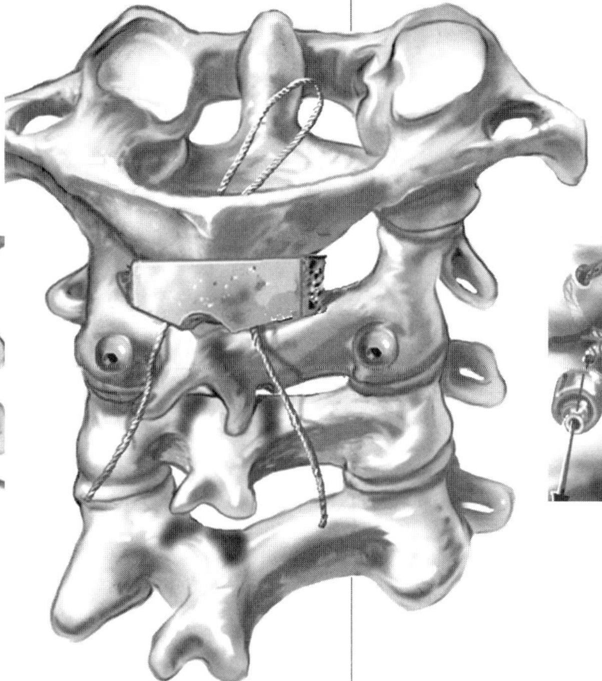

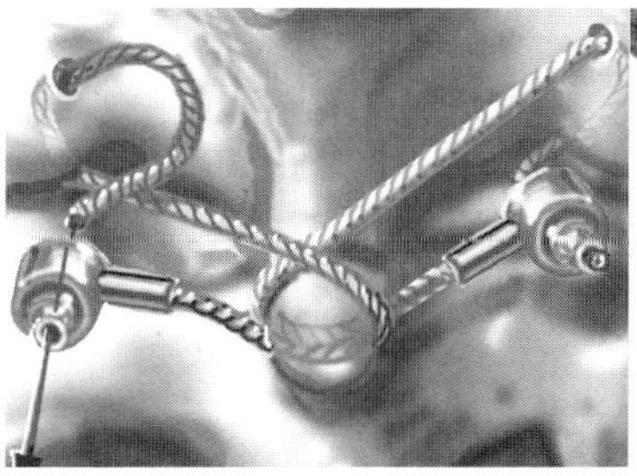

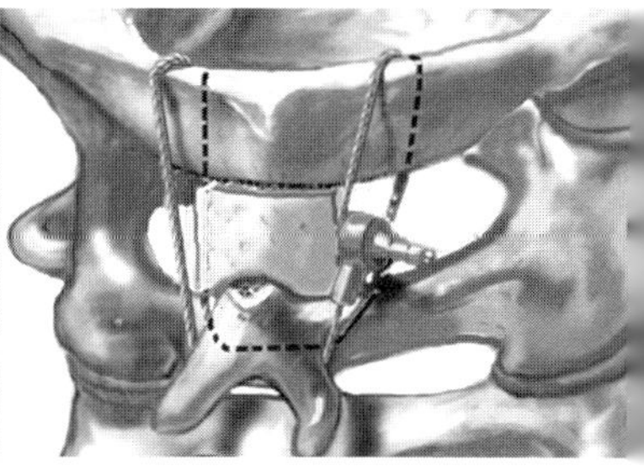

Posterior Cable Techniques

Although some posterior cable techniques are described in this chapter for historical significance, wire fixation of the posterior elements still offers the surgeon a viable option for fusion. In some instances, such as C1-C2 fixation, the posterior tension band is still a critical part of the fusion. Interspinous wiring is still an excellent option to close down a fractured facet complex, although it is now usually supplemented with lateral mass fixation. Graft wiring is also still an option, particularly in the pediatric population, because the lateral masses can be too small for screw fixation.

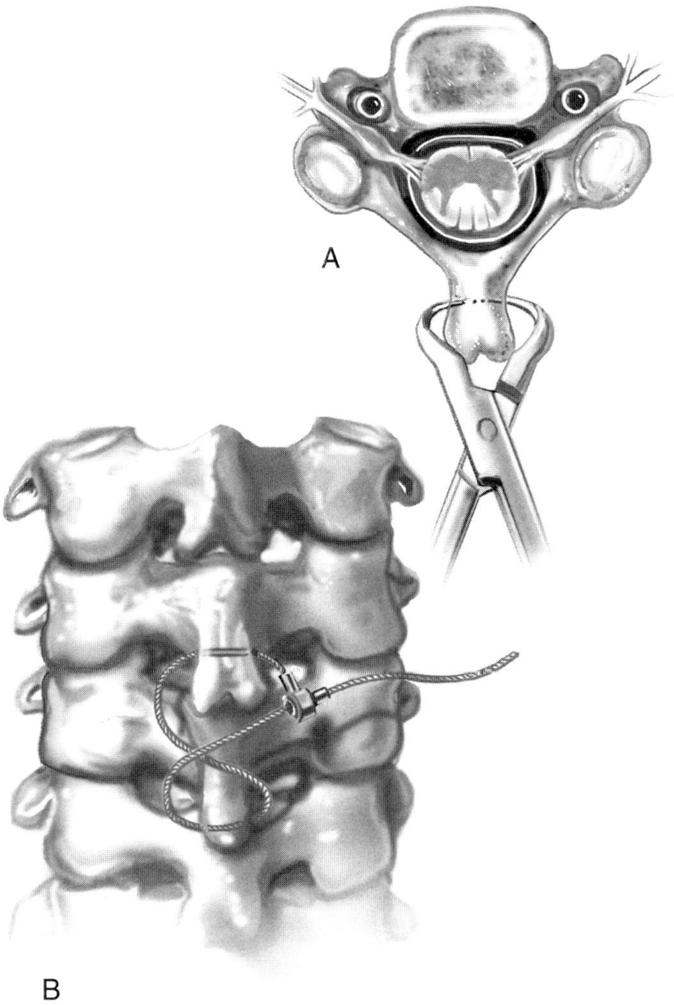

Figure 15-1, A and B. **A,** Interspinous wiring or cable techniques allow for reconstruction of a posterior tension band after lateral mass fixation or act as a stand-alone construct for a unilateral facet joint fracture. To facilitate interspinous wiring, a towel clamp or right-angled dental drill bit is used to create a hole through the spinous process. To place this hole, the surgeon must have a mind's eye view of where the cervical spinal cord is. The hole should be placed in the rostral position of the spinous process. The pilot hole should be placed at a depth slightly above the junction of the lamina/spinous process junction so as to avoid inadvertent dural puncture due to a deep lead hole. For placement of the wire through the spinous process, a hole large enough to accommodate a cable should be made. **B,** The cable should first be placed through the superior spinous process lead hole and then carried through the interspinous space and around the opposite side of the inferior spinous process. To complete the loop, the cable is looped back through the interspinous space, and the hat is secured over the cable. Using a tensioner, appropriate tension is applied to restore the posterior tension band.

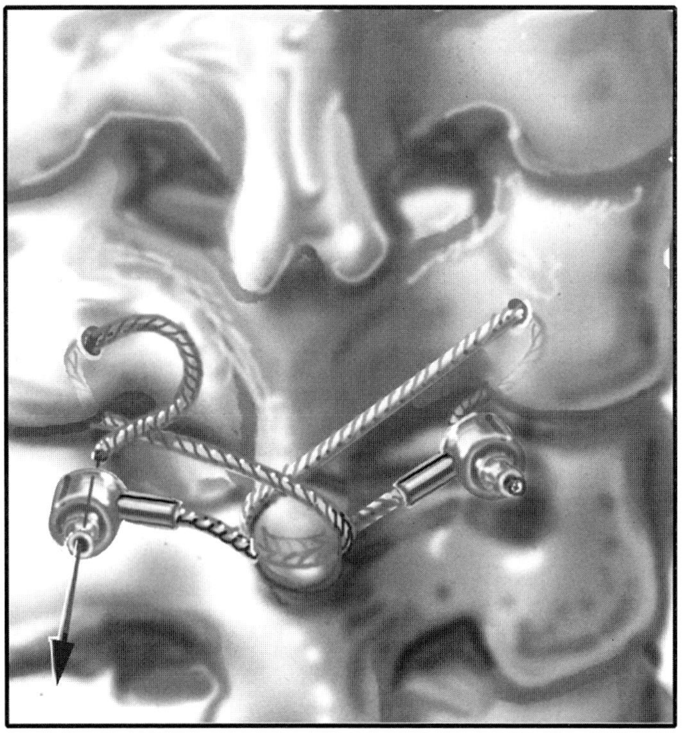

Figure 15-2. An alternative to interspinous wiring is facet-to-spinous process wiring. This technique can also be used for unilateral instability; however, fractures at the facet joint may make cable placement difficult. A right-angled dental drill bit is used to place an entry hole perpendicular through the superior and inferior facet joint. A Penfield dissector can be placed into the facet joint to prevent drilling too deep. The cable is then passed through the path via the pilot holes and the spinous process.

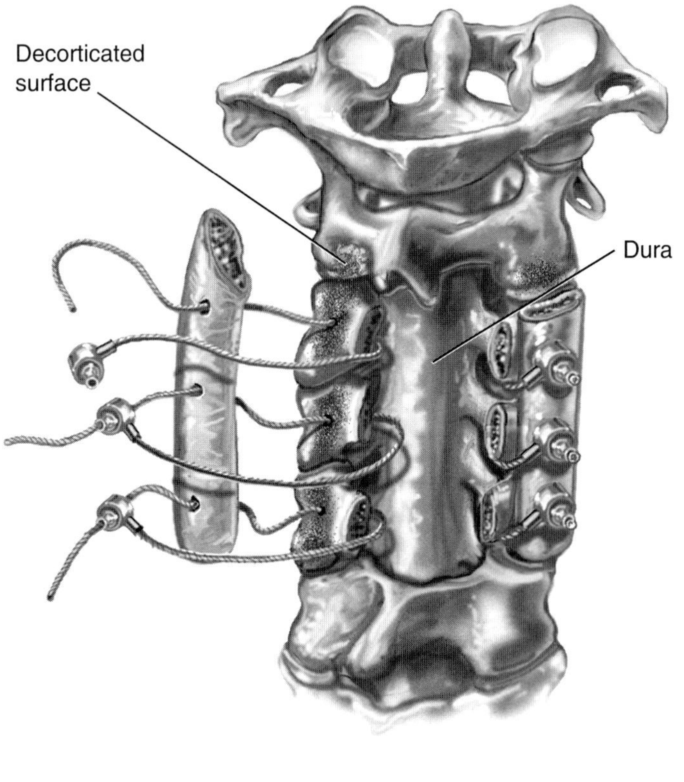

Figure 15-3. Facet wiring techniques can also be used to secure autograft. This is particularly useful in applying autologous rib graft to the facet joints. This technique can be used in lieu of posterior plates or screw rod constructs if they are not available. Decortication of the lateral masses and facet joints is performed with a drill bit. The cable is then passed through the graft and the facet joint and tightened down with the tensioner. This can be performed in conjunction with a posterior cervical decompression or as a fusion alone.

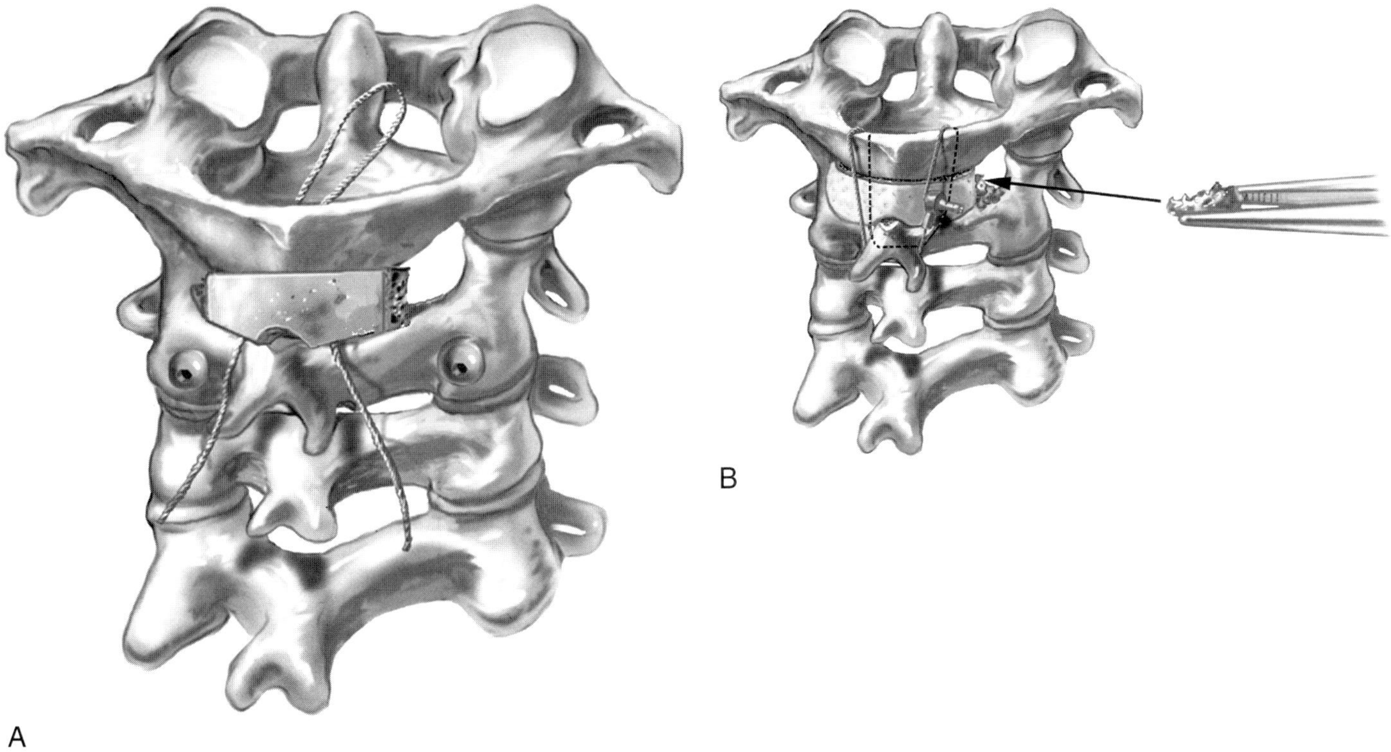

Figure 15-4, A and B. A, C1-C2 fusion options include a Sonntag-type posterior tension band fixation. A Sonntag fusion involves a looped cable passed under the C1 ring and lassoed around the spinous process of C2. A customized autologous graft is placed between the previously decorticated C1-C2 interspace. The cable is then tightened to secure a cancellous-to-cancellous bone surface. The cable not only holds the graft in place but also allows for adequate compression. **B,** Morselized autograft can be packed into the lateral portion of the fusion to augment arthrodesis.

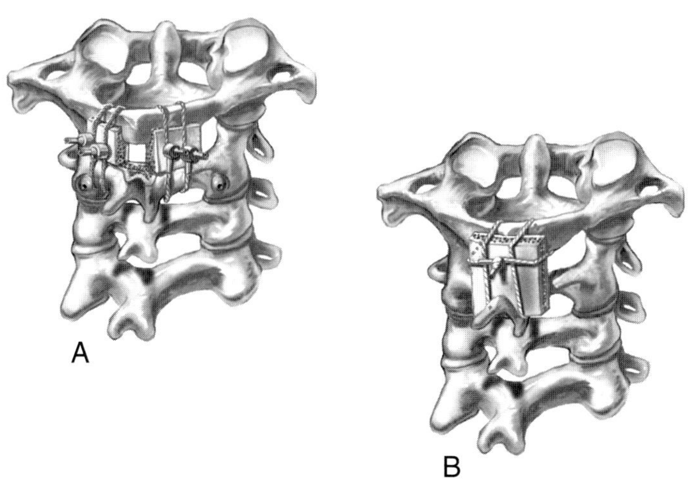

Figure 15-5, A and B. A, Other posterior tension band options for C1-C2 include bilateral autograft secured with double cables under C1 and C2 representing the classic Brooks-type fusion. **B,** The Galle-type fusion can also be used by placing a bone graft in a crossed wire technique. Although both techniques have shown valid fusion rates, biomechanical studies suggest that the Sonntag is a superior tension band construct. These techniques can be used alone or in conjunction with C1-C2 transarticular screw fixation. The addition of transarticular screws to the posterior tension band constructs increases the fusion rate from the 80% range with tension band alone to the 95% to 98% range with combined tension band and screw fixation.

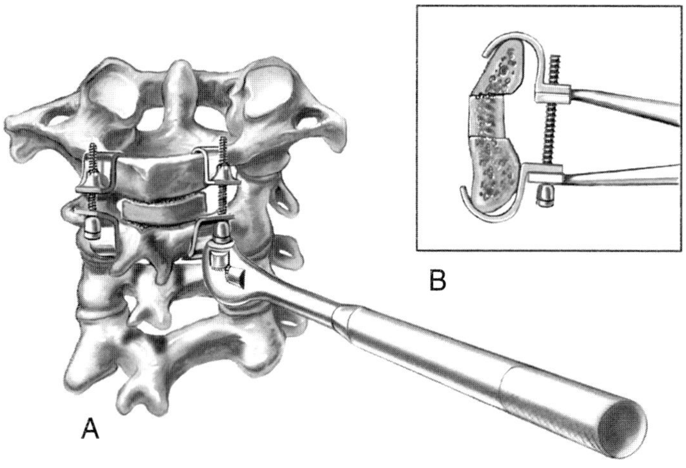

Figure 15-6, A and B. Posterior C1-C2 clamp techniques including the Halifax clamp can also be used to secure a posterior tension band with autograft at the C1-C2 junction.

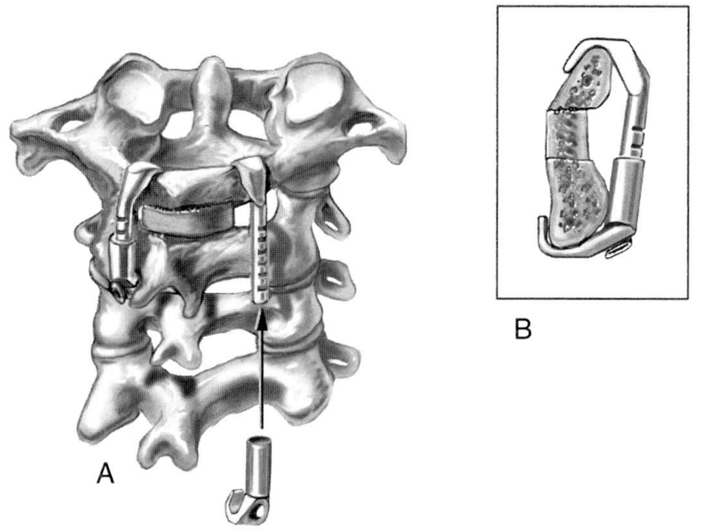

Figure 15-7, A and B. The Apofix clamp system also allows for an excellent tension band construct in the placement of autographs between C1 and C2. We have found this system to be more successful with fewer mechanical complications than the older Halifax system. An important point with the Apofix system is that the bone graft width should be made significantly smaller than a typical Sonntag-type fusion. If the bone graft is too wide, it is difficult to affix the Apofix clamps onto the C1 and C2 lamina. We typically use a square-shaped bicortical graft and then pack smaller morselized portions of bone in the lateral aspect of the fusion site.

COMMON PITFALLS

Figure 15-8. A common pitfall for interspinous wiring is placement of the cable hole too posterior on the spinous process or too close to the interspinous ligament. If poor purchase is made in this area, the cable can pull through the bones and become dislodged, thus requiring another interspinous cable hole to be made.

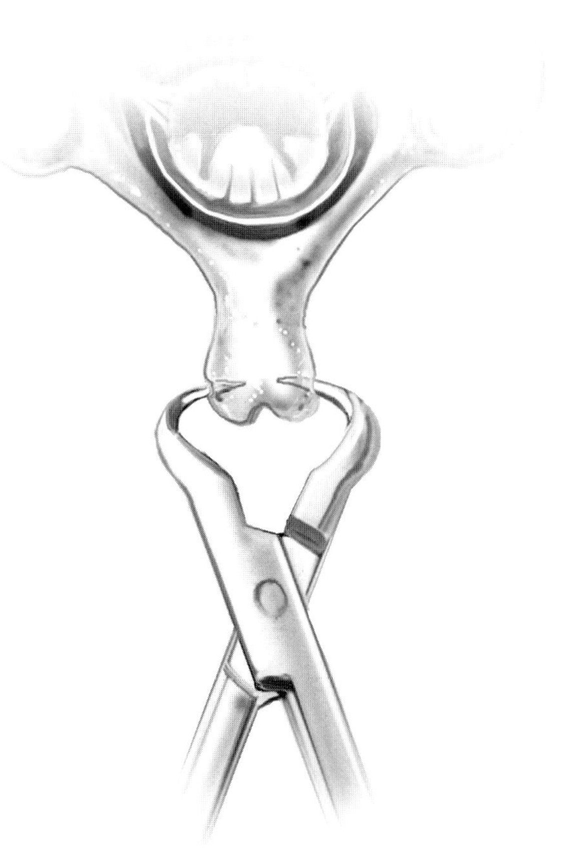

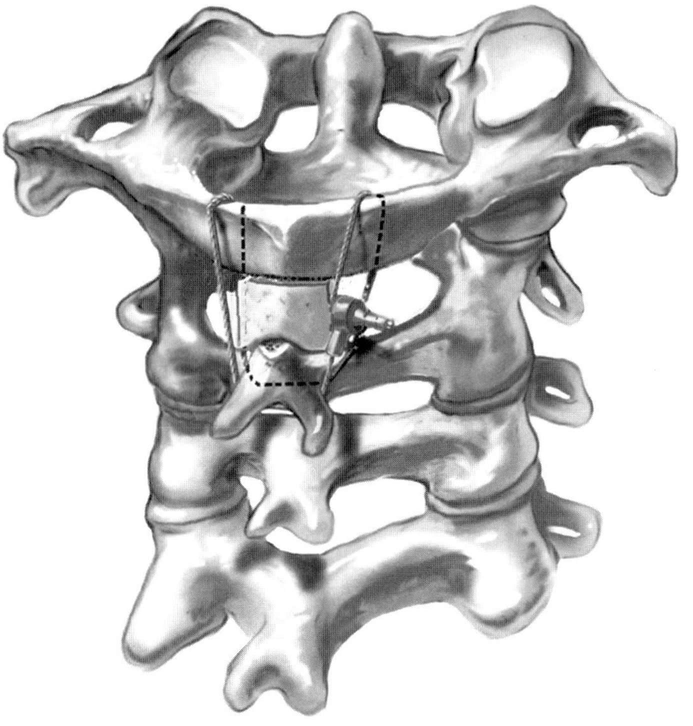

Figure 15-9. A pitfall of the posterior C1-C2 cable technique is customizing too short a graft. If the bone graft is too short for the Sonntag-type fusion, it may not be tightly opposed to the C1-C2 cancellous interface. The other problem with a graft that is too short is that if overtightening of the cable is used to better secure the graft, the C1-C2 relationship may change with overcompression. With a Sonntag fusion, the bone graft should also be wider than it is tall for proper capture of the bone graft by the lateral cables.

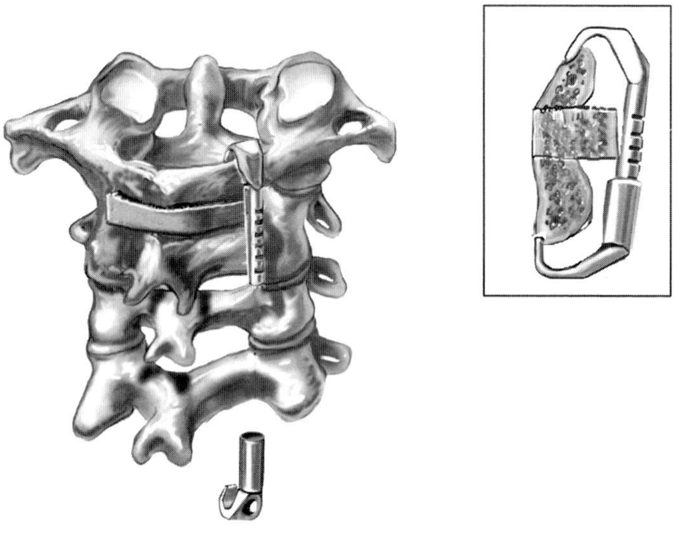

Figure 15-10. If too large a bone graft is placed when using the Apofix system, it can be difficult to anchor the clamps under C1 and C2.

POSTOPERATIVE RESULTS

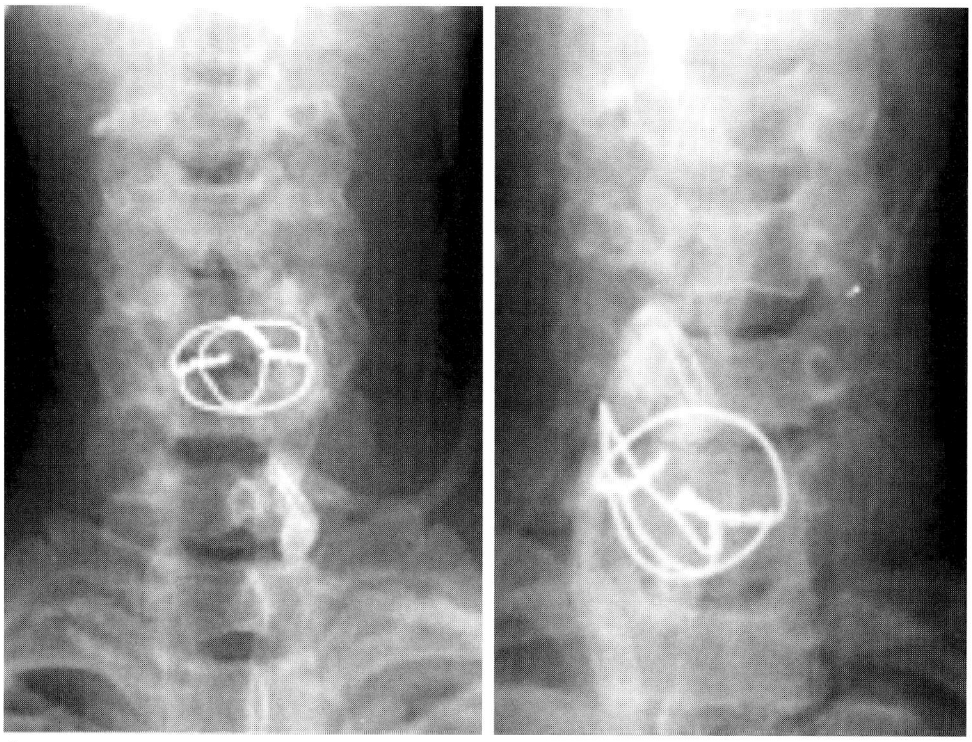

A B

Figure 15-11, A and B. Anterior-posterior (AP) spine x-ray demonstrating interspinous wire fixation **(A)** and facet-spinous process wiring **(B)**.

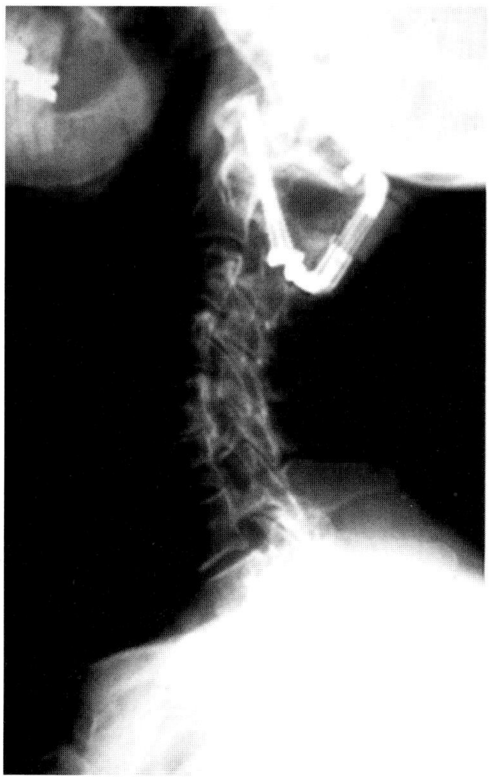

Figure 15-12, A and B. Lateral C spine x-rays demonstrating successful C1-C2 arthrodesis utilizing C1-C2 transarticular screws and an Apofix C1-C2 posterior clamp fixation,

CHAPTER

XVI

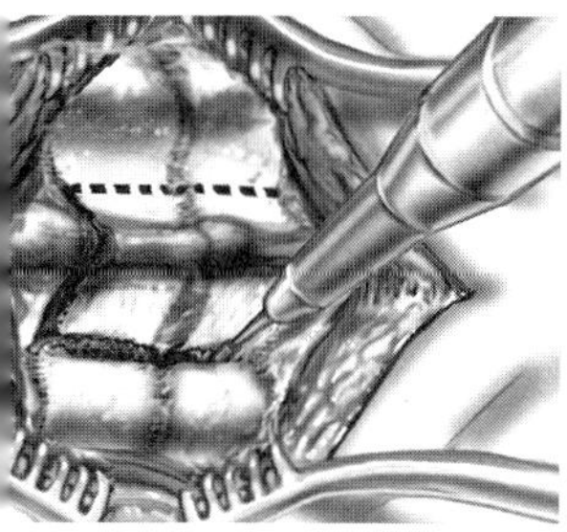

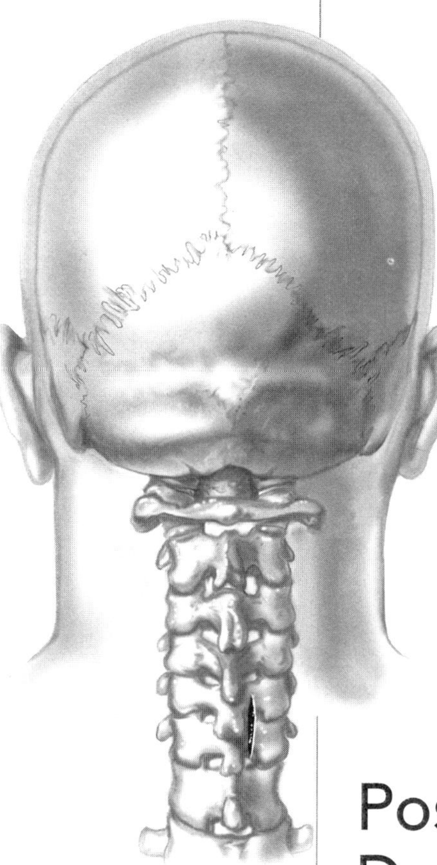

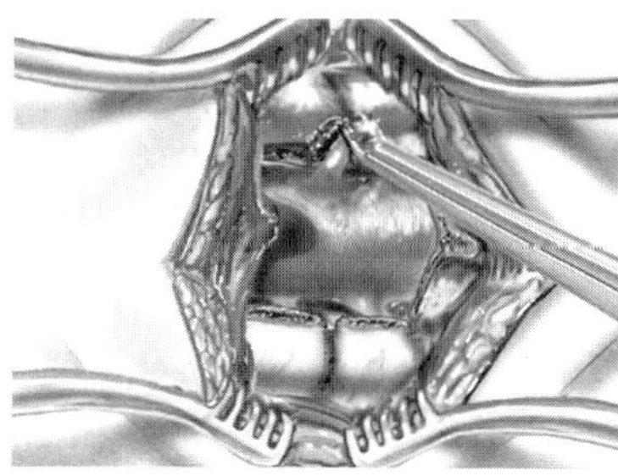

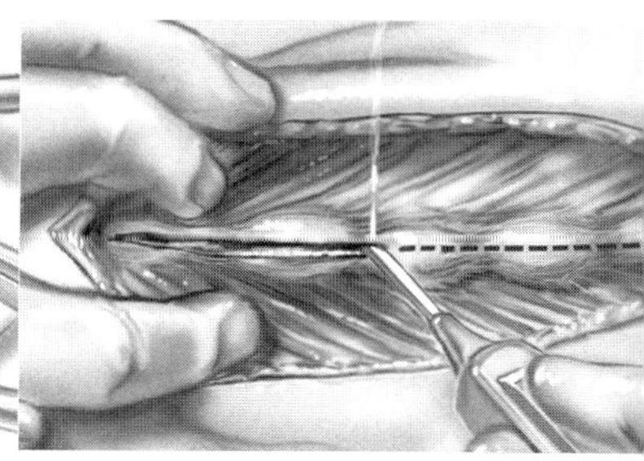

Posterior Decompression: Laminoforaminotomy, Laminectomy, and Laminaplasty

Laminoforaminotomy is a posterior decompression technique for cervical foraminal stenosis and for small soft lateral disc fragments that are compressing cervical nerve roots and causing symptomatic cervical radiculopathy refractory to conservative therapy. Posterior laminoforaminotomy is one of the oldest spinal procedures for radiculopathy and offers the potential advantage of preserving motion because it does not require a cervical fusion. In selected patients, this procedure produces excellent results with a minimal complication rate. The only drawbacks to this procedure include a higher recurrence rate and the potential for postoperative deltoid weakness in patients with C4-C5 pathology.

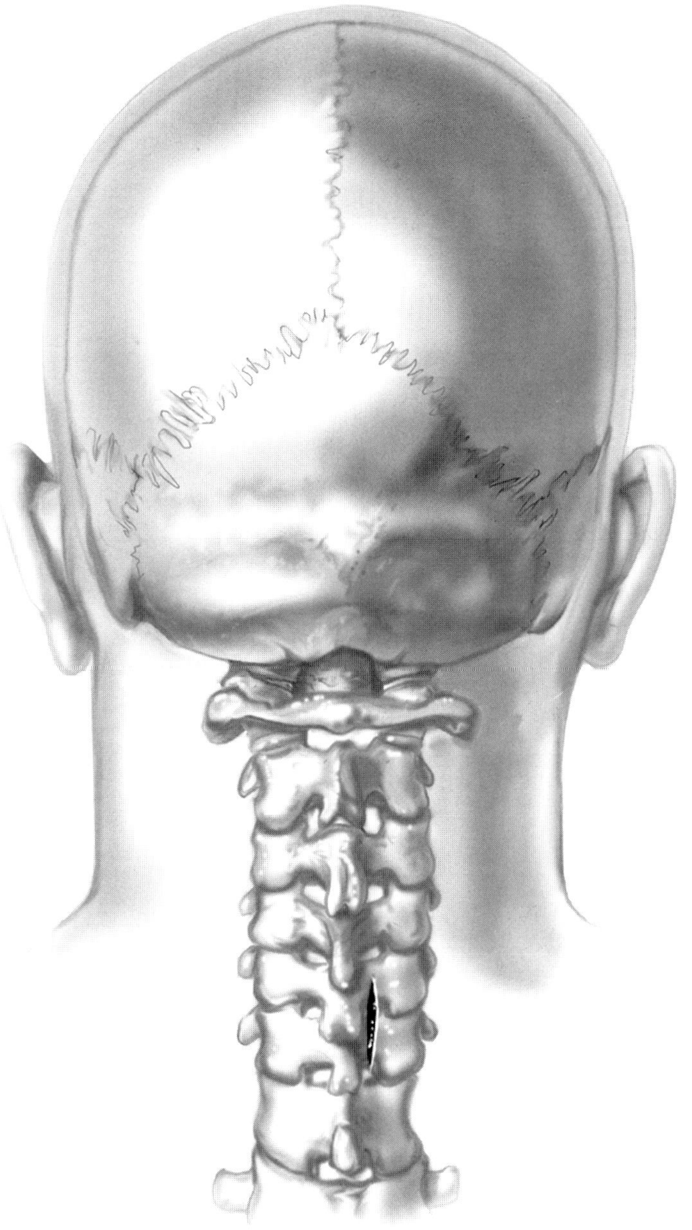

Figure 16-1. To minimize incision length, a preoperative postpositional radiograph should be obtained to mark the incision directly over the appropriate facet joint. After the appropriate skin level has been identified and marked, a 2-cm incision is made on the lateral border of the spinous process on the affected side. Dissection is carried down using monopolar subperiosteal technique to expose the appropriate nerve root exit zone at the level of the facet joint. An alternative is to use a tubular retraction system for a minimal access approach.

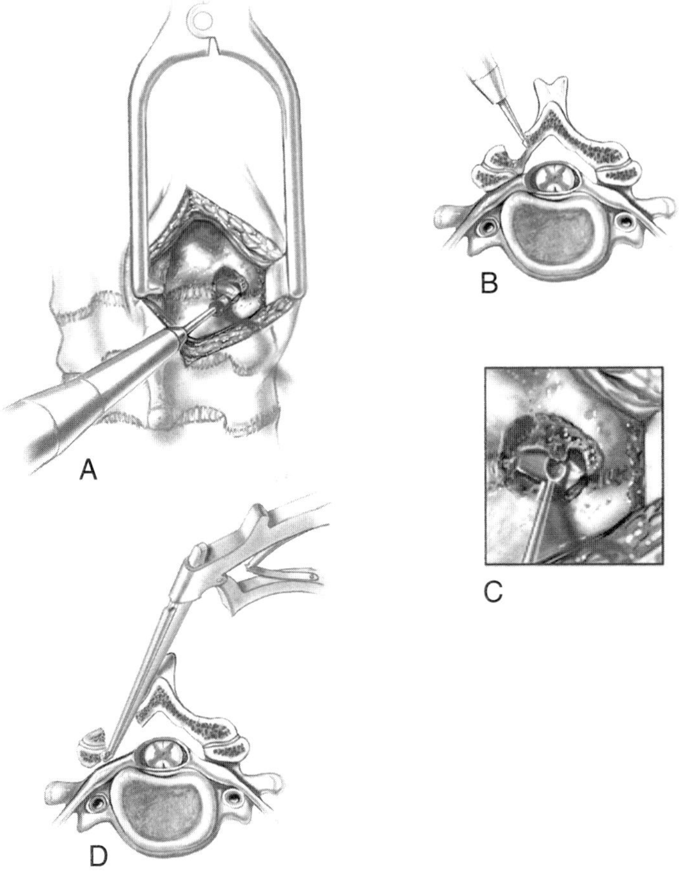

Figure 16-2, A–D. A second intraoperative radiograph should be obtained, and the exposed facet joint should be marked to confirm the appropriate level **(A).** A matchstick drill bit is used to drill a small hole that incorporates 50% of the superior lamina and 50% of the inferior lamina extending out to, but not more than, 50% of the facet joint on that side. The bone is thinned down using an eggshell drilling technique **(B** and **C).** The remaining cortical surface is removed either with a curette or a Kerrison rongeur. The yellow ligament is identified and opened with a right-angled nerve hook or an up-angled curette. The ligament is removed, and the lateral edge of the dura and exiting nerve root are visualized. Dural veins are coagulated and divided, and the facet joint is undercut to decompress the nerve root. Fifty percent of the facet joint must be preserved to maintain joint integrity **(D).** A 1- to 2-mm Kerrison rongeur is used to open the distal foramen without compromising the more superficial joint. If a soft disc fragment is seen compressing the nerve root on magnetic resonance scan, the shoulder of the nerve root is dissected free, and epidural veins are coagulated. The disc fragment can be removed with a right-angled nerve hook.

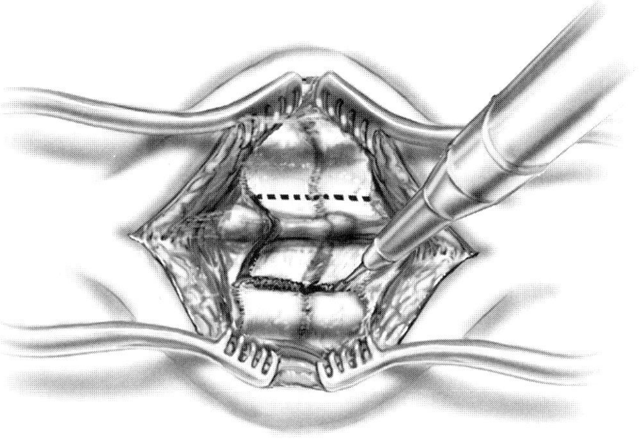

Figure 16-3. When a posterior laminectomy short-segment decompression is planned, an incision of an appropriate length is made over the affected segment. The dissection is carried down with a monopolar subperiosteal technique, and a self-retaining retractor is placed. The appropriate segment is identified and cleaned of all soft tissues, and the laminar-facet line is identified. A mini matchstick drill bit is used to drill a trough bilaterally to disarticulate the lamina from the facet complex. Alternatively, a small foot-plated drill can be used to create the bone cuts.

Figure 16-4. The posterior elements are then removed. The spinal cord is decompressed, and the dural veins are coagulated.

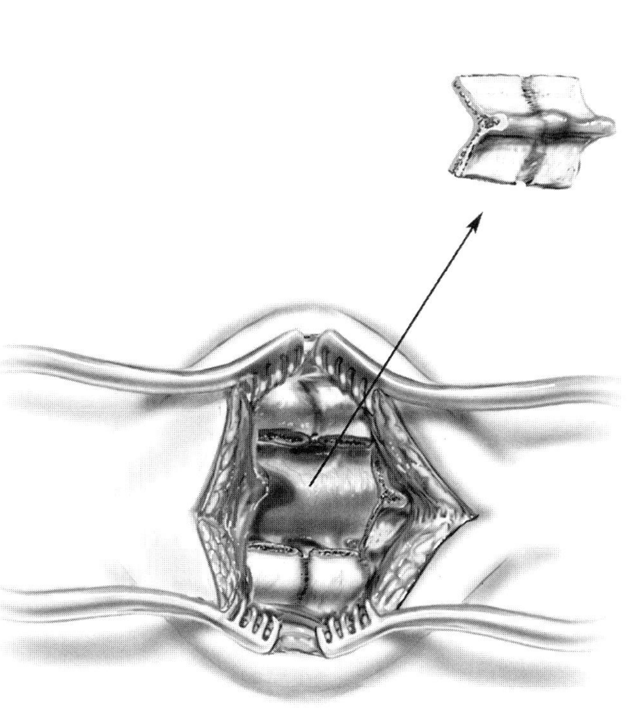

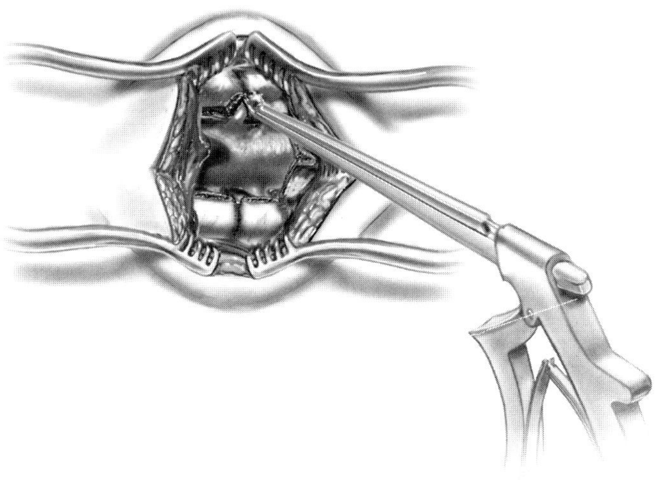

Figure 16-5. A 1- or 2-mm Kerrison rongeur can be used to extend the foraminotomy for nerve root decompression in patients with symptomatic radiculopathy.

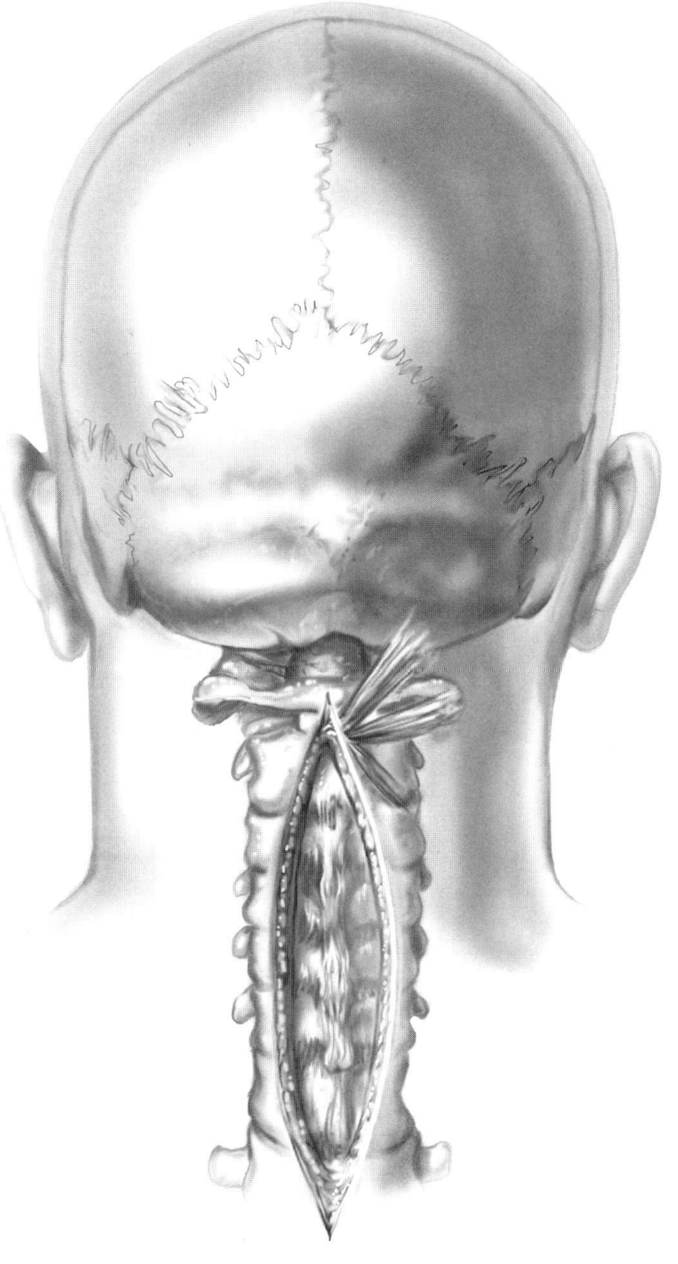

Figure 16-6. In longer-segment decompressions, a longer incision is planned to give adequate exposure with more decompression. The lateral portions of the facet joints do not need to be exposed for a decompression, and this tissue should be preserved to maintain a vascular supply to the facet complex.

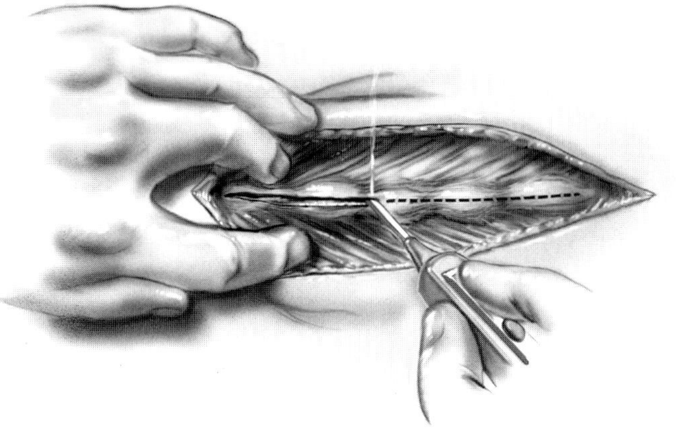

Figure 16-7. Before placing a self-retaining retractor, we have used a finger retraction technique to expose the posterior elements.

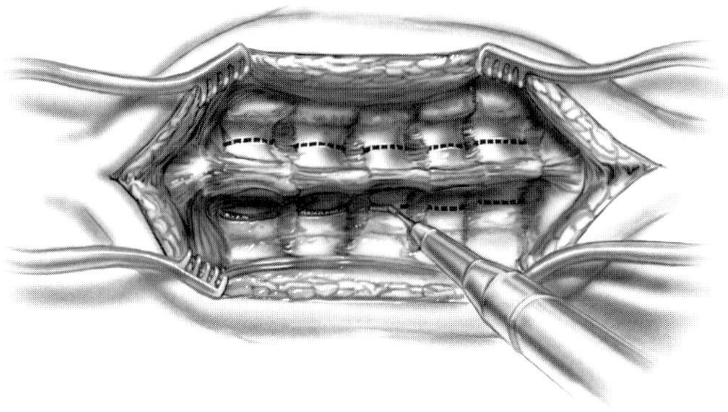

Figure 16-8. The lamina facet line is identified, and the trough is drilled with a mini matchstick drill bit along the lateral border of the lamina. This maneuver is performed bilaterally, thus disarticulating the lamina and spinous processes from the facet complex. The facet complex must be preserved during the decompression to maintain stability.

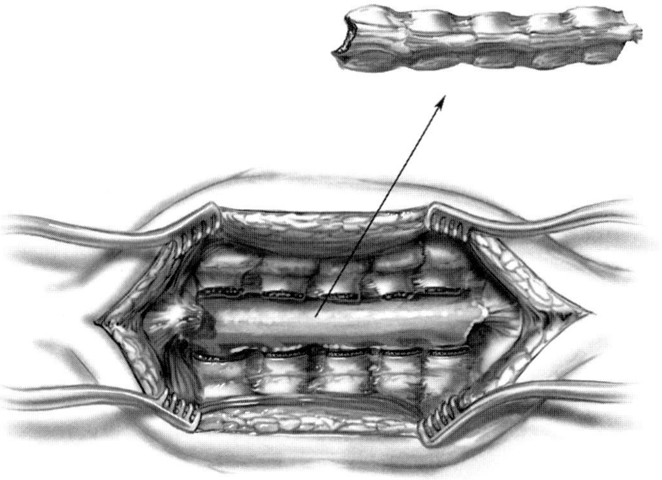

Figure 16-9. The posterior elements are then removed, and epidural veins are coagulated with bipolar cautery. A 2-mm Kerrison or 4-0 up-angled curette is helpful to ensure complete bone removal.

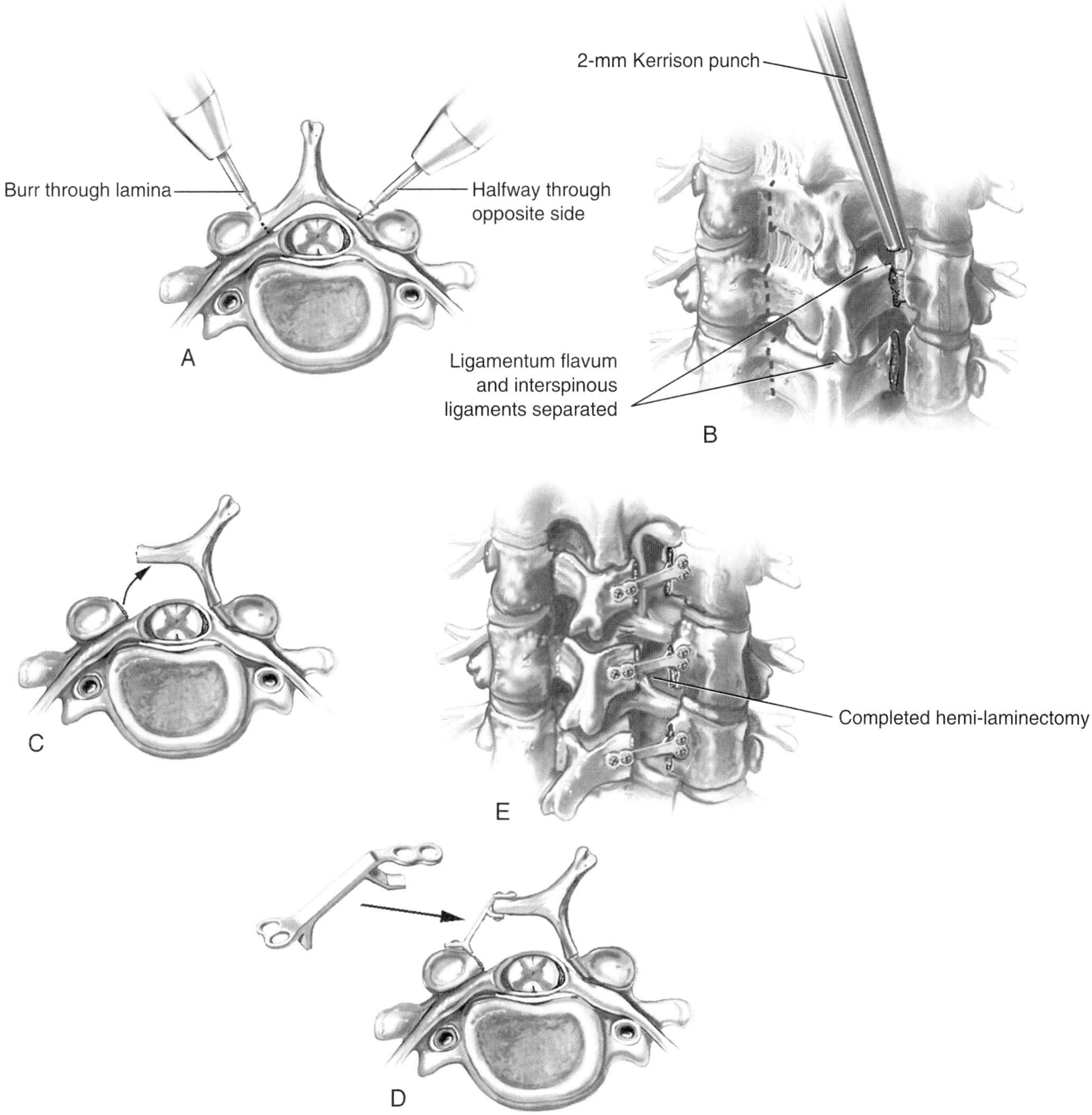

Figure 16-10, A–E. Laminoplasty is an alternative option for providing a posterior cervical decompression with anatomical preservation. **A** and **B**, This technique involves using the mini matchstick drill bit to disarticulate one side of the lamina from the facet joint complex. The contralateral side is also drilled only halfway through the cortical margin. The disarticulated side is then cleaned of soft tissue and remaining bone removed with a 2-mm Kerrison rongeur. **C**, The posterior elements are then rocked posteriorly, thus creating a greenstick fracture on the partially drilled side. **D** and **E**, Either bone graft or a laminaplasty device is placed to maintain the open-book position of the posterior elements. This can be secured to the lamina and facet joints with screw fixation. This technique allows for enlargement of the spinal canal without removal of the posterior tension band.

COMMON PITFALLS

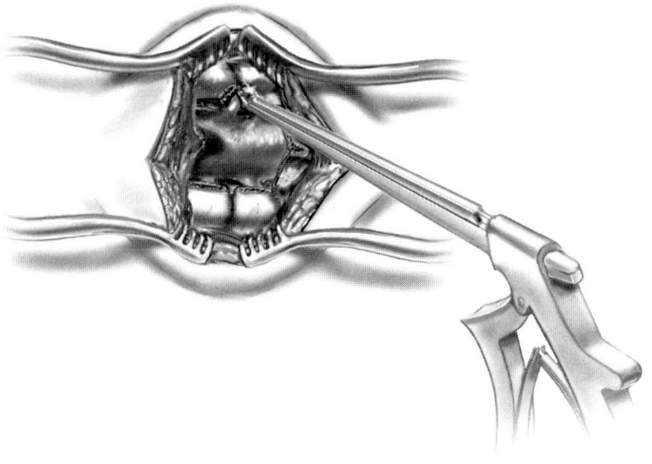

Figure 16-11. One common pitfall is to create a laminectomy that is too wide by violating the facet joints or by doing bilateral extensive foraminotomies at one level. It is important that at least 50% of the facet joints are preserved when performing a multilevel laminectomy. The symptomatic root can be decompressed with a foraminotomy, but care must be taken to preserve the majority of the facet joint. If the facet joint is not preserved, the patient has a higher likelihood of cervical instability.

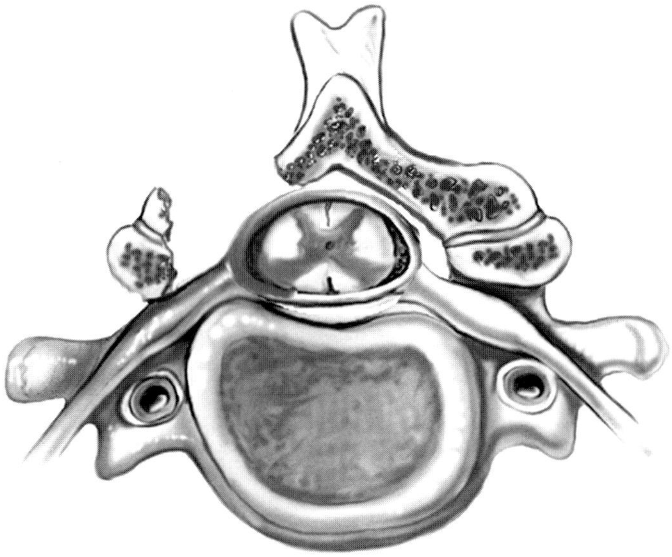

Figure 16-12. Another pitfall in posterior approaches is creating a facetectomy that is too wide when performing a laminoforaminotomy. If more than 50% of the facet joint is drilled out, there is a higher likelihood for instability and recurrent radiculopathy. To enlarge a foraminotomy, the foramen must be undercut with a 1- to 2-mm Kerrison rongeur, with the exception of the C4-C5 level (see next page).

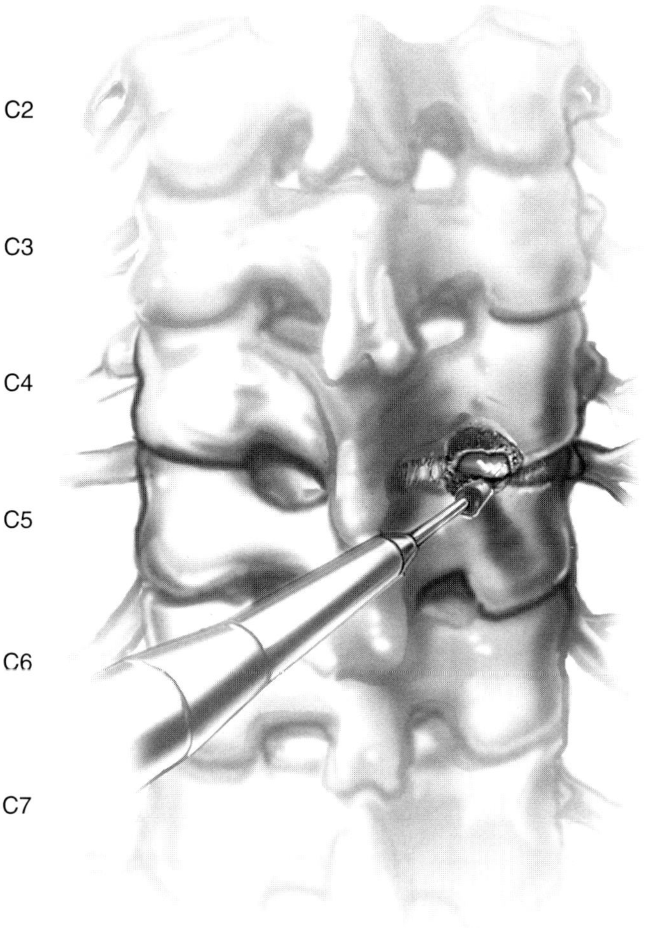

Figure 16-13. C5 radiculopathies that are approached posteriorly are of special concern. The C5 nerve root seems to be more sensitive to manipulation from either an anterior or posterior approach. For this reason, great care is exercised in decompressing the C5 nerve root during a C4-C5 laminoforaminotomy. A mini matchstick drill bit is used to drill out the foraminotomy almost completely. Then, using a small, forward-angled curette, the cortical rim is removed. It is important to avoid placement of any large Kerrison rongeur on the C4-C5 foramen; this would put the C5 nerve root at risk for manipulation, irritation, and subsequent deltoid weakness.

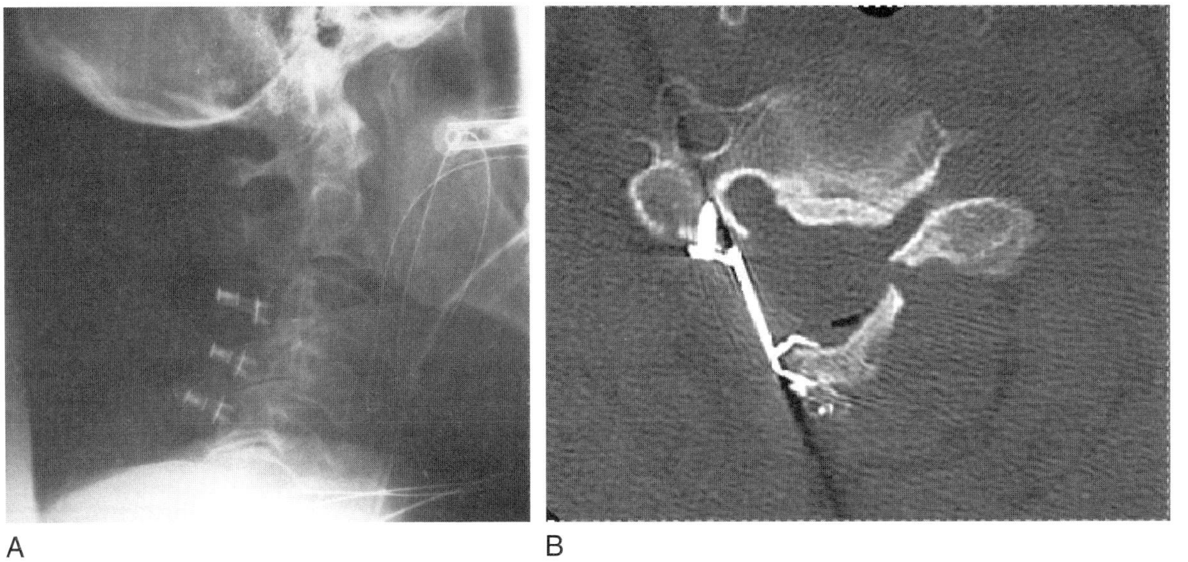

Figure 16-14, A and B. **A,** Lateral cervical spine radiograph demonstrating laminoplasty instrumentation. **B,** Axial computed tomography (CT) scan demonstrating an open door laminoplasty with subsequent enlargement of the spinal canal with preservation of the majority of the posterior element anatomy.

CHAPTER

XVII

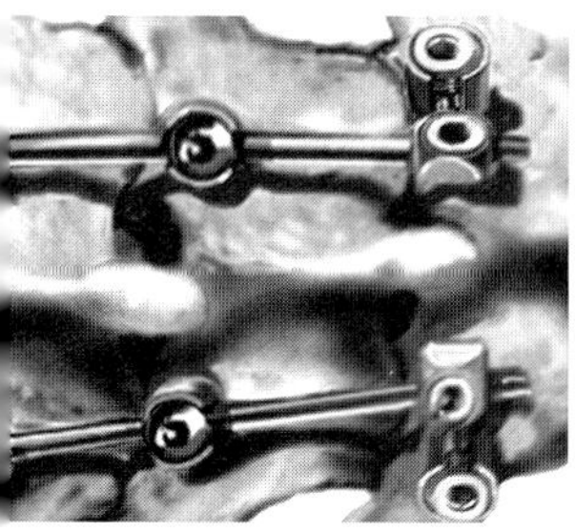

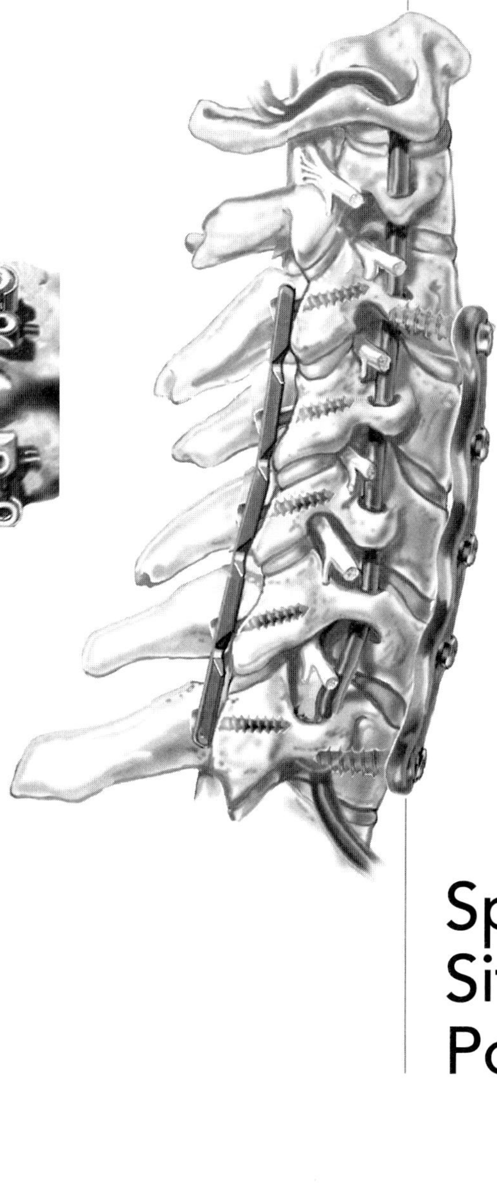

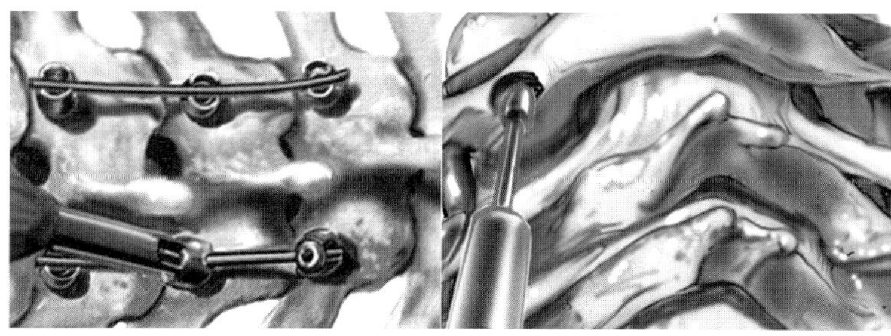

Special Situations: Posterior

This chapter describes certain unique fusion techniques used to incorporate junctional segments and special screw fixation strategies. The first section covers incorporation of C2 into fusion constructs. C2 can be captured either by pars or pedicle fixation for upper cervical arthrodesis or for long-segment subaxial cervical spine constructs.

The next section discusses hybrid technologies used to marry junctional segments in certain long constructs. The last section discusses special considerations for combined anterior posterior arthrodesis.

C2 PARS AND PEDICLE SCREWS

The anatomy of the C2 pars intraarticularis and adjacent structures is not amenable to lateral mass screw fixation. Therefore, when incorporating C2 in a fusion construct, either a C2 pars screw or a C2 pedicle screw must be used. A C2 pars screw incorporates the same entry point and trajectory as a C1-C2 transarticular screw. The length of the screw is shorter, however, and does not traverse across the C1-C2 joint.

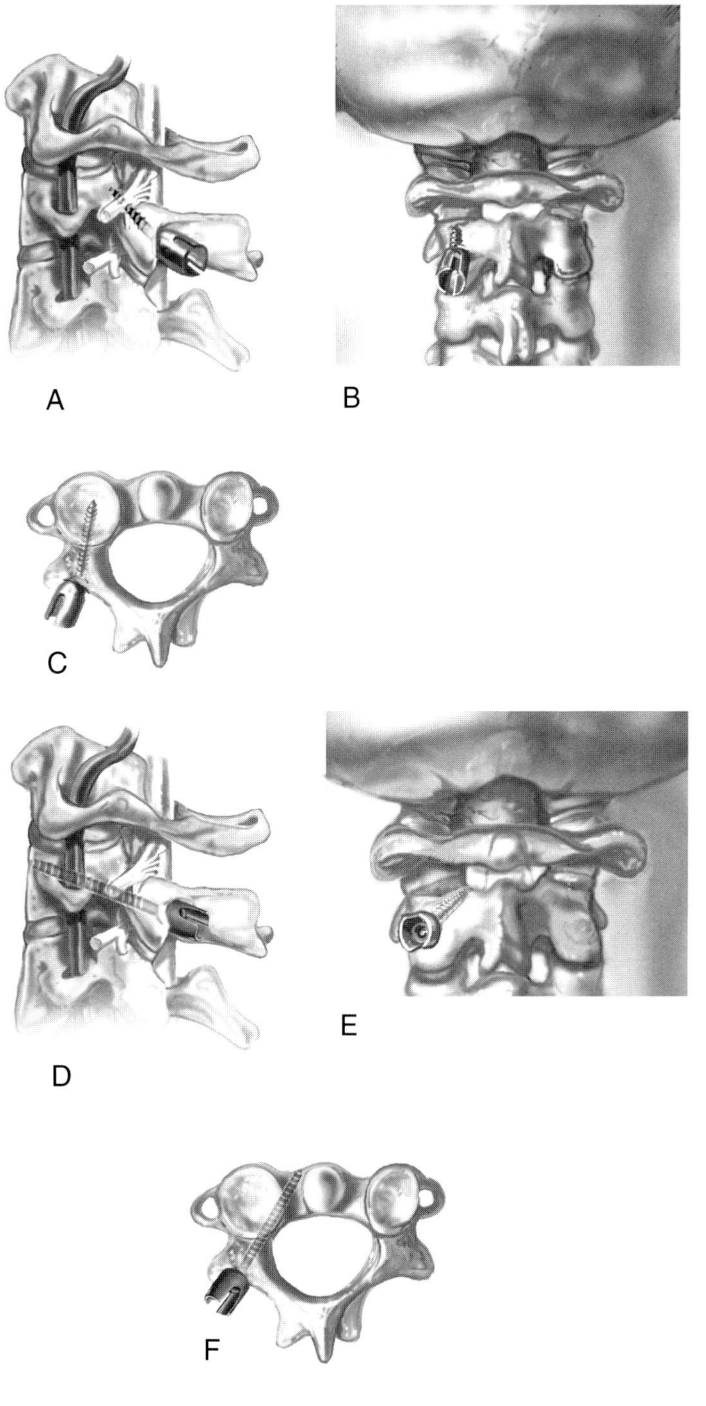

Figure 17-1, A–F. Lateral **(A)**, posterior-anterior **(B)**, and axial **(C)** schematic of C2 pars intraarticularis screw placement. Note the screw length (short of the C1-C2 joint space) and trajectory (identical to C1-C2 transarticular screw). Lateral **(D)**, posterior-anterior **(E)**, and axial **(F)** schematic of C2 pedicle screw placement. Note the longer screw length and more medial trajectory compared with C2 pars intraarticularis screw placement.

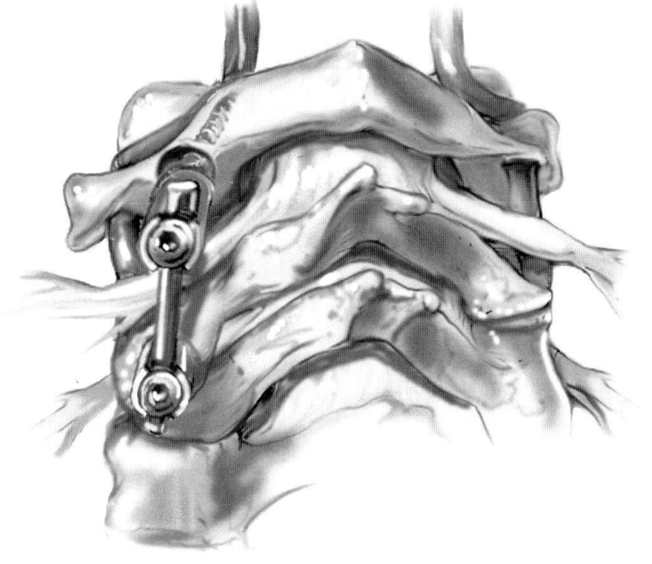

A

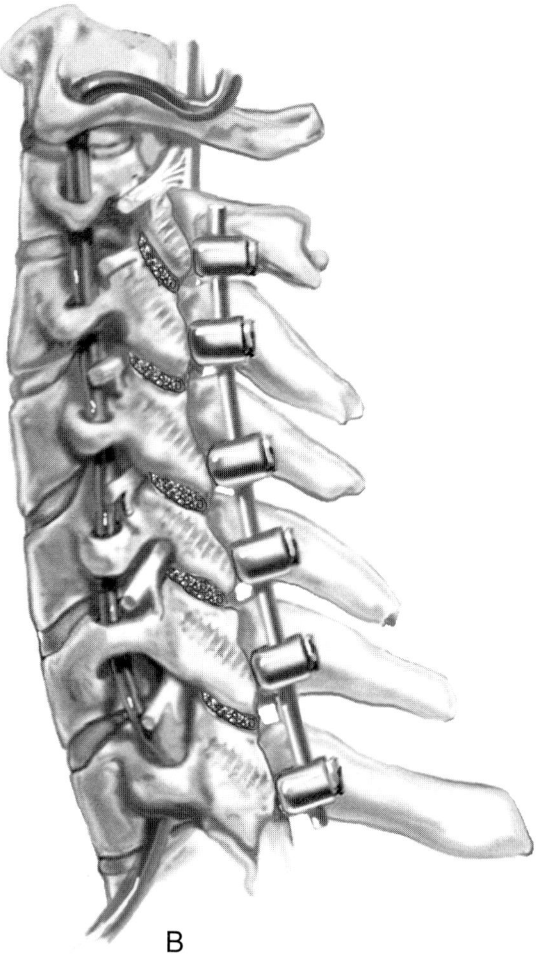

B

Figure 17-2, A. Incorporation of C2 in an upper cervical construct.

Figure 17-2, B. Incorporation of C2 in a lower cervical construct.

C1-C2 SCREW FIXATION USING C1 LATERAL MASS SCREWS

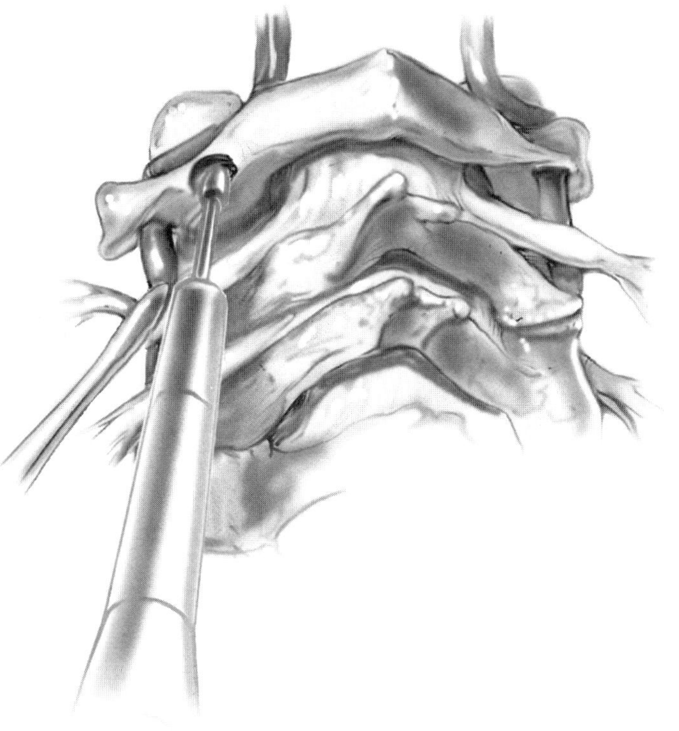

Figure 17-3. Placement of C1 lateral mass screws allows for another option in the treatment of C1-C2 instability in addition to C1-C2 transarticular screw fixation. The level of dissection and exposure is similar to the exposure for C1-C2 transarticular screw fixation. Once adequate exposure is obtained, a small inferior portion of the C1 lateral mass is removed with a drill to expose the entry point for the C1 lateral mass screw. The C2 nerve root is retracted inferiorly. The entry site is above the C2 pars.

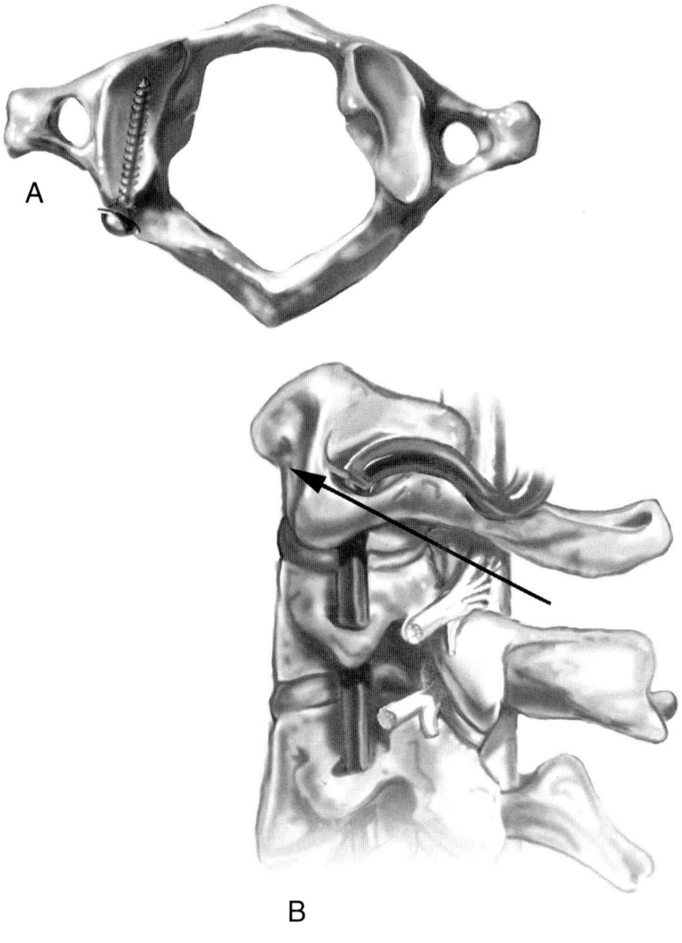

Figure 17-4, A and B. Ten to fifteen-degree lateral to medial direction is the desired trajectory to capture the C1 lateral mass. The vertebral artery lies lateral and rostral to this trajectory. The rostrocaudal direction is approximately a 0- to 10-degree angulation. A lateral C-arm is used, with the screw aimed at the C1 tubercle on lateral C-arm flurograph. Screw length is determined by preoperative computed tomography (CT) scan and is typically 35 mm in length.

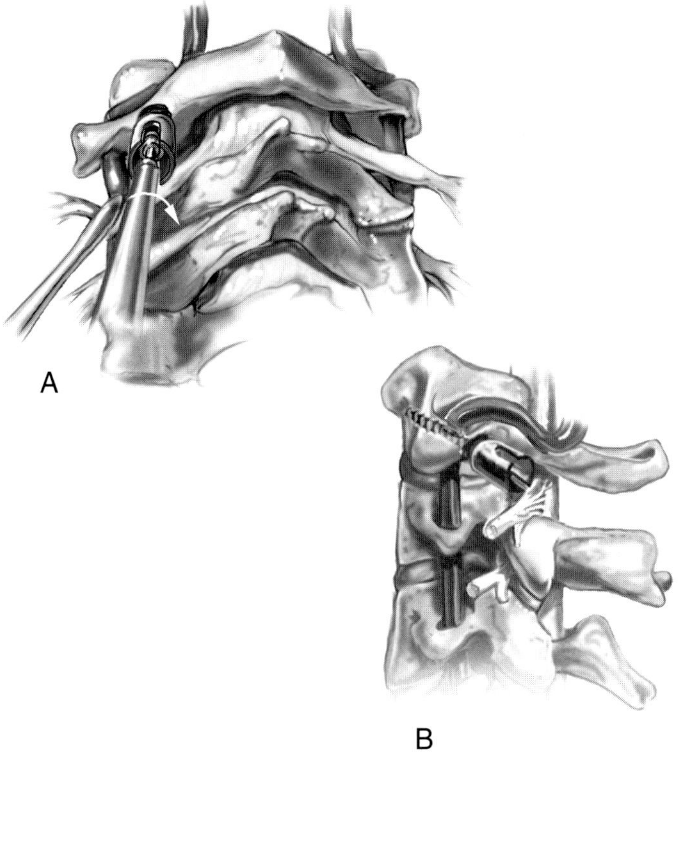

Figure 17-5. Once the appropriate site is marked, drilled, and tapped, a polyaxial screw is placed above the C2 nerve root. The polyaxial head should be left long enough so that it doesn't apply pressure to the C2 nerve root. Screw length is typically 35 mm.

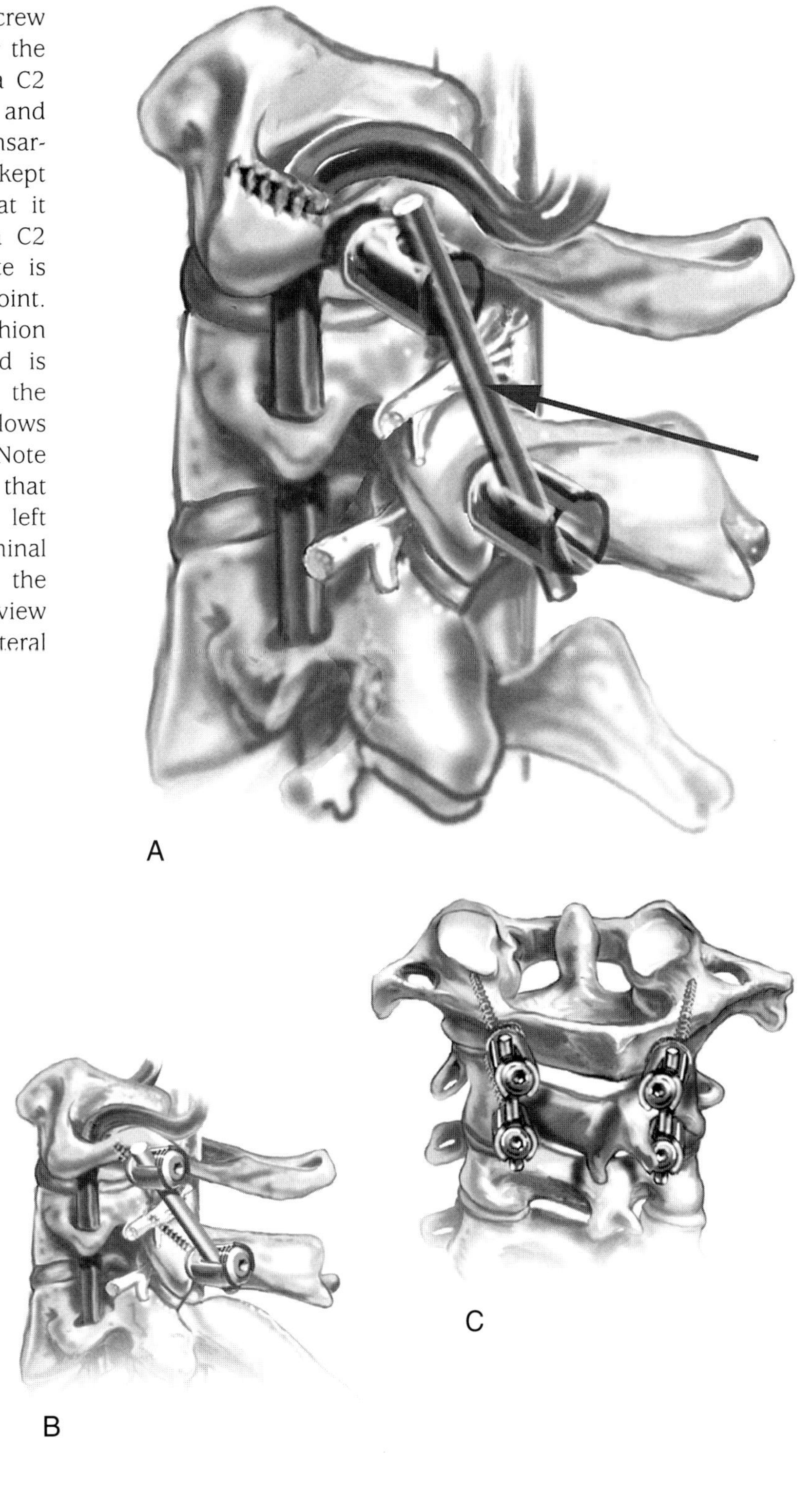

Figure 17-6, A–C. **A,** Either a C2 pars screw or a C2 pedicle screw can be placed for the capture of the inferior C2 complex. If a C2 pars screw is planned, screw trajectory and entry points are identical to the C1-C2 transarticular approach. The screw is simply kept shorter at approximately 18 mm so that it does not traverse the C1-C2 joint. If a C2 pedicle screw is planned, the entry site is 5 mm lateral to the medial C2-C3 facet joint. The screw is directed in a more medial fashion to capture the C2 pedicle. **B,** The rod is then attached to the polyaxial head of the screw. The polyaxial mechanism allows for more freedom in attaching the rod. Note that the polyaxial screw head in C1 that captures the lateral mass must be left proud to allow room for adequate foraminal volume so that it does not compress the exiting C2 nerve root. **C,** Posteroanterior view of bilateral C1-C2 fixation via a C1 lateral mass/C2 pedicle screw fixation.

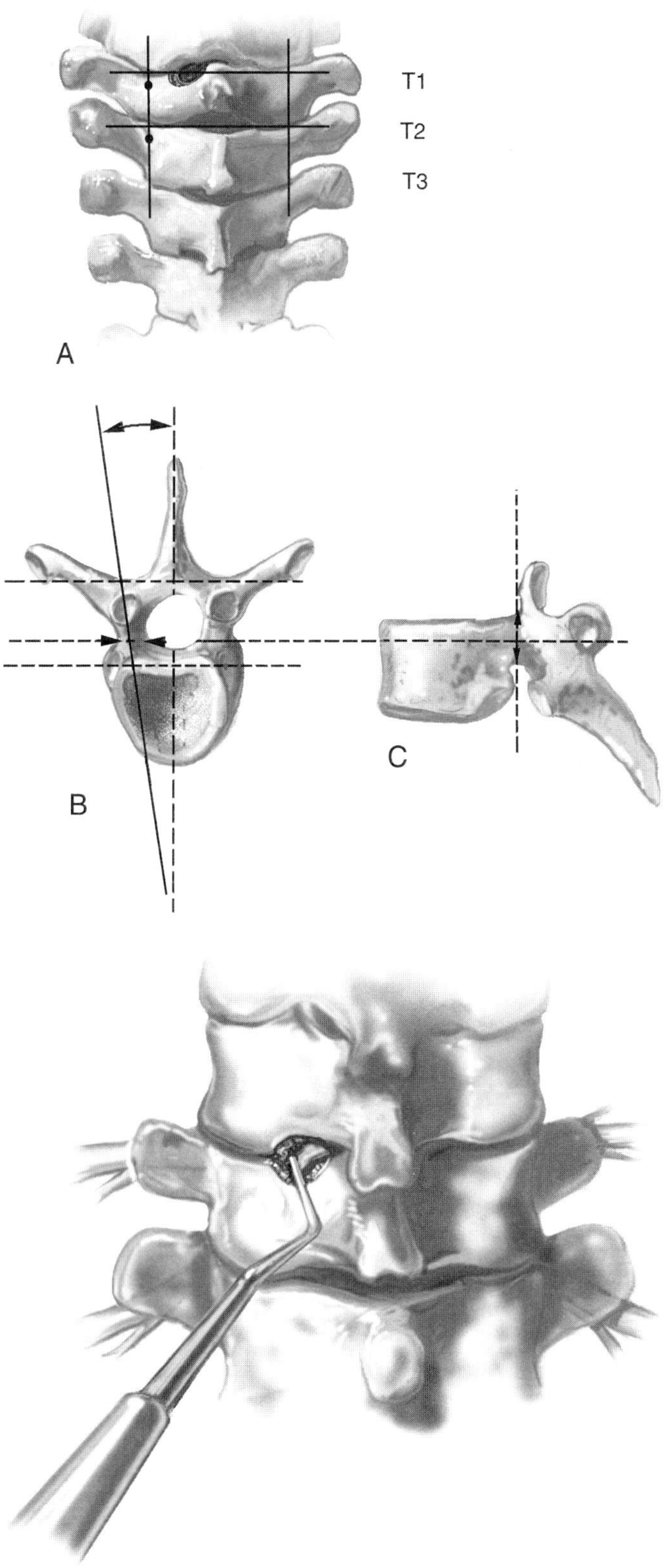

LOWER CERVICAL AND UPPER THORACIC PEDICLE SCREW FIXATION

Cervical pedicle screw fixation in the C6 or C7 vertebral body may be necessary if the lateral mass anatomy is too small to accommodate lateral mass screw purchase. We have found this to be the case in a significant portion of C7 lateral masses but rarely needed to place a pedicle screw at C6. Pedicle screw placement incorporates significantly different angles for trajectory than lateral mass screw fixation. Cervical pedicle screw fixation should be performed ipsilateral to the side of the patient, and placement should be angled 25 to 30 degrees medially perpendicular to the rostrocaudal plane.

Figure 17-7, A–D. **A, B,** and **C,** In long-segment cervical constructs adjacent to the cervicothoracic junction, it is sometimes necessary to incorporate T1 or T2 to prevent a junctional instability. Entry sites for upper thoracic pedicles are located 1 mm below and in the middle of the superior facet. Because there is variation in anatomy, we recommend using either spinal navigation or a laminoforaminotomy technique to palpate the medial pedicle wall before drilling and screw placement. Thoracic pedicle screws should be placed on the ipsilateral side of the patient with a trajectory of 25- to 30-degree medial angulation. **D,** After the laminoforaminotomy is performed, a Woodson dissector is used to palpate the medial pedicular wall. The surgeon can then double-check the anatomical entry point and begin screw placement in the T1 or T2 pedicle.

CERVICOTHORACIC FUSION

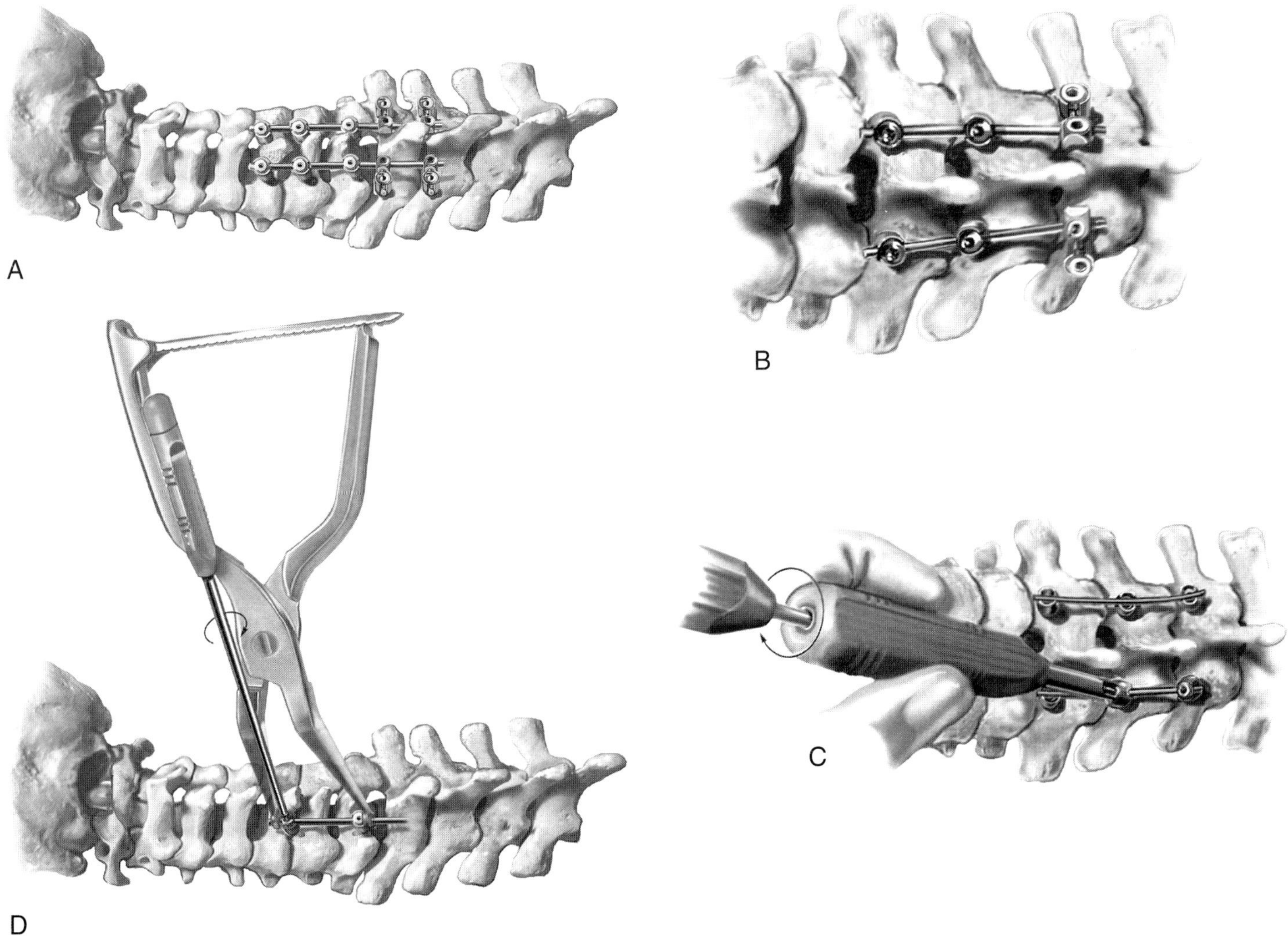

Figure 17-8, A–D. In bridging the cervicothoracic junction, varied pedicle and lateral mass entry points can present a problem for the surgeon marrying these segments together. Fortunately, the polyaxial screw head fixation system allows for a certain amount of "forgiveness" when incorporating the screws to the rod. **A,** A polyaxial screw head with long screw constructs allows for a medial or lateral tilt of the head to accommodate variability of screw placement. Offset connectors can also be used to couple the rod to the screw's large mediolateral offset. **B,** Rods can then be placed into the polyaxial screw heads. **C,** The top-loading screws can be attached with the rod pusher. **D,** Compression or extension devices can then be used in the direction of the scoliosis to correct deformity. Top-loading screws can be tightened for any temporary or permanent locking mechanism.

OCCIPITAL AND CERVICOTHORACIC FUSION

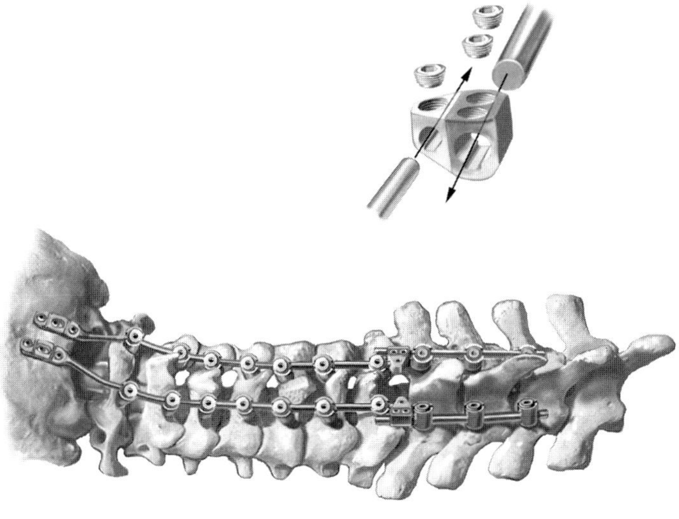

Figure 17-9. The occipital-cervical and cervical-thoracic junction can be incorporated in long constructs using the polyaxial rod system. Chapters 12 and 14 describe the screw entry sites for capture of the occipital bone as well as the lateral masses of the cervical spine. Upper thoracic pedicles have been described earlier in this chapter. Using the polyaxial screw heads in the cervical and thoracic region and the cortical screws in the occipital bone, a plate rod system is coupled together with the use of a hybrid plate rod system from the occipital-cervical region. The occipital-cervical rod is left long and can then be married to the thoracic screws through the use of a domino connector. Top-loading screws are placed to tighten constructs. Cross-links can be applied as needed either to the cervical or thoracic region.

REEXPLORATION CONSIDERATIONS

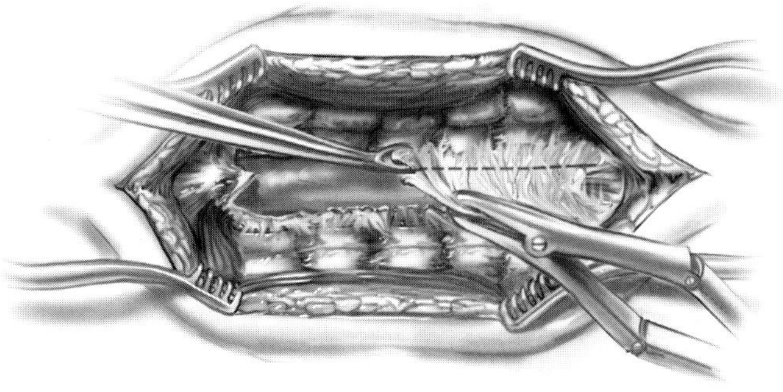

Figure 17-10. Reexploration for either posterior cervical decompression or fusion procedures is rare in our experience. It may be related to the tendency to deal with these failures from an anterior approach. It also may suggest that there is a very low complication rate with the majority of decompressive posterior cervical procedures. Rarely, in some patients, a "postlaminectomy membrane" can form and cause recurrent compression and myelopathy. An important point to remember in a posterior reexploration is that the lateral mass bony anatomy is the safest area to dissect. ("Bone is home.") Once the adequate bony landmarks have been cleared, the postlaminectomy membrane can be captured with a Kerrison rongeur and a large Ruggles-type curette. The Ruggles-type curette can dissect the scar tissue from the lateral masses, where the tissue is normally adherent.

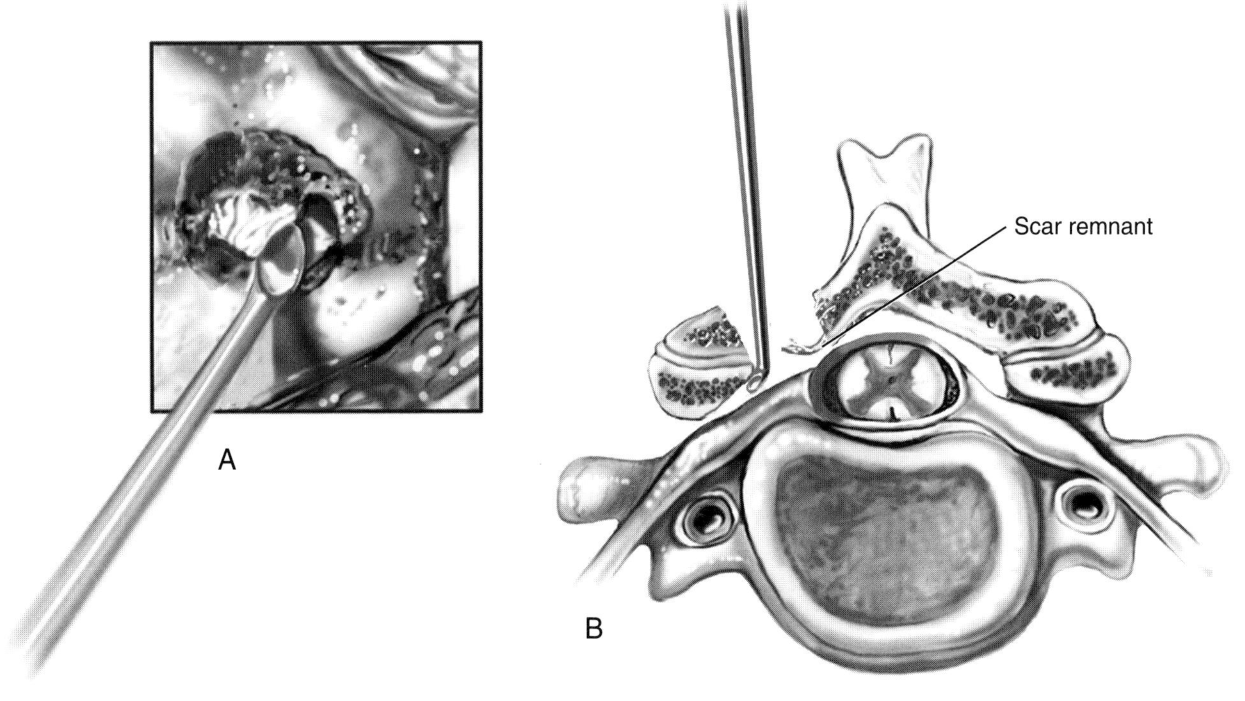

Figure 17-11, A and B. Exploration of a laminoforaminotomy. In our experience, this is rarely a problem. It probably represents our tendency to approach recurrent radiculopathy that previously was treated with a posterior approach by performing an anterior cervical discectomy and fusion. If, however, a reexploration foraminotomy is contemplated, the dissection, again, should be centered on carefully dissecting the scar tissue away from the bone. The soft tissue points must be dissected and sharply divided with a scalpel or sharp curettes. Once the lateral border of bone is dissected with a straight curette, a forward-angled curette can extend to the foramen where the virgin epidural space exists. The laminotomy can then be widened safely lowering the risk of a dural rent or nerve root injury.

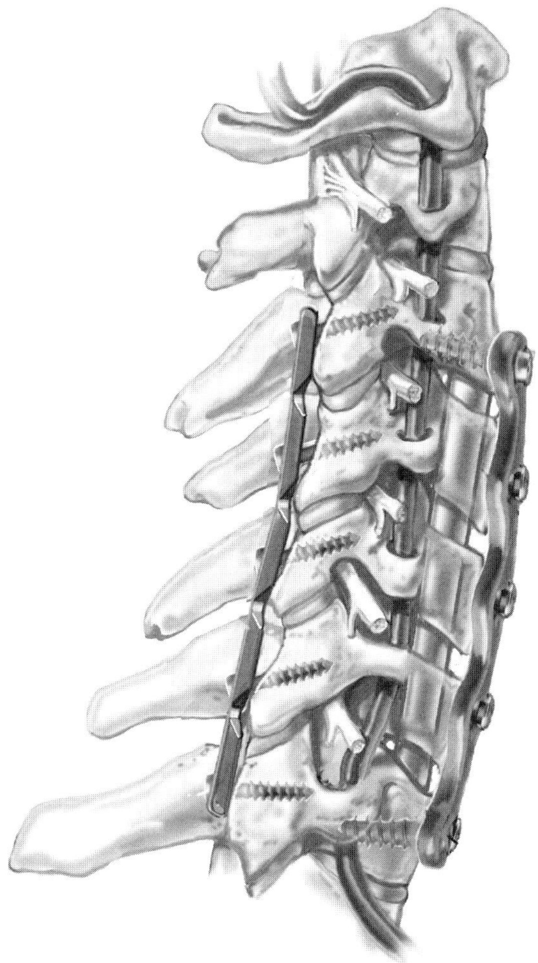

CONSIDERATIONS FOR COMBINED ANTERIOR-POSTERIOR CERVICAL FUSION

Figure 17-12 There is much controversy regarding the need for combined anterior-posterior (AP) or 360-degree fusion procedures of the cervical spine. In general, our experience has shown that isolated anterior or posterior fixation is adequate in treating short segment pathologies (1 or 2 levels). In patients with multilevel pathology, a combined AP reconstruction and arthrodesis with fixation should be considered.

COMMON PITFALLS

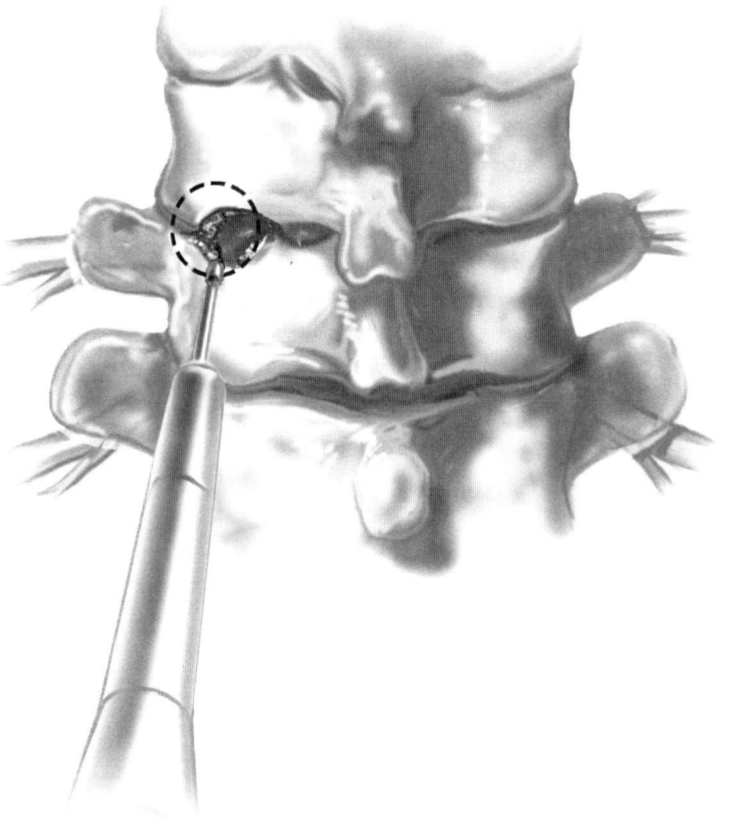

Figure 17-13. When exposing the T1 and T2 thoracic pedicles via laminoforaminotomy, a common pitfall is to begin the drilling too far laterally and thereby inadvertently drilling the medial portion of the thoracic pedicle. It is important, when the upper thoracic pedicles are being exposed, that the laminoforaminotomy begin medially and then be directed laterally to visualize the medial pedicular wall.

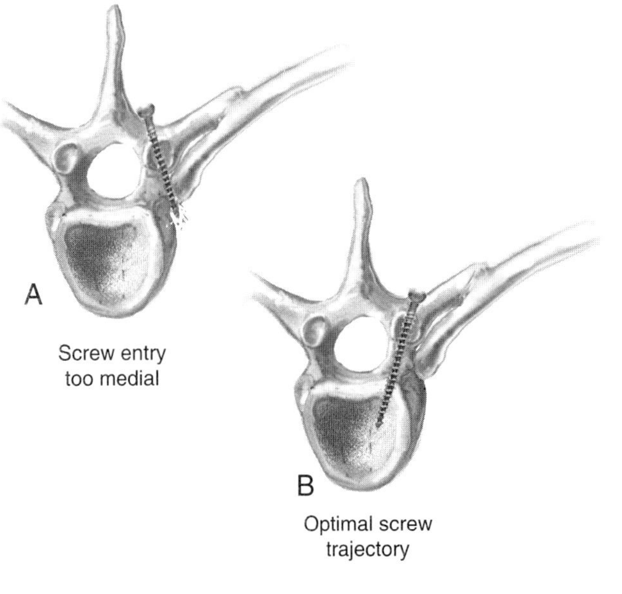

Figure 17-14, A and B. **A,** Entry of thoracic pedicle screw too far medially. When an upper thoracic pedicle is being placed, a lateral entry point is critical to initiate a medially directed screw. The tendency is to begin screw placement too medial and have a lateral breakout of the screw. There is still adequate purchase with a lateral breakout because usually the screw heads enter the costovertebral joint, which also has stability. **B,** The ideal trajectory, however, is lateral to medial at 25 to 30 degrees to get optimal bony purchase.

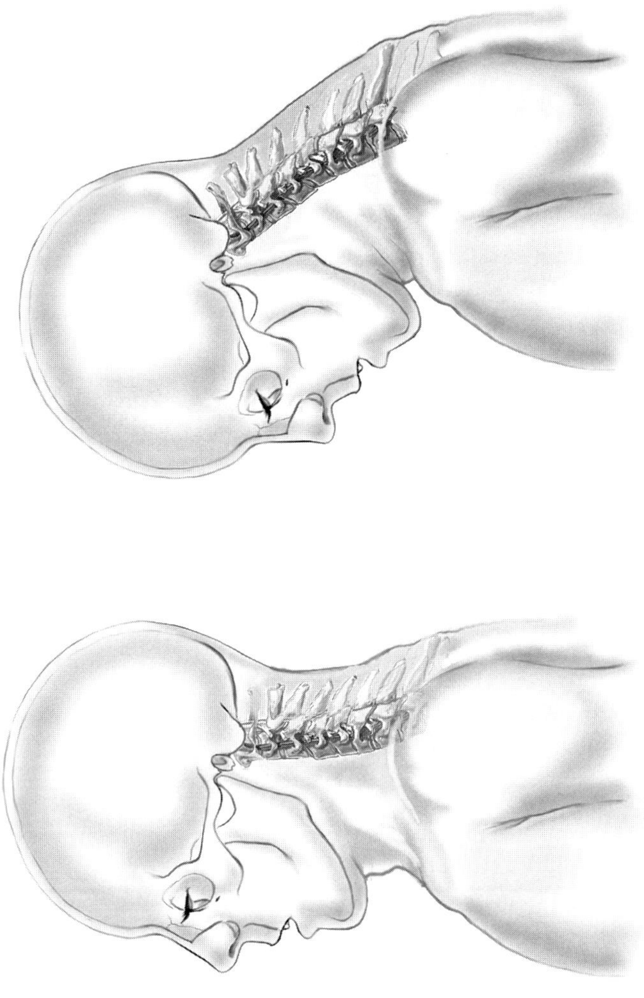

Figure 17-15. Positioning. It is critical in occipitocervicothoracic fusions to preserve sagittal balance as much as possible. We have found that patients who have been fused in a slightly flexed or military tuck position can have trouble swallowing. The dysphagia results from altered mechanics with the head in the tucked position. Therefore, before proceeding with preparation and draping of the surgical field, a C-arm or lateral view radiograph should be obtained to best visualize the proper amount of sagittal balance in the patient. This can be altered with adjustments of the skeletal head holder. This can also be adjusted intraoperatively under C-arm guidance in unstable patients before screw rod fixation.

POSTOPERATIVE RESULTS

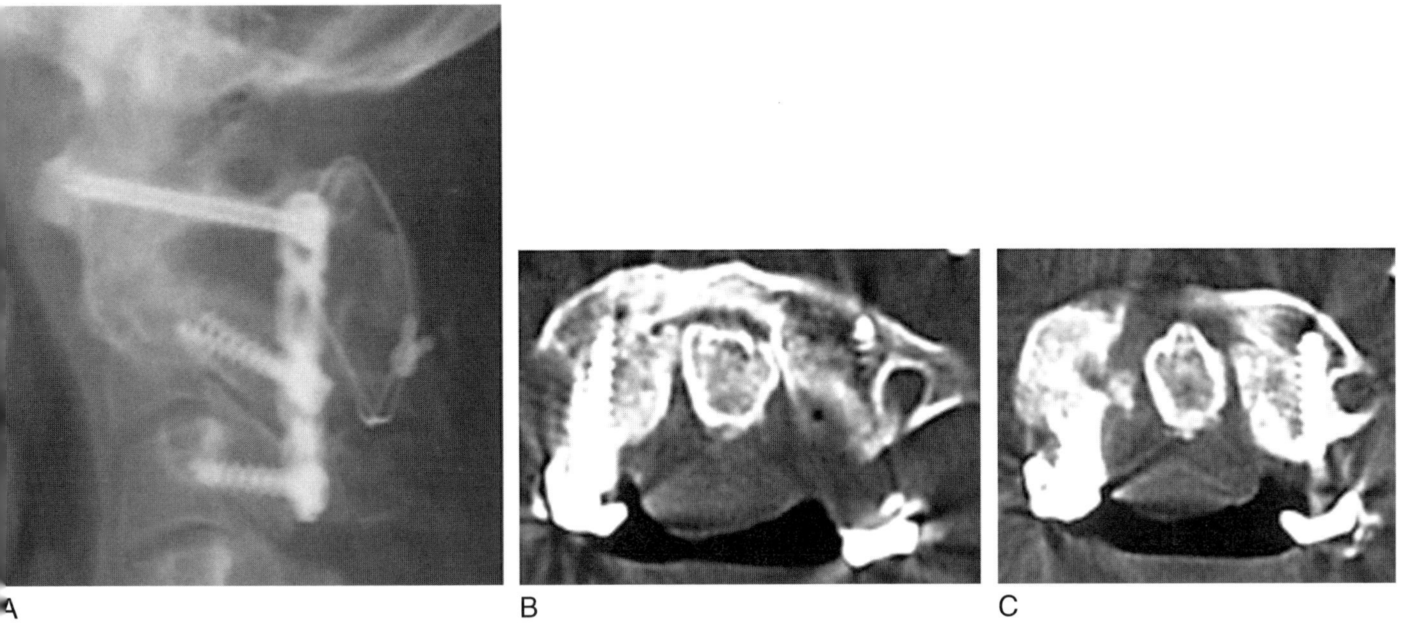

Figure 17-16, A–C. **A**, Lateral cervical radiograph demonstrating a C1-C3 posterior arthrodesis and screw fixation capturing C1 with C1 lateral mass screws, C2 with pars intraarticularis screws, and C3 with lateral mass screws. Note a posterior tension band has also been placed. **B** and **C**, Axial computer tomography scan showing capture of C1 with C1 lateral mass screws.

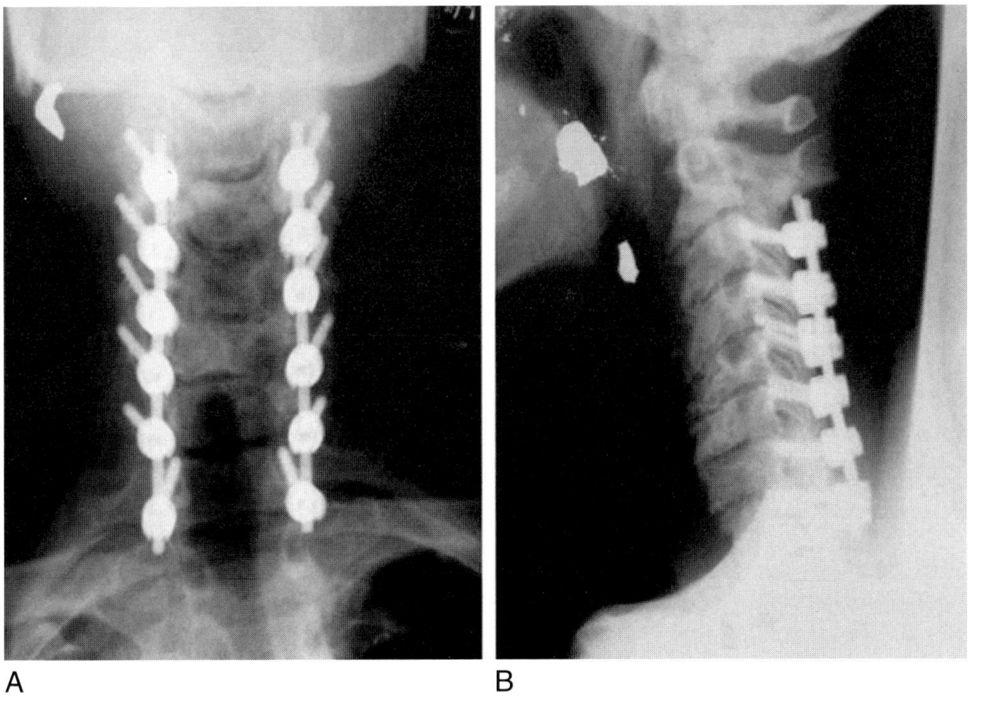

Figure 17-17, A and B. AP **(A)** and lateral cervical spine radiograph **(B)** demonstrating C3-C7 posterior instrumentation. C3-C7 lateral masses have been captured with lateral mass screws, and T1 has been captured with T1 pedicle screws.

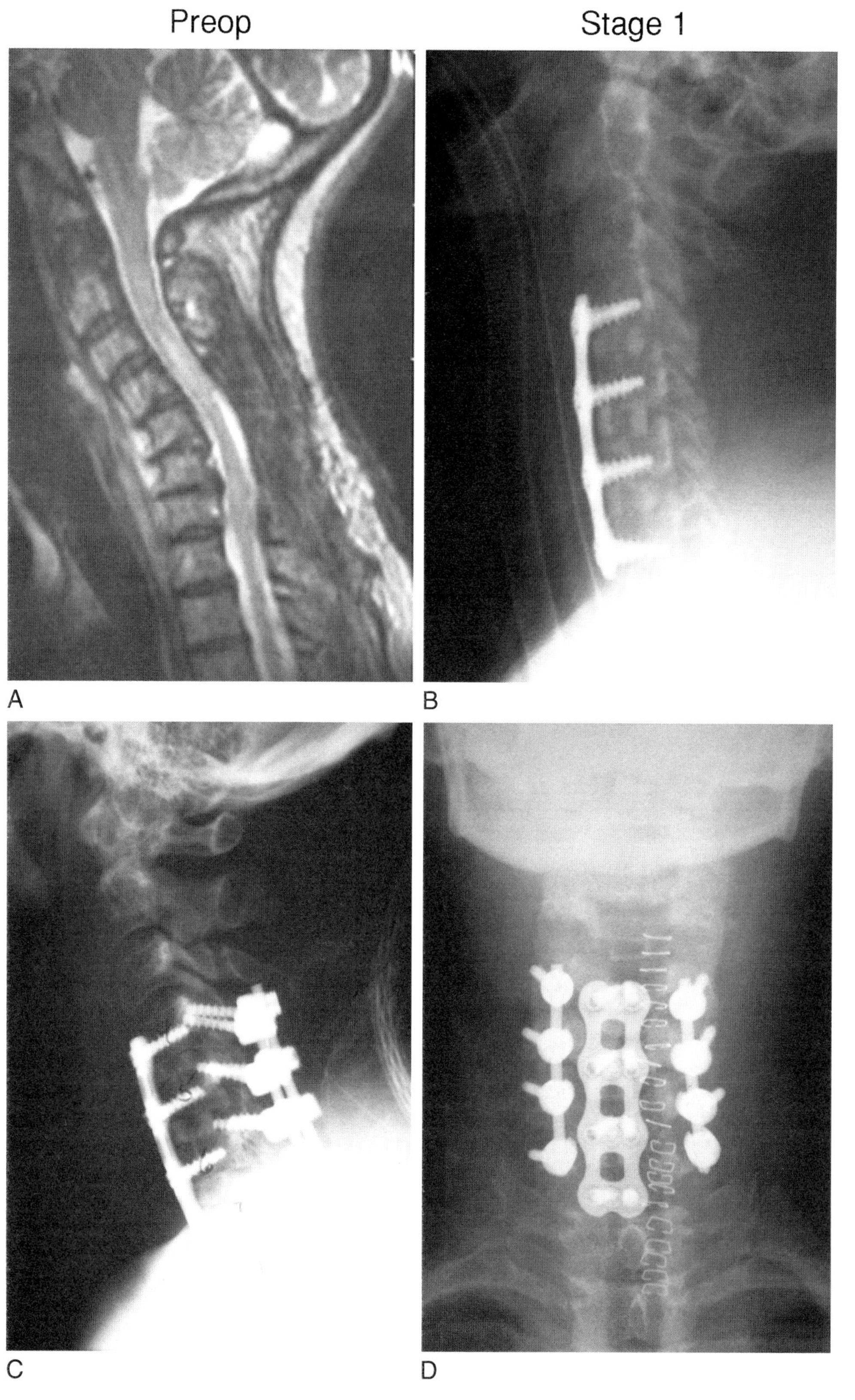

Figure 17-18, A–D. **A,** Lateral long TR MRI image demonstrating a post-laminectomy kyphosis. **B,** Lateral cervical spine radiograph demonstrating an anterior reconstruction with improvement of kyphosis after multilevel anterior cervical discectomies and fusion using allograft Smith Robinson type spacers and plate fixation (Stagel-anterior). **C,** Lateral spine radiograph demonstrating supplemental posterior lateral mass fixation to "protect" the anterior construct and to increase the chances for fusion (Stagel-posterior). **D,** AP lateral cervical spine radiograph demonstrating anterior plate fixation with supplemental posterior lateral mass fixation.

CHAPTER XVIII

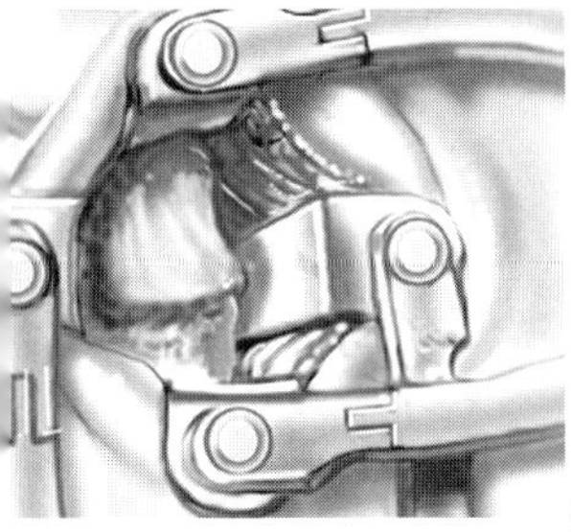

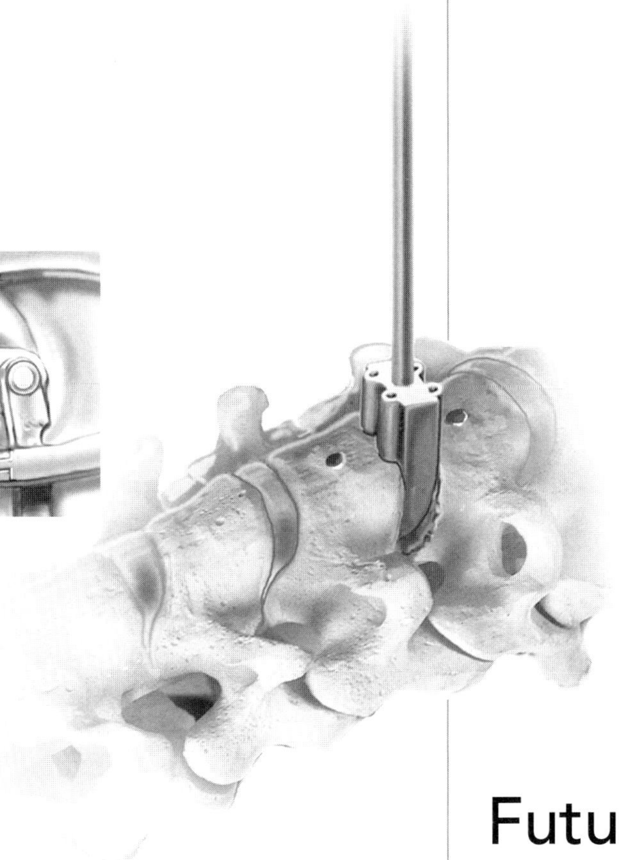

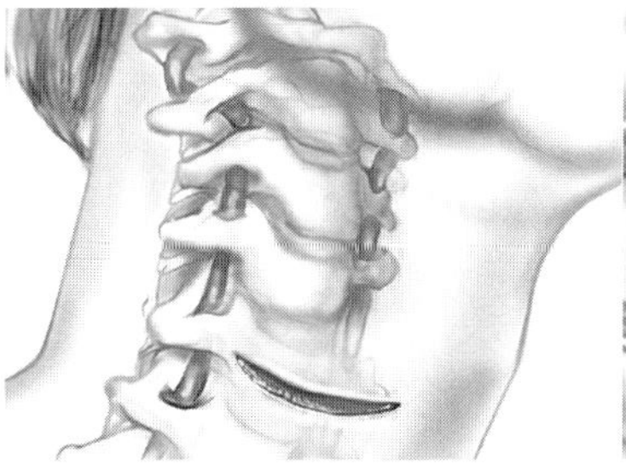

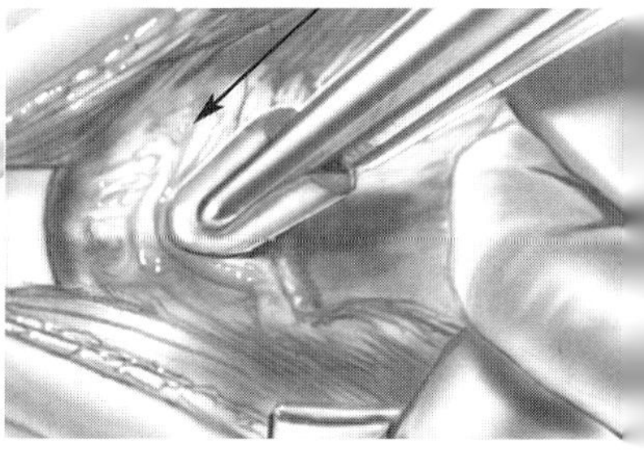

Future Technologies

PRESTIGE LP ARTIFICIAL CERVICAL DISC REPLACEMENT

Cervical arthroplasty using a metal-on-metal prosthesis was first performed in 1991 in Bristol, England. The Bristol/Cummins disc has had considerable clinical and radiographic success with up to 14 years of follow-up. Flexion-extension films have demonstrated motion maintenance on long-term follow-up. The next generation of metal-on-metal cervical prosthesis, the Prestige disc, was first introduced in 1998, and this has evolved into a lower-profile implantable device with more streamlined implantation equipment.

Indications for cervical arthroplasty continue to be defined and are beyond the scope of this chapter. Many factors must be taken into account and include the patient's age, range of neck motion, joint stiffness, and a history of prior cervical surgery. This chapter will deal with the surgical technique for implantation of the Prestige LP disc.

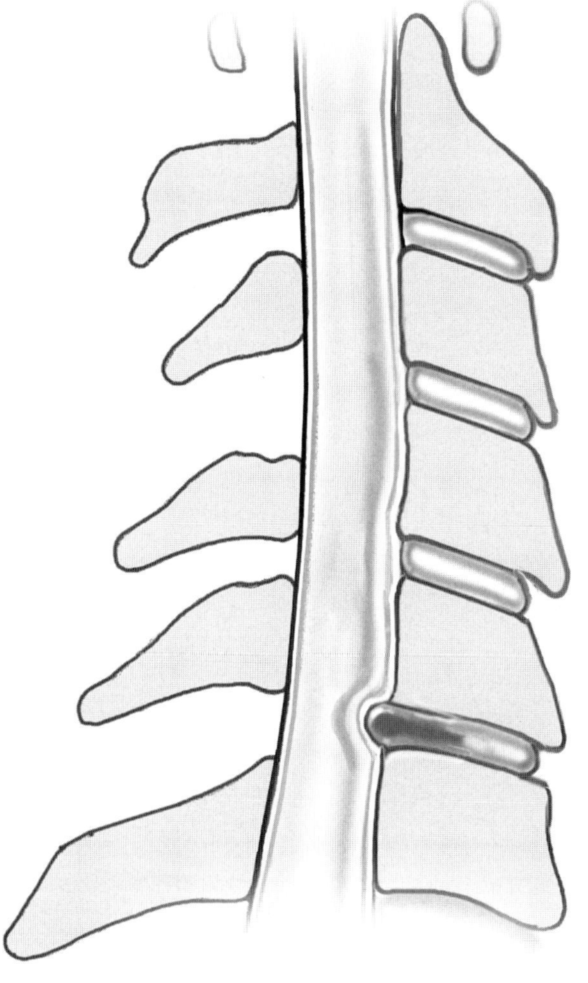

Figure 18-1. Ideal patients for this disc replacement include those with single-level disease in the midcervical region. Patients with central or lateral disc herniations causing either radiculopathy and/or cord compression are also potential candidates. A preoperative computed tomography (CT) or a magnetic resonance image (MRI) scan with a parallel-slice protocol is important for templating. The smaller of the two vertebral body end plates is selected and measured at the target disc space. CT imaging is preferred. When measuring, do not include bone spurs or ridges that will be removed in the subsequent gardening or decompression process. One can adjust for magnification factors with the Prestige LP prosthesis template. The selected size should be used only as a guide in selection of the size-specific instrumentation and implant. Templating will determine the appropriate footprint of the implant but not the height of the implant. Ultimately, the implant size must be based on clinical judgment, disc space preparation, and trials.

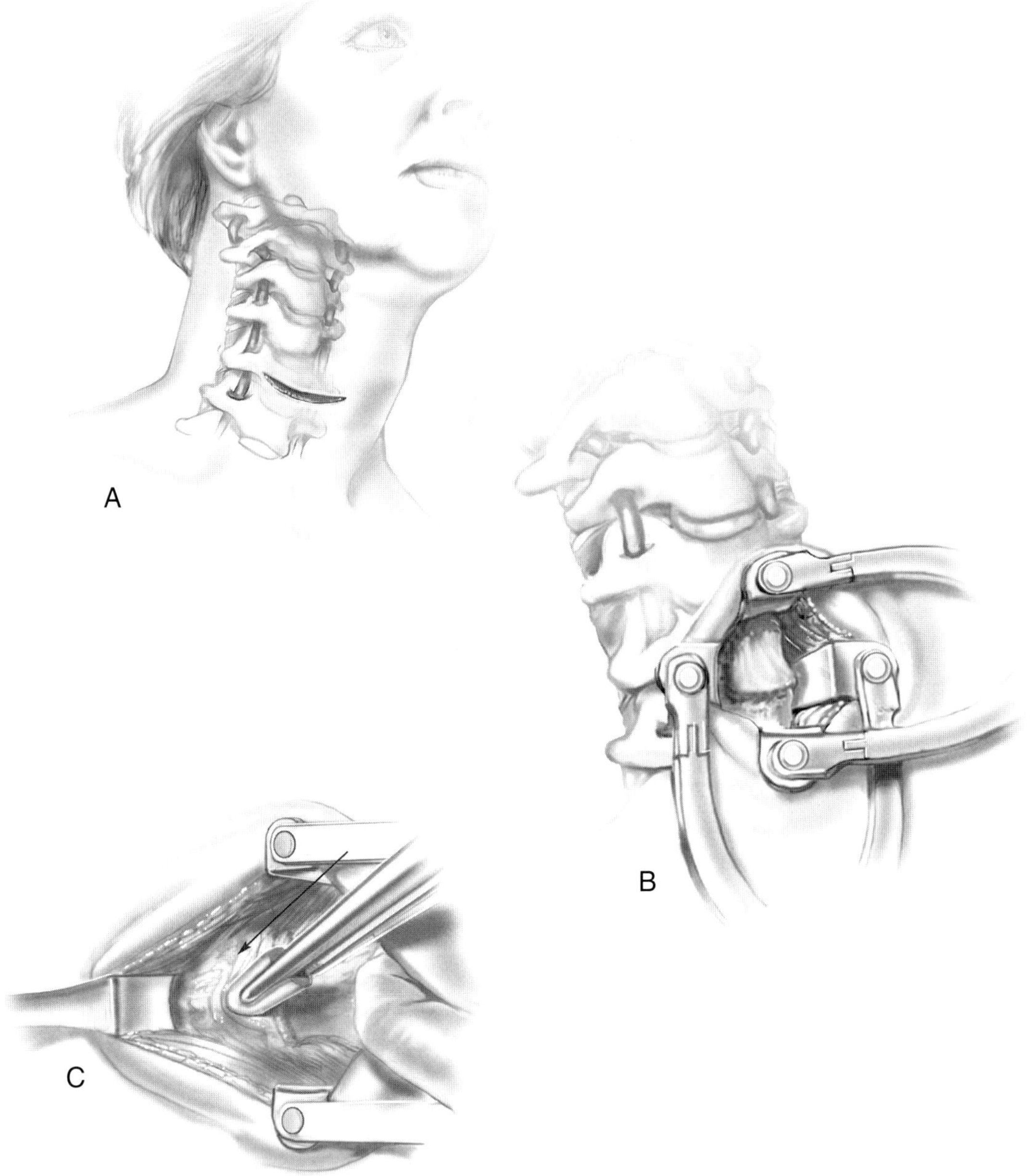

Figure 18-2, A–C. The patient is placed in a supine position with the head in a neutral orientation. A small roll should be placed under the posterior cervical area to support and maintain cervical lordosis. For lower cervical exposures, the shoulders should be taped or pulled down to secure better visualization of the lower cervical spine on fluoroscopy. A transverse incision is made at the appropriate level **(A)**, and the level is identified by fluoroscopy or x-ray. The vascular dissection plane is developed between the trachea and the esophagus medially and the carotid sheath laterally. The anterior vertebral column is exposed, and the longus colli muscles are dissected in a subperiosteal fashion with either a Kittner dissector or monopolar cautery. The retractors are then placed **(B)**, and the vertebral bodies can be cleaned of any soft tissue **(C)**.

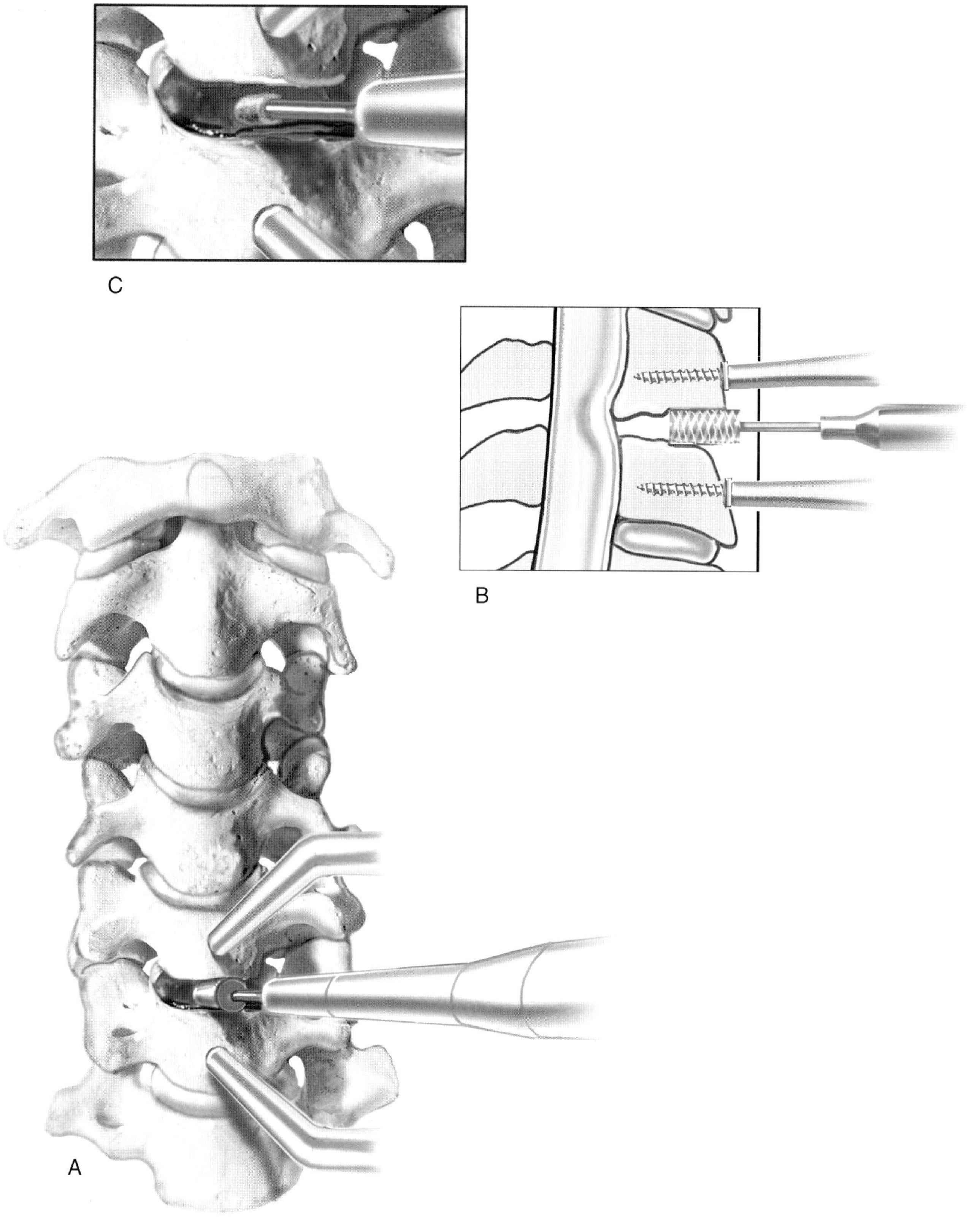

Figure 18-3, A–C. A radical anterior cervical discectomy is performed at the appropriate level. Disc material and cartilage are removed in a standard fashion, and the posterior longitudinal ligament is exposed. The vertebral body distraction pins are positioned midline in the vertebral bodies, and distraction is dialed in to enlarge the disc space and reestablish lordosis. A high-speed drill can be used for removal of the posterior disc and osteophytes to achieve decompression. The posterior longitudinal ligament is removed, and the dura is identified. A barrel bit is used to enlarge the discectomy site and create parallel end plate surfaces. It is important to remove only cartilaginous end plates to avoid excess bone removal.

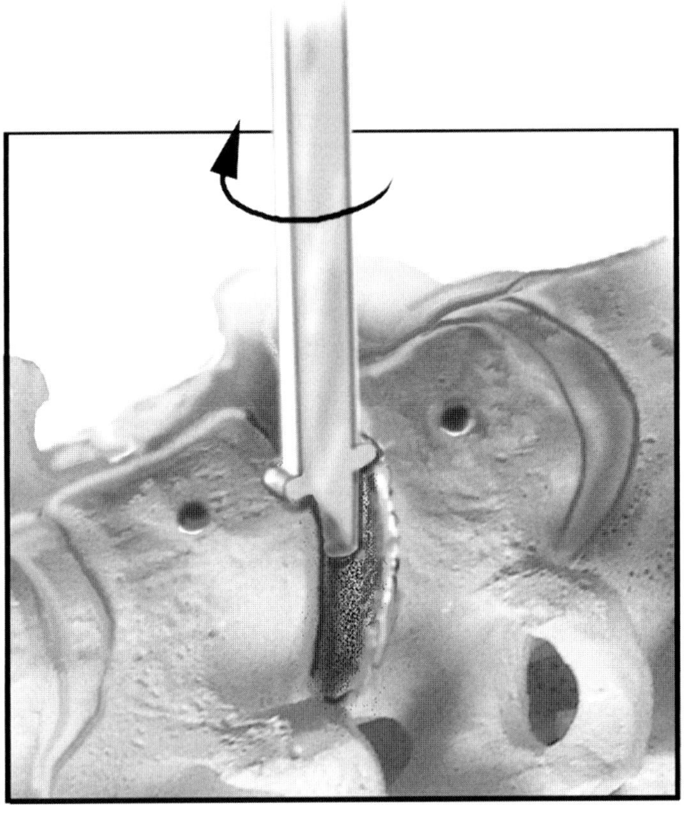

Figure 18-4. After the discectomy and decompression are complete, the distraction pins are removed, and the vertebral body distraction is relaxed. The end plates are prepared, and a shim distractor is placed to assist in the introduction of instruments into the disc space for end plate preparation without external distraction.

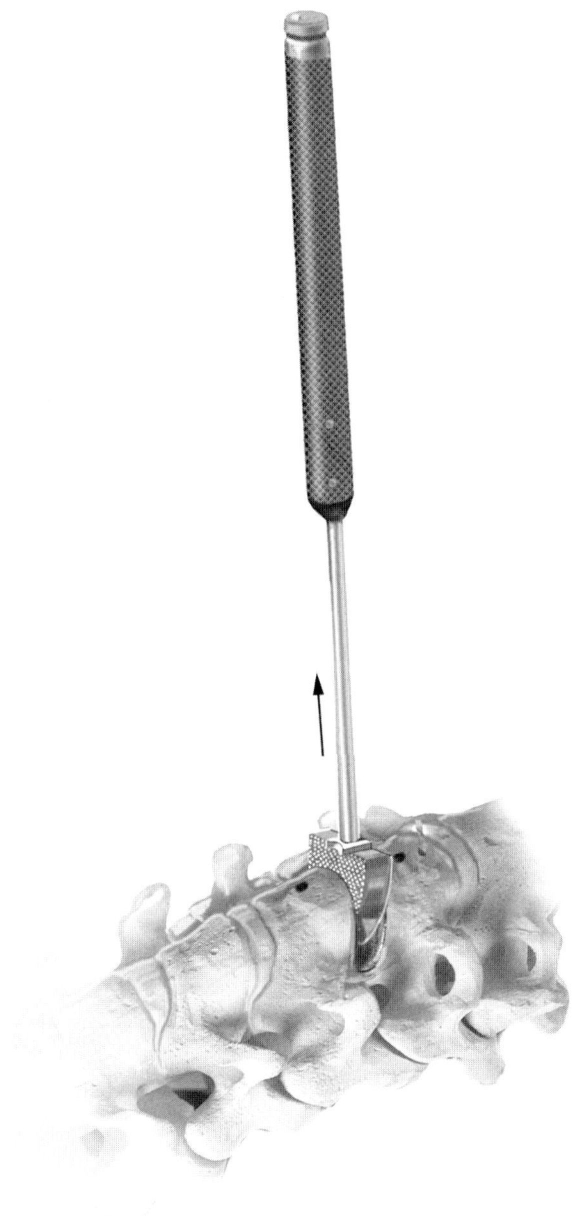

Figure 18-5. A templated rasp can also be used to prepare the end plates. The rasp should have maximal end plate contact and should be introduced into the disc space with a positive stop position superiorly to prevent the rasp from entering the disc space too deeply. Rasping will remove any intrusions that might remain after parallel end plate preparation.

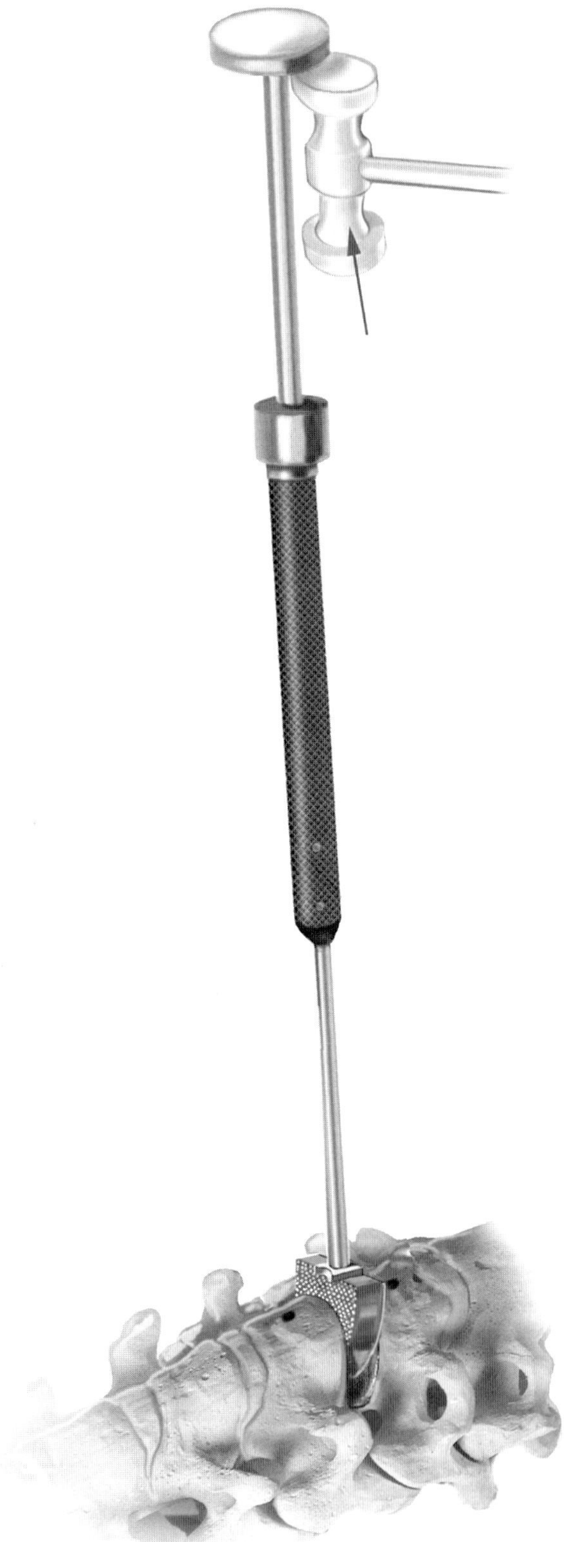

Figure 18-6. Sometimes the rasp can fit so snugly that it is difficult to remove with manual traction, and a reverse slap hammer action can be used.

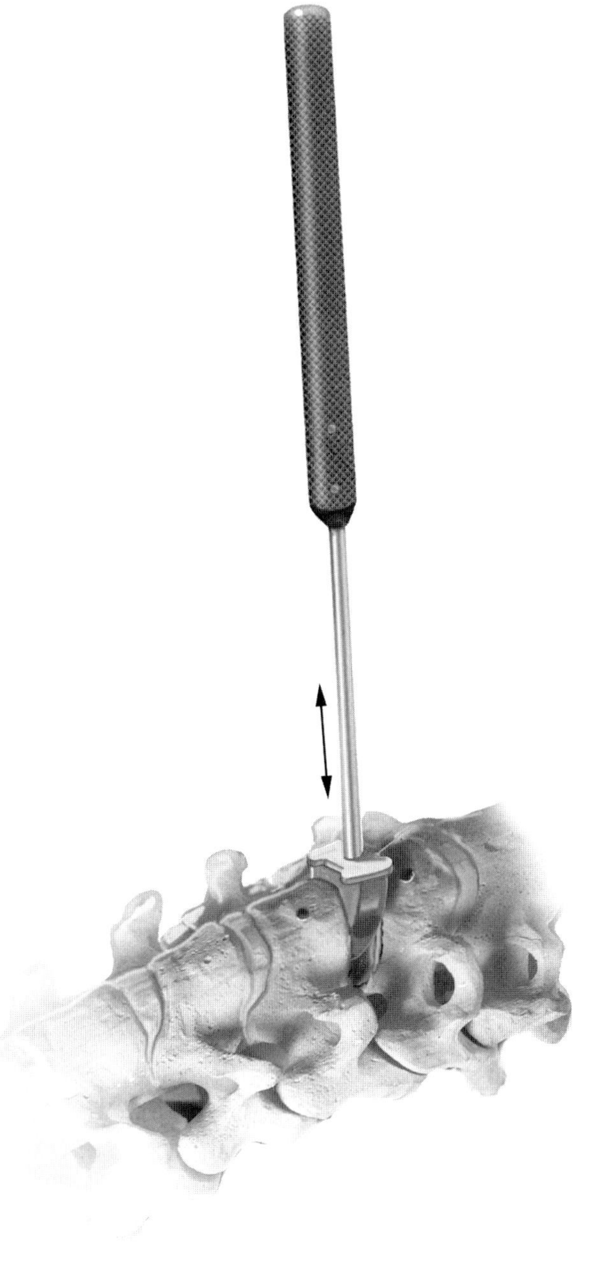

Figure 18-7. After adequate end plate preparation, the implant trial is introduced to confirm the size of the prepared disc space. The size dimensions of the implant trial should precisely match the end plate interfacing dimensions of the implant. The implant trial will measure the disc space height and depth and should fit snugly without distracting the disc space. If there is any difficulty in placing the implant trial during insertion, a smaller trial or additional end plate preparation must be considered. Once the implant trial is in position, it should be checked with lateral fluoroscopy. On fluoroscopic imaging, the prepared end plates must be in complete contact with the flat portions of the implant trial, and the posterior tip of the trial must reach the posterior aspects of the disc space. The implant trial has four anterior tabs that match the anterior tabs of the Prestige LP cervical disc. The anterior vertebral body surfaces must not have any protruding bone that would interfere with the placement of the trial tabs, which must be flush with the anterior surface.

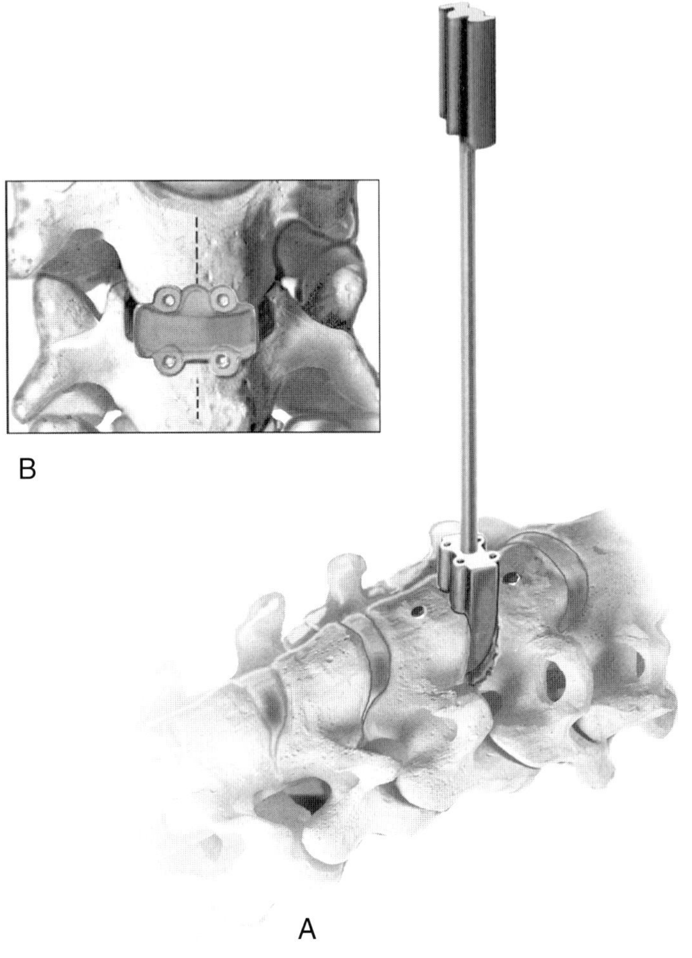

Figure 18-8, A and B. **A,** After the implant trial has been placed, the corresponding rail cutter guide is used to prepare the implant fixation channels into the end plates. The rail cutter guide is gently impacted into the prepared disc space. The guide must be centered on the midline of the vertebral bodies. **B,** The rail cutter guide must be impacted until all four drill guide ports on the head of the guide touch the anterior surface of the spine.

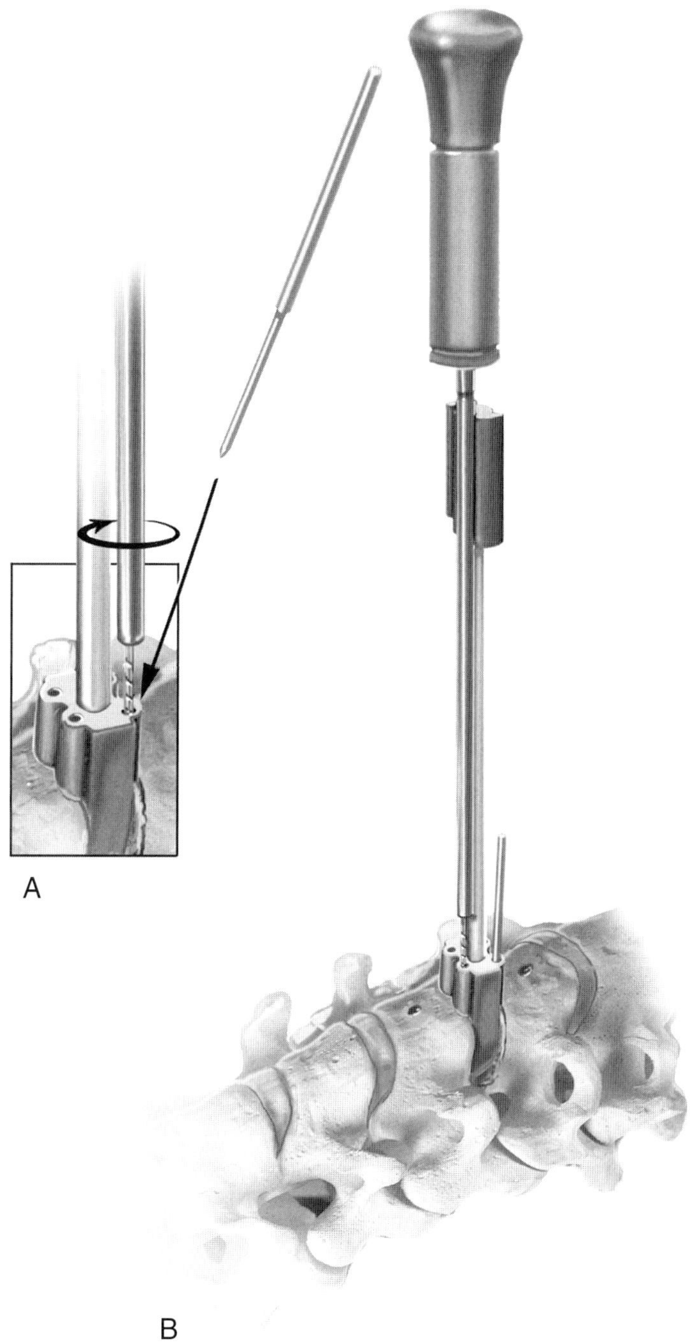

Figure 18-9, A and B. The rail cutter bit is attached to the drill bit handle. The rail cutter bit is then inserted into one port on the rail cutter guide, with the shaft of the bit resting in the corresponding slot at the top of the rail cutter guide. The first fixation channel is drilled into the end plate. While the rail cutter guide is held firmly in place, the drill bit is removed, and a temporary fixation pin is placed in the channel. The next channel is drilled in the contralateral port, and the second fixation pin is placed. The process is repeated for the third and fourth, and the fourth channel is drilled. The fixation pins and cutter guide are removed. Each properly prepared end plate should have two parallel channels as shown. If this is not the case, one should double-check and ensure that the end plates were properly paralleled, and this step should be repeated.

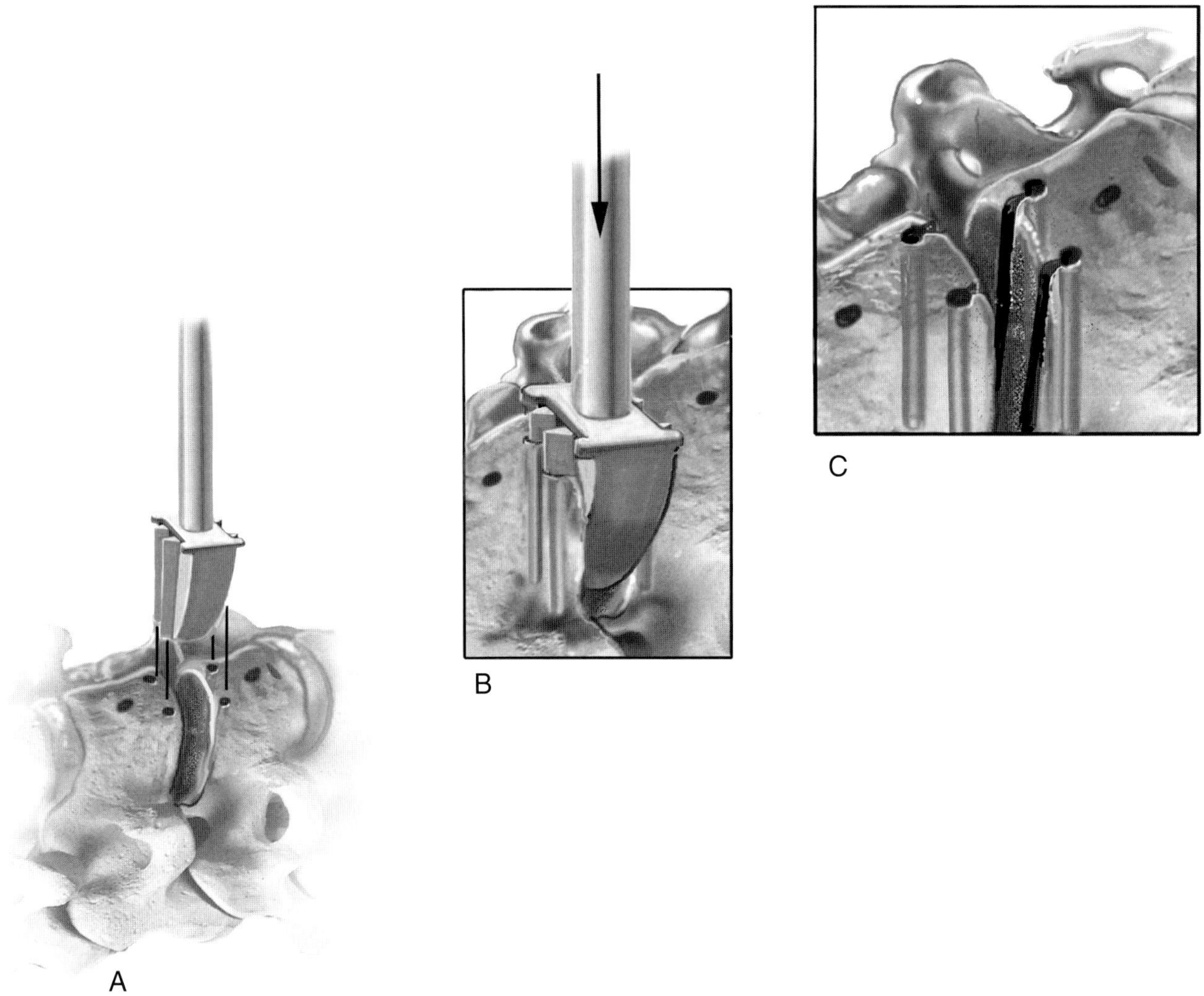

Figure 18-10, A–C. **A,** The four cutting blades of the rail punch are aligned into the four ports made by the rail cutter. **B,** The disc space is gently tapped into until the depth stops contact with the anterior surface of the spine. **C,** This should complete the preparation of the four channels into the end plates as shown.

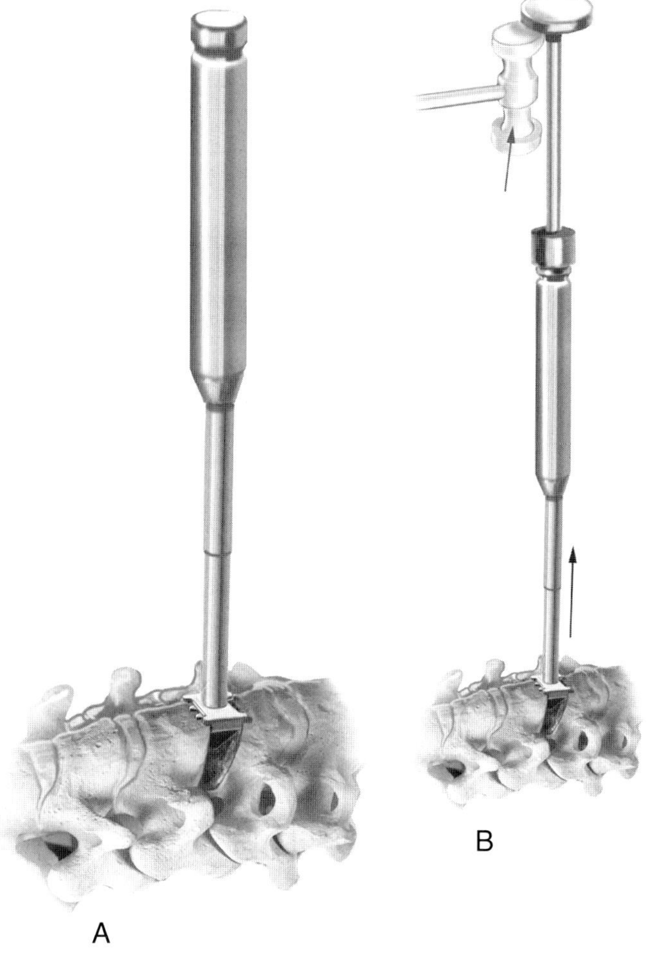

Figure 18-11, A and B. Macroscopic view of the channel cutting **(A)** and the removal of the rasp **(B)**.

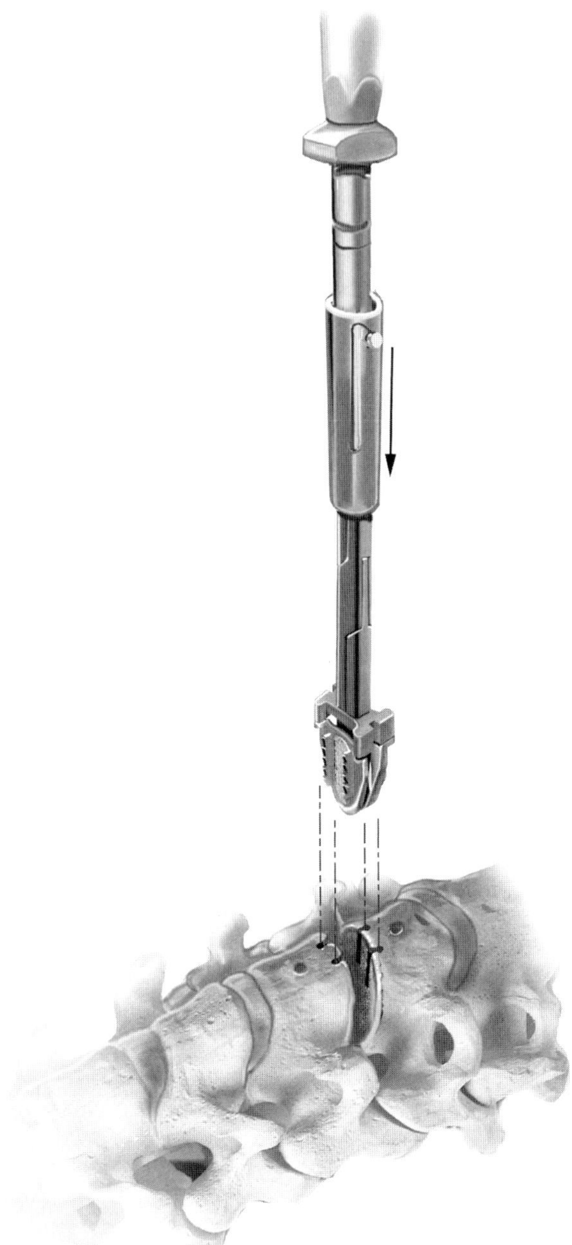

Figure 18-12. The appropriately sized Prestige LP disc is placed into the corresponding slot of the loading block. The ball portion of the implant should be superior. The Prestige LP cervical disc is attached to the implant inserter via the placement of the four inserter prongs into the ports on the anterior disc tabs and advancement of the outer sheath toward the disc. With the ball portion of the prosthesis positioned superiorly, the Prestige LP disc rails are aligned with the channels on the end plates.

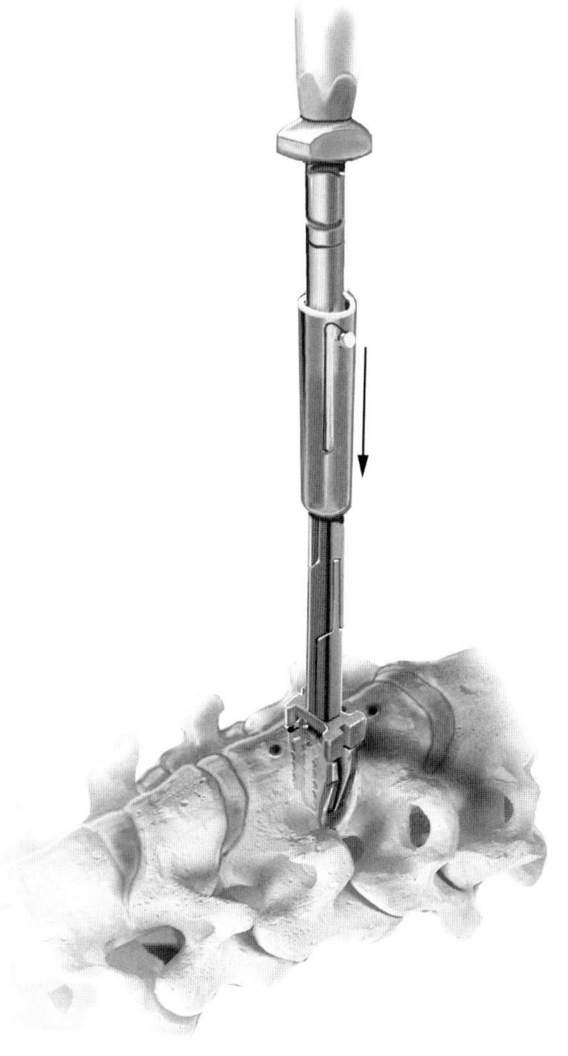

Figure 18-13. The prosthesis is inserted into the prepared disc space. One then gently taps into the space with a mallet until the anterior tabs come into contact with the anterior surface of the vertebral bodies. If the anterior surfaces are not exactly level, a slight gap may remain between the tabs and the anterior surface on either the inferior or superior body. This is acceptable.

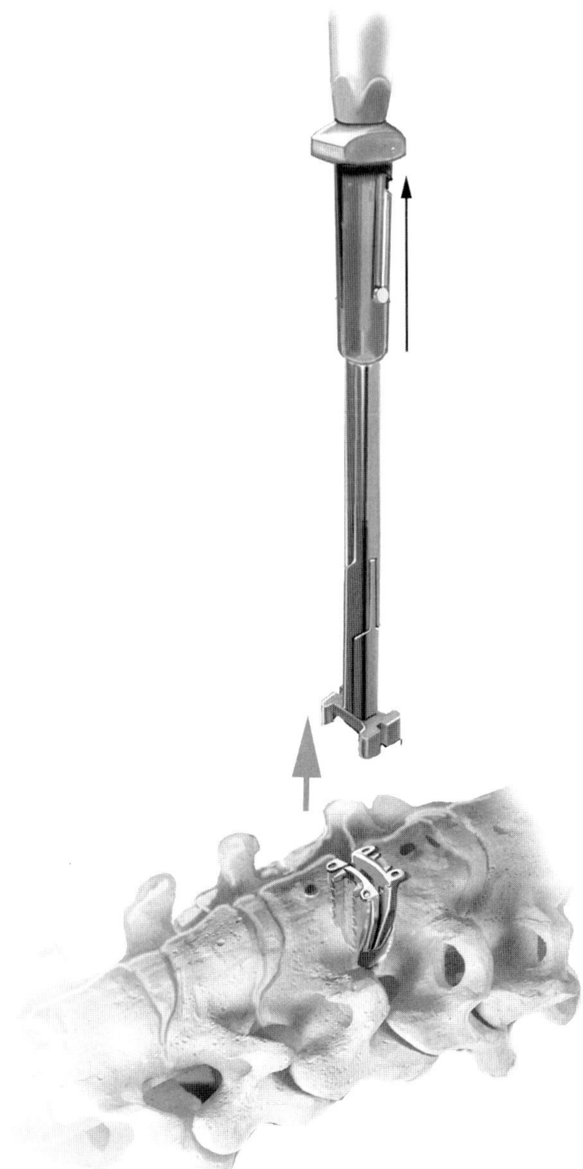

Figure 18-14. The anterior sheath is slid back, and the inserter is gently removed. If necessary, the final impactor is used to fully seat the disc by aligning it with the anterior aspects of the implant and gently tapping with the mallet.

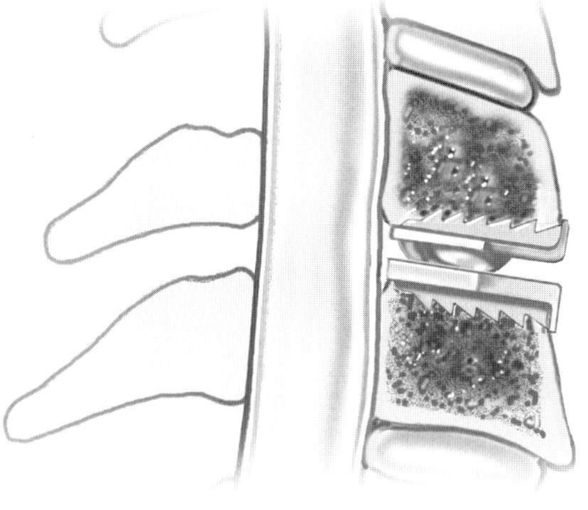

A

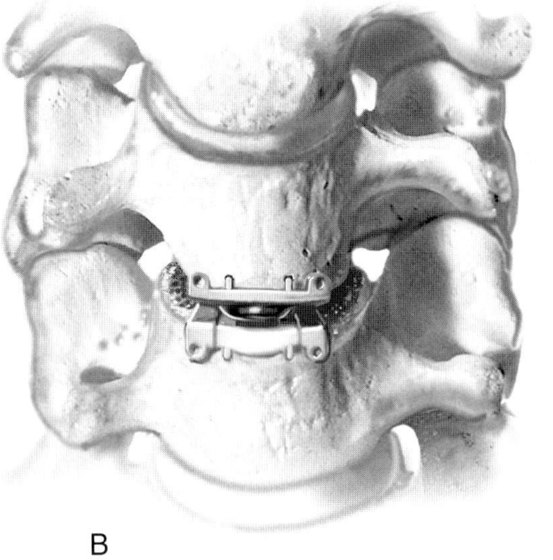

B

Figure 18-15, A and B. After final disc insertion, lateral and anteroposterior radiographs can be taken to verify proper placement. The surgery is completed using standard anterior cervical disc closure procedures. If the disc is in a suboptimal position, or if there is some reason the implant must be removed, the Prestige LP cervical disc can be separated from the end plate with a drill to create a space between the implant and the end plate. It can then be removed using forceps.

POSTOPERATIVE RESULTS

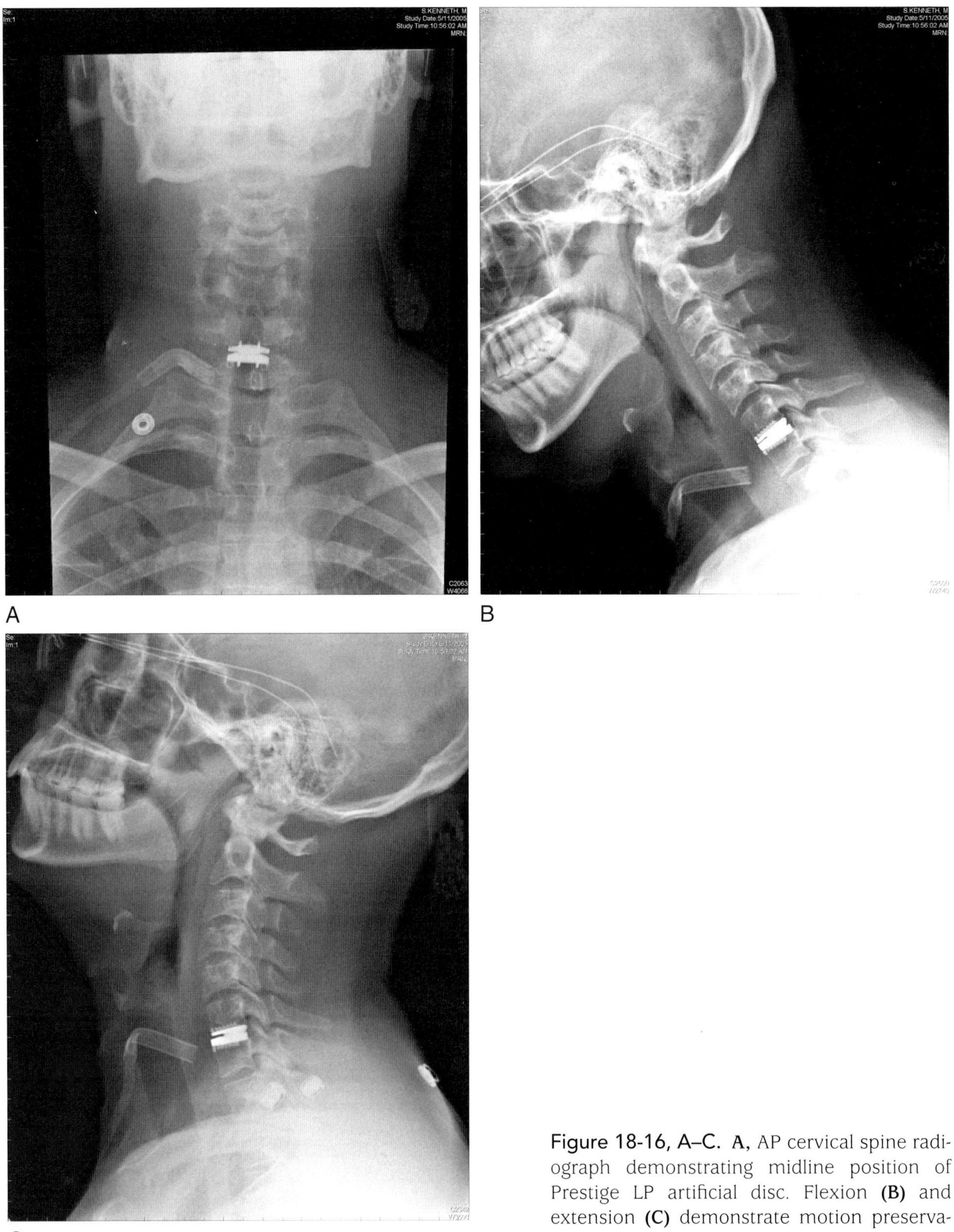

Figure 18-16, A–C. **A,** AP cervical spine radiograph demonstrating midline position of Prestige LP artificial disc. Flexion **(B)** and extension **(C)** demonstrate motion preservation at the operated segment.

Index

Page numbers in *italics* indicate illustrations.